# Vagina

# 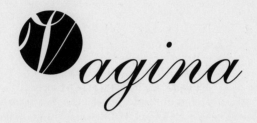agina

## A New Biography

---

# Naomi Wolf

*An Imprint of HarperCollinsPublishers*

Grateful acknowledgment is made to reprint the following lyrics: "Press My Button," words and music by Lil Johnson. Copyright © 1941 by Universal Music Corp. Copyright renewed. All rights reserved. Used by permission. Reprinted by permission of Hal Leonard Corporation. "Don't You Make Me High," words and music by Louisa Barker, Daniel Barker, and J Mayo Williams. Copyright © 1938 by Universal Music Corp. Copyright renewed. All rights reserved. Used by permission. Reprinted by permission of Hal Leonard Corporation. "I Need a Little Sugar in My Bowl," words and music by Clarence Williams, J. Tim Byrmn, and Dally Small. Copyright © 1932 by Universal Music Corp. Copyright renewed. All rights reserved. Used by permission. Reprinted by permission of Hal Leonard Corporation. "If You See My Rooster," words and music by Minnie McCoy. Copyright © 1933 Universal Music Corp. Copyright renewed. All rights reserved. Used by permission. Reprinted by permission of Hal Leonard Corporation.

The names and identifying characteristics of some of the individuals featured throughout this book have been changed to protect their privacy. Any resemblance to actual persons, living or dead, is purely coincidental.

HarperCollins books may be purchased for educational, business, or sales promotional use. For information please write: Special Markets Department, HarperCollins Publishers, 10 East 53rd Street, New York, NY 10022.

FIRST EDITION

Designed by Leah Carlson-Stanisic

Library of Congress Cataloging-in-Publication Data has been applied for.

ISBN 978-0-06-198916-2

12  13  14  15  16   OV/RRD   10 9 8 7 6 5 4 3 2 1

FOR A.

*How strange and awful it seemed to stand naked under the sky! How delicious! She felt like some new-born creature, opening its eyes in a familiar world that it had never known.*

—KATE CHOPIN, *THE AWAKENING*

# Contents

# Acknowledgments

This book could not have been written without the help of many others, especially the many distinguished scientists, researchers, counselors, and physicians whom I interviewed. They shared their time and expertise generously in order to inform non-scientists about women's health and sexuality. In order of their appearance in the book, I am very grateful to Dr. Deborah Coady of Soho OB/GYN in New York City; Nancy Fish of the same practice; Dr. Ramesh Babu of New York University Hospital; Dr. Jeffrey Cole of the Kessler Center for Rehabilitation in Orange, New Jersey; Dr. Burke Richmond of University of Wisconsin School of Medicine and Public Health, Madison, Wisconsin; Katrine Cakuls in New York City; Dr. Jim Pfaus of Concordia University in Montreal, Quebec; medical writer Dr. Julius Goepp; and Dr. Basil Kocur of Lenox Hill Hospital in New York City. Interviewing the scientists has been extremely inspiring in terms of witnessing their commitment to advancing the understanding of women's sexuality, and interviewing the physicians has been similarly inspiring in terms of witnessing their sincere dedication to advancing the treatment of women's sexual health. Many of these scientists and physicians read the manuscript in various versions, and I thank them wholeheartedly again for their time, which has many demands upon it, and for their valuable feedback. Any errors, of course, are my own.

I am grateful to Caroline and Charles Muir and Mike Lousada, who took time to inform me about the history and practice of Tantra.

Warm thanks are due also to the many women and men who shared their personal stories, whether under their own names or with pseudonyms.

I am deeply indebted to my brilliant editors Libby Edelson and Daniel Halpern of HarperCollins and Lennie Goodings of Virago. I could not have had more perceptive, challenging, and insightful readers and commentators. Thanks also to Michael McKenzie and Zoe Hood. The copyeditor, Laurie McGee, was meticulous and patient. Rashmi Sharma provided admirable help with research materials. John and Katinka Matson and Russell Weinberger of Brockman, Inc., my agents, also read versions of the manuscript and provided much-appreciated commentary.

My deepest gratitude, as always, is for my family—parents, partner, and children.

# *Vagina*

# Introduction

## WHAT IS THE VAGINA?

*W*hy write a book about the vagina?

I have always been interested in female sexuality, and in the history of female sexuality. The way in which any given culture treats the vagina—whether with respect or disrespect, caringly or disparagingly—is a metaphor for how women in general in that place and time are treated. And there have been as many ways of seeing the vagina—what students of intellectual history call "constructs"—as there have been cultures. When I began this journey, I thought that if I looked at the vagina from these different historical perspectives, I would learn a great deal about women, both as sexual subjects and as members of communities; this investigation would surely illuminate where we are today. (Also, since I am a woman and I like pleasure, I was eager to learn things I might not know about female sexuality.) I thought I would find the truth about the vagina by studying all of these "constructs." I believed that some would prove to be basically accurate, and others, deeply inaccurate. But I now believe that all of them are only partially true, and that some constructs—including our own—are thoroughly subjective and full of misinformation.

Is the vagina a pathway to enlightenment, as it was for Indian practitioners of the Tantra? Or a "golden lotus," as Chinese Tao philosophy maintained? Is it the "hole" that the Elizabethans saw it as being? Or the test site for female maturity, an organ whose response separates the women from the girls, as Sigmund Freud believed?

Or is it what American feminists from the 1970s and on claim it to be: a not-so-important organ subordinated to the more glamorous clitoris? Or is it what contemporary mass-produced pornography says it is: a "hot," but essentially interchangeable, orifice, available visually by the thousands to anyone with a modem? Or is it what right-on sex-positive 2000s postfeminism says it is: a zippy pleasure producer for lusty women that demands dial-up satiation, from the texting of random partners for "booty calls," to high-tech vibrating electronics?

I read books such as evolutionary biologists Christopher Ryan and Cacilda Jethá's *Sex at Dawn;*[1] I reread sociologist Shere Hite's *The Hite Report: A Nationwide Study of Female Sexuality;*[2] I studied histories of the vagina such as *The Story of V: A Natural History of Female Sexuality* by cultural historian Catherine Blackledge;[3] and I looked at the latest research on female orgasm, from scientific databases such as *The Archives of Sexual Behavior.* I journeyed to laboratories where some of the most cutting-edge neurobiological research is being done on the role of female sexual pleasure—such labs as that of Dr. Jim Pfaus, at Concordia University in Montreal, Quebec, where landmark experiments are establishing that female sexual pleasure plays an important role in mate selection even among lower mammals.

I began to feel that all these books, articles, and destinations offered only pieces of the puzzle.

For personal as well as for intellectual reasons, I began to realize that the real headline is one that is rarely talked about, outside of a small circle: that there is a profound brain-vagina connection that seemed to me to contain more of the truth of the matter than anything else I was exploring. This book's germ started as a historical and cultural journey, but it quickly grew into a very personal and necessary act of discovery. I needed to learn the truth about the vagina because of a glimpse I had, by accident, into a dimension of its reality that I had never seen before.

Due to a medical crisis, I had a thought-provoking, revelatory experience that suggested a possibly crucial relationship of the vagina to female consciousness itself. The more I learned, the more I understood the ways in which the vagina is part of the female brain, and thus part of female creativity, confidence, and even character.

As I learned about the neuroscience and physiology behind what I had experienced, the connections between the female brain and the vagina introduced themselves into my understanding of other issues that women face. Once I had evidence that these connections were real, I felt that they held the key to much that had happened to women throughout history. I also felt that information about these connections—and the insights they afforded into female sexuality and selfhood—were important to bring to women today, and indeed to anyone who cares about women, because they can help us understand and value ourselves so much better.

As part of this investigation, I also wanted to hear what men had to say about their feelings about the vagina—apart from the two-dimensional story that our porn-saturated culture tells us. As I began to talk about what my subject was, scores of men of my acquaintance responded to my questions about their relationship to the vagina with hearteningly endearing answers. Often, though not always, a look of something like adoration or even love would appear in the expressions of men who were willing to describe their feelings about this part of a woman. The feelings these men described, though neither the men nor their words were random samples, were far from demeaning or pornographic.

To my surprise, many heterosexual men who were willing to talk to me about how they really felt expressed a kind of holistic (that is, not merely sexual) *gratitude* for the vagina, and they did not stress aspects of pleasure in isolation from what they often characterized as a sense of relief and joy at being so completely "accepted" and so fully "welcomed." Indeed, *acceptance* and *welcome* were two words that came up again and again in heterosexual men's discussions with me. Their responses made me think that women underestimate the importance to men of women's acceptance of them.

Of course, we can assume that some of these responses were mediated by the fact that a woman was asking the question; but the fact that so many men struck the same emotional tenor over and over again, made me believe that there was some truth here. When I described the connections I was finding between the vagina and other kinds of creativity and well-being, some men replied that these possible connections conformed to some of their own experiences with the women in their lives.

That initial set of insights about the brain-vagina connection, and the more subtle truths I derived from it about female emotional and sexual responses, altered my own life, my relationship, and my way of seeing, for the better. It made me feel, in a new way—no disrespect to men—incredibly *lucky* to be a woman, and it helped me to understand better exactly *why* women are lucky to be in their bodies.

———

One source of discomfort about being a woman in this culture is that the language we have with which to talk about our bodies, and about the vagina in particular, is so very awful. The common misreading of the vagina as "mere flesh" is a major reason for this discomfort. Female sexual pleasure, rightly understood, is not just about sexuality, or just about pleasure. It serves, also, as a medium of female self-knowledge and hopefulness; female creativity and courage; female focus and initiative; female bliss and transcendence; and as medium of a sensibility that feels very much like freedom. To understand the vagina properly is to realize that it is not only coextensive with the female brain, but is also, essentially, part of the female soul.

As I grew to better understand these aspects of the vagina, I began to put questions to women and to researchers that explored the connection between the vagina and female creativity, confidence, and the sense of connection to things and to people. The answers I received confirmed to me that I was heading in the right direction.

Before I began my research, many aspects of the vagina in history and in society had been mysterious to me: from the question of why so many women writers and artists had had their bursts of greatest creativity after a sexual awakening; to why some women tend to become addicted to love; to why heterosexual women are so often existentially torn between a bad boy/good man attraction; to—on a darker note—why the vagina has been targeted for abuse, violence, and control for most of Western history.

The more I learned about the neurology of the vagina and the biochemistry it releases in the brain, the more these mysteries, which had seemed all my life to be cultural, cleared up for me. Once one understands what scientists at the most advanced laboratories and clinics around the world are confirming—that the vagina and the brain are essentially one network, or "one whole system," as they tend to put it, and that the vagina mediates female confidence, creativity, and sense of transcendence—the answers to many of these seeming mysteries fall into place.

In the first section of the book, I explore the ways in which the vagina has been severely misunderstood. By looking at recent science, and asking questions in person and online, I found that the vagina's experiences can—on the level of biology—boost women's self-confidence, or else can lead to failures of self-confidence; can help unleash female creativity, or present blocks to female creativity. These experiences can contribute to a woman's sense of the joyful interconnectedness of the material and spiritual world—or else to her grieving awareness of the loss of that sense of interconnectedness. They can help her experience a state of transcendental mysticism that can affect the rest of her life—or leave her at the threshold of that state, intuiting that there is something "more." This latter experience, in turn, can lead not only to a decrease in her desire for sex, but can also risk a tincture in the rest of her life of what can only be called "existential depression" or "despair."

The second section of this book explores how social control of the vagina, and of women's sexuality, has been a vehicle to control women's minds and inner lives throughout the history of the West.

The third section of this book looks at the contemporary scene, and shows how modern pressures, such as the prevalence of pornography, are desensitizing both men and women in relation to the greater "life" of the vagina.

The final section of the book explores how to "reclaim the

Goddess"—that is, how to reframe our sense of the vagina, in relationship to ourselves and to our lovers, in the context of its actual neurological task of being a mediator and protector of women's highest, most joyful, and most unbroken sense of self. I will look at what women really need—for sexual happiness and fulfillment, but also for overall well-being—based on new neuroscience, as well as on what I learned from several Tantric masters, who spend their days healing or awakening women who are sexually and emotionally wounded or dormant.

Most of the examples in this book, especially about the physiology of female arousal and orgasm, will have implications that are inclusive for women of any sexuality—gay, straight, bisexual, and so on. But one of my primary themes is the exploration of heterosexual women's physical and emotional interactions with men. Some of the scientific studies focus directly on the physiology of heterosexual intercourse.

This focus on my part is not because I think that lesbian and bisexual arousal, orgasm, relationships, or mind-body connections are any less fascinating than are their heterosexual counterparts. It is because, rather, I believe (especially now) that female sexual responses, and the female mind-body connection, are so complex and so worthy of careful, individualistic attention that I do not believe that the politically correct approach of lumping all female experience together, with a nod to categories, can do justice to these variations. I believe, rather, that parallel questions about the physiology of lesbian and bisexual eros, the lesbian and bisexual mind-body connection, and the question of the vagina in lesbian and bisexual contexts, all deserve entire books of their own.

Nor are these questions directed only to women currently in relationships; while, as noted, many examples center around lovemaking, these insights apply, first of all, to women's sexual relationships with themselves.

## WHAT IS "THE GODDESS"?

Throughout this book, I will be referring to a state of mind or a condition of female consciousness I will call, for ease of reference, but also for the sake of the echo, "the Goddess." I don't mean to summon up in your mind crunchy-granola, 1970s images of pagan Goddess worship on all-female retreats in state parks, nor am I intending a simplistic, pop-culture shorthand for "self-esteem." Rather, I am carving out rhetorical space that does not yet exist when we talk about the vagina, but which refers to something very real.

Psychologist William James established a school of study known as "biological consciousness"—that is, the exploration of how the physical body affects states of mind. In 1902, James brought out his classic, *The Varieties of Religious Experience*.[4] In this book, on which I am basing part of my argument, he explores the role of the transcendent experience—which many people have had only in hints or glimpses, but which current research shows that most people have experienced to some degree—in healing traumatized or depressed lives.[5] Without making claims for the objective nature of "God" or "the Sublime," James addressed the issue of neurology as a substratum for these common mystical experiences. He made the case that when the brain experiences the states that correspond to those concepts, even though these may be physically-based experiences, nonetheless, transformation of a person is possible: "as a matter of psychological fact, mystical states of a well-pronounced and emphatic sort are usually authoritative over those who have them."[6]

James believed that these mind-states—which he and we call "mystical," and which the poet William Wordsworth described as a sense we all have, at moments, of familiarity with a "glory" that is elsewhere—are available to us through the doorway of the subconscious.[7] "Mystical states indeed wield no authority due simply to their being mystical states . . . they tell of the supremacy of the ideal, of vastness, of union, of safety and of rest. They offer us *hypotheses*, hypotheses which we may voluntarily ignore, but which as thinkers we cannot possibly upset."[8] These states are transient and passive, but James pointed out that as a result of experiencing such states of consciousness, great healing, great creativity, and even great happiness often entered people's lives. Were many people indeed happier, more loving, and more creative as a result of even momentary experiences of "God" or "the Sublime," whether or not those mind-states were caused by "mere" biochemistry? James made the case that they were.

Even before the latest neuroscience showed that the female orgasmic brain reveals activity that leads to a kind of loss of ego boundaries, a mystical or trancelike experience—perhaps not identical to what James was investigating, but not so different in its effect—scientists have known that there is a long-established link between orgasm and the release of opioids in the brain. Opioids—a form of neuropeptide—produce the experience of ecstasy, transcendence, and bliss. Sigmund Freud, in his 1930 book *Civilization and Its Discontents,* referred to what Romain Rolland had identified as "the oceanic feeling." Rolland had used the phrase to refer to the emotional tenor of religious feeling, the "oceanic" sense of limitlessness. Freud called this longing infantile.[9]

But Freud was a man; and recent science may indicate that, at least in orgasm, women may experience this oceanic feeling in a unique way. Recent MRI research, by Janniko Georgiadis and his team, showed in 2006 that regions of the female brain that have to do with self-awareness, inhibition, and self-regulation go quiet for women briefly during orgasm.[10] This can feel to the woman involved like a melting of boundaries, a loss of self, and, whether exhilaratingly or scarily, a loss of control.

Generally, many neuroscientists over the past thirty years have confirmed that James was biochemically correct: there are indeed changes in the brain that correspond to the experience of "the Sublime." Tremendous benefits—a greater sense of love, compassion, self-acceptance, and connectedness—have been shown in people who have cultivated those states of mind, as psychologist Dan Goleman's work on "emotional intelligence," in his 1995 book with that name, and the Dalai Lama's work on meditation, have shown. Western researchers have also demonstrated that meditative bliss states can involve opioid release. All women, as we will see, are potentially multiorgasmic; so the mystical or transcendental potential of female sexuality described above also allows women to connect often, and in a unique way, even if just for brief moments, with experiences of a shining, "divine," or greater self (or nonself, as Buddhists would say) or with a sense of the connection among all things. Producing the stimulation necessary for these mind-states is part of the evolutionary task of the vagina.

Philosophers have spoken for centuries of "a God-shaped hole" in human beings—the longing human beings feel to connect with something greater than themselves, and which motivates religious and spiritual quests. As seventeenth-century philosopher Blaise Pascal put it: "What else does this craving, and this helplessness, proclaim but that there was once in man a true happiness, of which all that now remains is the empty print and trace? This he tries in vain to fill with everything around him, seeking in things that are not there the help he cannot find in those that are, though none can help, since this infinite abyss can be filled only with an infinite and unchangeable object; in other words by God himself." [11]

Scientists have teased out the fact that this longing, this hunger to fill an "infinite abyss," is a neural capability we are all born with, an innate ability to experience and connect with something that feels, subjectively, like transcendence. The Dalai Lama's work on meditation, along with that of Dan Goleman, Lama Oser, and the E. M. Keck Laboratory for Functional Brain Imaging and Behavior, suggests that specific sites in the brain light up when subjects experience a meditative state; Stanford neuroscientists, too, are finding the neurology of bliss. [12] Typically, in this mind-state, one feels, among other things, that all is well with oneself and with the universe, and the vexations and limitations of the ego fall away. Artists have produced some of humanity's greatest works of music, painting, and poetry following such experiences.

So I will make the case throughout this book that there is a version of this connection with "the Sublime"—even if it, too, like

Rolland's "oceanic feeling," is simply a neurological trick of our magically complicated human brain wiring—that women can experience during and after certain moments of heightened sexual pleasure. I maintain that this feeling is critically linked to an experience of self-love or self-respect, and a sense of freedom and drive. This is why the issue of whether or not female sexuality is treated with love and respect is so very crucial. Such moments of heightened sexual sensibility lead to a woman's awareness that she is in a state of a kind of perfection, in harmony with and in connection with the world. In that state of consciousness, the usual inner voices that say the woman is not good enough, not beautiful enough, or not pleasing enough to others, are stilled, and a great sense of a larger set of connections— even a sense of what I will call, for lack of a better term, a Universal or Divine Feminine—can be accessed.

Major creative insights, and powerful work, can emerge after an experience of transcendence of this kind. I do believe that when women learn to identify and cultivate an awareness of "the Goddess," defined in this way, their behavior toward themselves, and their life experiences, change for the better—because self-destructiveness, shame, and tolerance of poor treatment cannot live in harmony with this set of feelings.

But I would argue, less literally, that "the Goddess"—a gendered sense of self that is shining, without damage, without anxiety or fear—inheres in every woman, and that women tend intuitively to know when they have glimpsed it or touched upon it. When women realize the spark of "the Goddess" in themselves, healthier, more self-respecting, and other sexual behavior follows. The vagina serves, physiologically, to activate this matrix of chemicals that feel, to the female brain, like "the Goddess"—that is, like an awareness of one's own great dignity, and of great self-love as a woman, as a radiant part of the universal feminine.

The vagina may be a "hole," but it is, properly understood, a Goddess-shaped one.

*Does the Vagina Have
a Consciousness?*

## Meet Your Incredible Pelvic Nerve

---

*The poetic, the scientific, the erotic—why should the imagination care which master it served?*

—Ian McEwan, "Solar"

*S*pring 2009 was beautiful. I was emotionally and sexually happy, intellectually excited, and newly in love. But it was a spring in which I also, slowly, started to realize that something was becoming terribly wrong with me.

I was forty-six. I was in a relationship with a man who was extremely well suited to me in various ways. For two years, he had given me great emotional and physical happiness. I have never had difficulty with sexual responsiveness, and all had been well in that regard. But almost imperceptibly, I began to notice a change.

I had always been able to have clitoral orgasms; and in my thirties, I had also learned to have what would probably be called "blended" or clitoral/vaginal orgasms, which added what seemed to be another psychological dimension to the experience. I had always experienced a postcoital rush of good emotional and physical feelings. After lovemaking, as I grew older, usually, after orgasm, I would see colors as if they were brighter; and the details of the beauty of the natural world would seem sharper and more compelling. I would feel the connections between things more distinctly for a few hours afterward; my mood would lift, and I would become chattier and more energized.

But gradually, I became aware that this was changing. I was slowly but steadily losing sensation *inside* my body. That was not the worst of it. To my astonishment and dismay, while my clitoral orgasms were as strong and pleasurable as ever, something very different than usual was happening, after sex, to my *mind*.

I realized one day, as I gazed out on the treetops outside the bedroom of our little cottage upstate, that the usual postcoital rush of a sense of vitality infusing the world, of delight with myself and with all around me, and of creative energy rushing through everything alive, was no longer following the physical pleasure I had certainly experienced. I started to notice that sex was increasingly just *about* that physical pleasure. It still felt really good, but I increasingly did not experience sex as being incredibly emotionally meaningful. I wanted it physically—it was a hunger and a repletion—but I no longer experienced it in a poetic dimension; I no longer felt it as being vitally connected to everything else in my life. I had lost the rush of seeing the connections between things; instead, things seemed discrete and unrelated to me in a way that was atypical for me; and colors were just colors—they did not seem heightened after lovemaking any longer. I wondered: *What is happening to me?*

Although nothing else in my life was going wrong—and though my relationship continued to be wonderful—I began to feel a sense of depression; then, underneath everything, a sense of despair. It was like a horror movie, as the light and sparkle of the world dialed downward and downward—now, not just after lovemaking, but in everyday existence. The internal numbness was progressing. I could not pretend I was imagining it. An emotional numbness progressed inexorably alongside it. I felt I was losing, somehow, what made me a woman, and that I could not face living in this condition for the rest of my life.

I could not figure out, from anything I had researched, what could possibly be causing this incredible, traumatic loss. One late night, sitting by the cold iron woodstove, alone, frantic with questions, and feeling hopeless, I began literally bargaining with the universe, as one does in times of great crisis. I actually prayed, proposing a deal: if God (or whoever was listening; I would go with anyone who was willing to take the call) would somehow heal me—somehow restore what I had lost—and if I learned anything worth knowing in the process, I would write about it—if there was the least chance that what I had learned could possibly help anyone else.

With a heavy heart—afraid to hear that nothing could be done for me—I made an appointment with my gynecologist, Dr. Deborah Coady. In this I was extremely fortunate, since she is one of the very few physicians who specialize in the aspects of the female body that, it would turn out, I was being affected by: problems with the pelvic nerve.

Dr. Coady is a lovely woman in her forties, with soft light-brown hair that falls to her shoulders, and a face that has a certain expression of gentle fatigue and receptivity to others' pain. Because of her specialty in female pelvic nerve disorders, and, in particular, in one of its painful variants, which thankfully I did not have, called "vulvodynia," she often sees women who are experiencing a broad range of suffering. This has made her unusually careful and compassionate.

Dr. Coady examined me, asked questions in a quiet voice, and finally told me she believed I was suffering numbness from nerve compression. I was so panicked at this point about what I was losing in terms of the emotional dimensions of my life and my sexuality—and so terrified of losing any more—that she took me into her private office.

There, in an effort to reassure me, she showed me two "Netter images"—beautifully drawn full-color anatomical illustrations. Frank Netter was a gifted medical illustrator, whose images of various parts of the human body are visual classics, collected by some neurologists, gynecologists, and other specialists, to help them explain abstract medical realities, in a vivid way, to their patients.

The first image depicted the way that the pelvic nerves in

women branch out to the base of the spinal cord.[1] Another showed how a branch, which originates in the clitoris and dorsal and clitoral nerve, arches elegantly to branch to the spinal cord, while other branches curve sinuously, originating in the vagina and also in the cervix. The nerve branches from the clitoris and vagina go to the larger pudendal nerve, whereas the nerve branch originating from the cervix goes to the larger pelvic nerve.[2] All of this complexity, I would learn later, gives women several different areas in their pelvises from which orgasms can be produced, and all of these connect to the spinal cord and then up to the brain.

Dr. Coady suspected that my problem was a spinal compression of one of the latter branches.

But she wanted to assure me that because of the way women were wired, no matter how bad the spinal compression that she suspected I had might prove to be, I would never lose the ability to have an orgasm, from the clitoris. Minimally comforted, I left her office, with an appointment for an MRI, and a referral to Dr. Jeffrey Cole, New York's pelvic nerve man.

———————

I met with Dr. Cole at the Kessler Institute for Rehabilitation, which he helps to lead, in Orange, New Jersey. A calm, quietly amusing man, with an old-fashioned, reassuring manner, he had looked at my initial x-rays, had examined my posture as I stood before him, and then had urgently written me a prescription for a hideous black back brace.

Two weeks later, I went back for a follow-up visit with Dr. Cole. Azaleas were now in bloom—it was still the loveliest part of the spring—but I felt almost faint as I sped into the suburbs in the backseat of a battered taxi. I was also very uncomfortable, since, for the past two weeks, I had been wearing the prescribed back brace. It extended from above my hips to below my rib cage, and it made me sit up perfectly straight.

I was really scared to hear what Dr. Cole had to say, since I knew he now had my MRI results. The MRI, Dr. Cole informed me, showed that I had lower-back degenerative spinal disease: my verte-brae were crumbling and compressed against each other. I was very surprised, having never had any pain, or any problem with my back at all.

He startled me by showing me the additional x-rays he had taken during the last appointment; there was no way to miss or misread it: on "L6 and S1," my lower back, my spinal column was like a child's tower of blocks that had slid, at a certain point, exactly halfway off central alignment—so that half of each stack of vertebrae was in con-tact with the other, but half of each ended in space.

I dressed and sat in Dr. Cole's consultation office. He put me through an unexpectedly tough and direct interview: "Did you ever have a blow to your lower back?" "Did anything ever strike your lower back?" He said it was a serious injury and that I must have some memory of having sustained it. I repeated that I had no mem-ory of any such trauma. When I finally realized what he might also be asking, I confirmed that no one had ever hit me.

But after about five minutes of this back and forth, I realized that yes, I had indeed once suffered a blow. In my early twenties, I had lost my footing in a department store, fallen down a flight of stairs, and landed on my back. I hadn't felt much pain, but I had felt shaken. An ambulance had arrived; I had been taken to St. Vincent's Hospi-tal and x-rayed. But nothing had been found to be the matter, and I had been released.

Dr. Cole took in the information and ordered another series of im-ages—this time a more detailed x-ray. He also performed an uncom-fortable test in which he shot electrical impulses through needles into my neural network, to see what was "lighting up," and what had gone dark.

In our third meeting, also at the suburban facility, I was back on the exam table. Dr. Cole explained that the new set of x-rays had revealed exactly what the matter with me was. I had been born, he explained, with a mild version of spina bifida, the condition in which the spinal vertebrae never develop completely. The blow from twenty years before had cracked the already fragile and incompletely formed vertebrae. Time had drawn my spinal column far out of alignment around the injury, which was now compressing one branch of the pelvic nerve, one of the branches Dr. Coady had shown me in the Netter image—the one that terminated in the vaginal canal.

I had been unbelievably lucky never to have had any symptoms until then, he said. Given the severity of my injury, it was fortunate that, though I had increasing numbness, I had had no pain. Much though I disliked working out, it seemed that a lifetime of grudging exercise had strengthened my back and abdomen enough to have kept any worse symptoms from manifesting until then. But time had done its work: where the two sections of spine were misaligned, the pelvic nerve was entrapped and compressed, and the signals from one of its several branches were blocked from moving up my spinal cord to my brain. The neural impulses from that part of my body had "gone dark." I wondered if this had something to do with how I felt—or was not feeling—after sex, though I was too shy to ask. He explained that I would need to consider surgery to fuse the vertebrae, and to relieve the pressure on the nerve.

After I had walked for him so he could check my gait to make sure my legs had not been affected, and after he had measured my shoulders to be sure they were level, I mentioned to him—perhaps partly for a second opinion, for reassurance—that Dr. Coady had assured me that my clitoral orgasms would not be affected, even if the branch of the pelvic nerve that was injured did not ever get better. He agreed that that was correct; if the clitoral branch of the network were to be affected, it would have been so by then. The fact that that branch was unaffected was an accident of my wiring. And then he explained casually, "Every woman is wired differently. Some women's nerves branch more in the vagina; other women's nerves branch more in the clitoris. Some branch a great deal in the perineum, or at the mouth of the cervix. That accounts for some of the differences in female sexual response."

I almost fell off the edge of the exam table in my astonishment. *That's* what explained vaginal versus clitoral orgasms? *Neural wiring?* Not culture, not upbringing, not patriarchy, not feminism, not

Freud? Even in women's magazines, variation in women's sexual response was often described as if it were predicated mostly upon emotions, or access to the "right" fantasies or role playing, or upon one's upbringing, or upon one's "guilt," or "liberation," or upon a lover's skill. I had never read that the way you best reached orgasm, as a woman, was largely due to *basic neural wiring.* This was a much less mysterious and value-laden message about female sexuality: it presented the obvious suggestion that anyone could learn about her own, or his or her partner's, particular neural variant as such, and simply master the patterns of the special way it worked.

"Do you realize," I stammered, not self-possessed enough in my astonishment to consider that the debate I was about to describe might not have been as momentous to him as it was to me, "you've just given the answer to a question that Freudians and feminists and sexologists have been arguing about for decades? All these people have assumed the differences in vaginal versus clitoral orgasms had to do with how women were raised . . . or what social role was expected of them . . . or whether they were free to explore their own bodies or not . . . or free or not to adapt their lovemaking to external expectations—and you are saying that the reason is simply that all women's *wiring* is different? That some are neurally wired more for vaginal orgasms, some more for clitoral, and so on? That some are wired to feel a G-spot more, others won't feel it so much—that it's mostly physical?"

"All women's wiring is different," he confirmed gently, as if he were addressing someone who had become slightly unhinged. "That's the reason women respond so differently from one another sexually. The pelvic nerve branches in very individual ways for every woman. These differences are physical." (I would learn later that this complex, variegated distribution is very different from male sexual wiring, which, as far as we know from the dorsal penile nerve, is far more uniform.)

I was silent, trying to absorb what he had said. Women have so many judgments about themselves, I have found, based on how they do or don't reach orgasm. Our discourse about female sexuality, which pays no attention whatsoever to this neural reality, which is the very mechanism of female orgasm, suggests that if women have trouble reaching orgasm, it is by now, in our liberated moment, surely, somehow, their own fault: they must be too inhibited; too unskilled; not "open" enough about their bodies.

Dr. Cole tactfully cleared his throat. He courteously sought to turn my attention back to my own predicament.

———

Dr. Cole referred me to Dr. Ramesh Babu, a neurosurgeon at New York Hospital, and that, too, was a very lucky thing. Irrationally, perhaps, I was immediately reassured to find that Dr. Babu, a suavely dressed and charismatic physician from India, had on his shelves among his neuroscience texts the same small statue of Kwan Yin, the Chinese goddess of compassion, that I had at home on my own bookshelves. Dr. Babu offered me an apple and then hectored me firmly but kindly on the need to operate without delay. Scarily, he wanted to put a fourteen-inch metal plate, with a set of attached metal joints, into my lower back, and fuse the damaged vertebrae. Fortunately, his will was just as strong as mine.

I scheduled the surgery. After a four-hour operation, I awoke, hideously groggy, in a hospital bed, the owner of this metal plate contraption, which fastened the vertebrae of my lower back together with four bolts. I had a vertical scar down my back that my boyfriend—in an effort to reassure me—described, referring to the punk rock band, as "very Nine-Inch Nails." All these changes seemed like very minor issues compared with the hope I now had of regaining the lost aspects of my mind and of my creative life, via my now-decompressed pelvic nerve.

After three months I was allowed to make love again. I felt better but not completely recovered; I knew that neural regeneration, if it were to happen, could take many months. I continued to recuperate steadily for six months, eager but also scared to find out what would happen, if anything, to my mind once my pelvic nerve was really free of obstruction again. Would the nerve fully recover? And, more important—would my mind fully recover? Would I feel again that emotional joy, sense again that union among all things?

Thanks to Dr. Babu and perhaps to whoever in the cosmos may have taken my call, I had a complete neural recovery, which was not something any of the team had taken for granted. This particular kind of neural compression, though not unheard of, is seldom written about outside of medical journals, and I am a walking control group for the study of the effect of impulses from the pelvic nerve on the female brain. Because of how scant information is on this subject, I feel I owe it to women to put down on paper what happened next.

As my lost pelvic sensation slowly returned, *my lost states of consciousness also returned.* Slowly but steadily, as internal sensation reawakened, and as the "blended" clitoral/vaginal kind of orgasms that I had been more used to, returned to me, sex became emotional for me again. Sexual recovery for me was like that transition in *The Wizard of Oz* in which Dorothy goes from black-and-white Kansas to colorful, magical Oz. Slowly, after orgasm, I once again saw light flowing into the world around me. I began to have, once again, a wave of sociability pass over me after lovemaking—to want to talk and laugh. Gradually, I reexperienced the sense of deep emotional union, of postcoital creative euphoria, of joy with one's self and with one's lover, of confidence and volubility and the sense that all was well in some existential way, that I thought I had lost forever.

I began again, after lovemaking, to experience the sense of heightened interconnectedness, which the Romantic poets and painters called "the Sublime": that sense of a spiritual dimension that unites all things—hints of a sense of all things shivering with light. That, to my immense happiness, returned. It was enough for me to have glimpses of it once again from time to time.

I remember being again in the small upstairs bedroom of the little cottage upstate; my partner and I had just made love. I looked out of the window at the trees tossing their new leaves and the wind lifting their branches in great waves, and it all looked like an intensely choreographed dance, in which all of nature was expressing something. The moving grasses, the sweeping tree branches, the birds calling from invisible locations in the dappled shadows, seemed, again, all to be in communication with one another. I thought: it is back.

From this experience a journey began: to understand what had happened to my mind, and to better understand the female body and female sexuality.

———————

In the following two years, I learned a great deal more than I had known before—which was not difficult, as, like most women, I had known nothing at all—about the female pelvic nerve. And it turns out that in some ways it is the secret to everything related to femininity itself.

When I use the term *vagina* in this book, I am using it somewhat differently from its technical definition. The medical meaning of *vagina* is just "the introitus," the vaginal opening, one of many inadequate words related to this subject. I am using it, unless I specify otherwise, to mean something that we, weirdly, have no one single word for: that is, for the entire female sex organ, from labia to clitoris to introitus to mouth of cervix.

Even defined in that more inclusive way, we still tend to think of the vagina in limited terms: as the parts we can see and touch on the surface of our bodies, between our legs: the vulva, the inner labia, and the clitoris—or the parts we can touch when we explore inside our bodies with our fingers—the vaginal canal. We have been terribly misconceiving the vagina by restricting our understanding of it to these surfaces of the skin, and to these inward membranes.

The vulva, clitoris, and vagina are just the most superficial surfaces of what is really going on with us. The real activity is literally far, and far more complexly, *under* these tactile surfaces. The vulva, clitoris, and vagina are actually best understood as the surface of an ocean that is shot through with vibrant networks of underwater lightning—intricate and fragile, individually varied neural pathways. All these networks are continually sending their impulses to the spinal cord and brain, which then send new impulses back down through other fibers in the same nerves to produce various effects.

This dense set of neural pathways extends throughout the entire pelvis, far underneath that outer vulvar skin and inner vaginal skin (though this last phrase, too, is not, medically, technically accurate: the skin inside the vagina is called, in one of the many unpleasant terms we have to refer to something so lovely, *mucous membrane* or *mucosa*).

You can see from the Netter images online that your gorgeous, complicated netting of neural pathways is connected to your spinal cord.[3] These neural pathways are continually "lighting up," as neurologists put it, with electrical impulses—depending on what is happening to your clitoris, vulva, and vagina.

Let me use a second metaphor. Imagine that you found a tangle of seaweed on the edge of the shore and lifted it. The heaviest parts rest on the sand in a mesh, but some skeins extend vertically. This neural network is shaped like that: it looks like a tangled skein of a hundred thousand golden threads that has been drawn upward. The mass of it gathers in the pelvis, but strands from the same network extend upward to the spinal cord and brain. Netter image 3093 shows this.[4]

The pelvic nerve in humans branches out of sacral vertebrae numbers four and five, or S4 and S5, which are vertebrae in your lower back. From there, it branches again into the three far-reaching neural pathways, which I mentioned earlier, that extend throughout your pelvis: one originating in the clitoris; one in the walls of the vagina; and one in the cervix. Another network of nerves originates along your perineum and anus. Among the many incredible things about your incredible pelvic nerve and its lovely multiple branches is that, as we saw, *it is completely unique for every individual woman on earth—no two women are alike.*

As you can see from the Netter images, the female pelvic neural network is highly complex. Its intense complexity is a reason that there is so much variability in women's sexual wiring. In contrast, the male pelvic neural network, which concludes in a comparatively very regular, almost schematized, *grid* of neural pathways, a circle of pleasure around the penis, seems to be much simpler. This greater sexual neural complexity in women is because we have both reproductive and sexual parts, such as the cervix and uterus, that men don't have.

There are many more neural networks extending from the female pelvis into the spinal cord than extend from the networks in the penis to the spinal cord. You can see this in the Netter images titled "Innervation of External Genitalia" and "Perineum, Innervation of Female Reproductive Organs," and "Innervation of Male Reproductive Organs."[5] Clearly the female neural network is far more diffuse than the male and has a *lot* more going on: in women, there is a tangle of neural activity at the top of the uterus, at the sides of the vagina, at the top of the rectum, at the top of the bladder, at the clitoris, and along the perineum. There are fewer distinct tangles of neural activity in the male pelvis. (The perineum is the skin between your anus and your vagina: let me stress again that one entire and distinct sexual neural network originates for women right here in the perineum, and it is this sexual neural network that, as one physician who read this section pointed out with alarm, "is routinely cut during an episiotomy for a difficult delivery." As I reported in *Misconceptions: Truth, Lies and the Unexpected on the Journey to Motherhood,* in America and Western Europe, unnecessary episiotomies are routinely performed for normal deliveries that would not require them if it were not for the economics of hospital time pressures, and of the litigation pressures on hospitals as well. In America and Western Europe, unsurprisingly, many women report diminished sexual sensation after childbirth, and especially after undergoing an episiotomy, though they are almost never informed by hospitals or physicians that an episiotomy will sever a sexual nerve system.)[6]

By looking at the pattern of the neural networks in the Netter images, and in the illustrations here, you see that women are designed to receive pleasure, and experience triggers to orgasm, from skillful caressing and rhythmic pressure of all kinds over many, many parts of their bodies. The pornographic model of intercourse—even our culture's conventional model of intercourse, which is quick, goal-oriented, linear, and focused on stimulation of perhaps one or two areas of a woman's body—is just not going to do it for many women, or at least not in a very profound way, because it involves such a superficial part of the potential of women's neurological sexual response systems.

For some women, a lot of neural pathways originate in the clitoris, and these women's vaginas will be less "innervated"—less dense with nerves. A woman in this group may like clitoral stimulation a lot, and not get as much from penetration. Some women have lots of innervation in their vaginas, and climax easily from penetration alone. Another woman may have a lot of neural pathway terminations in the perineal or anal area; she may like anal sex and even be able to have an orgasm from it, while it may leave a differently wired woman completely cold, or even in pain. Some women's pelvic neural wiring will be closer to the surface, making it easier for them to reach orgasm; other women's neural wiring may be more submerged in their bodies, driving them and their partners to need to be more patient and inventive, as they must seek a more elusive climax.

Culture and upbringing definitely have a role in how you climax and can affect whether you climax easily or not, but that is not all there is to it. This discourse heaps vast unnecessary guilt and shame on millions of women or, conversely, depending on their tastes, leads them to feel slightly perverted. Do you feel like you're imposing on your lover because (unlike his last girlfriend) you really need that "extra" oral sex from him? Are you embarrassed that you may wish you could ask for stimulation of both orifices when you make love? Does it sometimes take you longer than you'd like to climax, or is climax sometimes even elusive? Hey: it may not be due to your grandmother who made sure you slept with your hands on top of the covers, or to those censorious nuns in middle school; you are not any less sexual a being, or even, necessarily, any more inhibited, than his last girlfriend. Whatever it is you like and need in bed—as a woman, with all that variability—these preferences *may just be due to your physical wiring.*

## *Your Dreamy Autonomic Nervous System*

---

*My heart flutters in my breast,*
*whenever I look quickly, for a moment—*
*I say nothing . . . my ears roar,*
*cold heat rushes down me,*
*I am greener than grass*
*to myself I seem*
*needing but little to die . . .*

—Sappho, "Fragment"

For women, sexual response involves entering an altered state of consciousness. This transformation depends on your dreamy autonomic nervous system, or what scientists call the "ANS." This system, which controls all the smooth muscle contractions in your body, contains both the sympathetic and parasympathetic divisions; it affects what your body does beyond your conscious control. The two divisions work in tandem. In women, the biology of arousal is more delicate than most of us understand, and it depends significantly on this sensitive, magical, slowly calmed, and easily inhibited system.

Arousal precedes orgasm, of course. In order for the pelvic neural network to do its crazy work, the autonomic nervous system first has to do *its* work. Researchers Cindy Meston and Boris Gorzalka discovered in 1996 that the female sympathetic nervous system (SNS) was crucially involved in whether or not female arousal was successful, or even possible.[1]

The autonomic nervous system prepares the way for the neural impulses that will travel from vagina, clitoris, and labia to the brain, and this fascinating system regulates a woman's responses to the relaxation and stimulation provided by "the Goddess Array," the set of behaviors a lover uses to arouse his or her partner. The ANS has to do with responses we can't consciously control: it manages many of the physical reactions that are connected to arousal and orgasm, including respiration, blushing, the flushing of skin, the filling of the corpora cavernosa—the spongy tissue in the vagina that engorges with blood to produce the "erection" of the clitoris—the filling of the vaginal walls with blood that is necessary for vaginal lubrication, the increase in heart rate, the dilation of pupils, and so on.

The brain affects the ANS, which in turn affects the vagina, which is why if you are a woman, you can think of a lover, become aroused, and find yourself wet. But the vagina also affects the brain, which in turn affects the ANS. It is a constant feedback loop. A positively experienced touch to the clitoris or vagina sends a signal to the ANS to stir up a complex series of subtle changes in the woman's body. That one touch, if it continues to be careful and skillful and responsive to the woman's reactions, changes a woman's breathing—causing her to start breathing more heavily, or panting; it raises her heart rate and thus her circulation rate, which in turn causes her skin to flush, her nipples to become erect, and her whole body to become more sensitive. Her raised heartbeat, if her lover's stimulation remains careful and attentive, sends blood shooting rhythmically into her vaginal blood vessels—the elaborate circulatory throughway distributed throughout the labia, around the vagina, and deep inside her pelvis—swelling them. This swelling expands both her inner and outer labia, which makes both layers of flesh more sensitive to pleasure; it engorges and extends the clitoris, allowing it to transmit pleasure far more keenly than otherwise; and it helps the walls of her vagina to become slick with lubrication.

This optimal activation of her ANS makes a woman eager for lovemaking and able to experience it in all its dimensions. But for this process to be complete, and thus truly fulfilling, the stimulation must be unhurried and carefully attuned to how the woman is responding. The process requires attention and time. And, as we will see, relaxation heightens the ideal activation of the ANS—and "bad stress" interferes with it.

"The full melting response" or "high orgasm" in women—which I would define (though our language around female sexual response is so inadequate) as that kind of orgasm that most intensely induces the most complete possible trance state and that most involves all the body systems, so that afterward the woman feels the most replete and also experiences the highest level possible for her of the positive brain chemicals' activities—is truly possible only when the ANS is optimally activated. In our culture we all know about engaging the pelvic neural network, which is what we are raised to think of when we think of "sex" (though our general understanding of even this network is, as we saw, too superficial). But full sexual and emotional release for women centers on an idea that is foreign to our discussion of sex: activation. The ideal is an activation of the whole female autonomic system—of respiration, lubrication, and heart rate—which in turn affects vaginal engorgement, muscular contraction, and orgasmic release: external stimuli as a woman thinks of sex elicit anticipator/dopamine release, and opioids and oxytocin are released by her orgasm. Most people in our culture are *not* raised to pay much attention to reading a woman's "activation" levels. If a woman's ANS response is ignored, she can have intercourse and even climax; but she won't necessarily feel released, transported, fulfilled, or in love, because only a superficial part of her capacity to respond has been made love to, or engaged.

The ANS also responds to a woman's sense of safety or danger. It sends the signals to the brain and then to the body that one is safe, so one can relax, eat, and digest; or relax and sleep; or relax and make love. The "relaxation response," a powerful phenomenon identified in the West by Dr. Herbert Benson in 1975 (but well known in many Eastern cultures), takes place when you relax to the point that your brain facilitates the ANS's healing work—and promotes the effectiveness of the things your body does that are not under your conscious control.[2] By now there are literally hundreds of studies showing the power of the relaxation response in bringing the human body and mind benefits ranging from better healing after surgery, to improved focus, to lower rates of heart disease.

Several recent studies show that the relaxation response is even more important to female arousal than we have realized before now. As we saw, Dr. Georgiadis and his team's MRI study showed that as a woman approaches closer and closer to orgasm, her brain centers for behavioral regulation become deactivated.[3] One could say that she actually becomes, biochemically, a wild woman or a maenad. She becomes so disinhibited and impervious to pain that it is as if she is in a state of altered consciousness. Women in "high" orgasm go more deeply into this trance state than at any other time. Judgment is suspended in this state, and women do not even feel pain in the same ways as in normal consciousness.

The ANS gets you to that point; it lets a woman relax, breathe deeply, flush, fill with blood in all the right places, get the high-focus energy of activated dopamine, and go eventually—safely—into the kind of trance state described above. Simultaneously she experiences the most intense kind of pelvic contractions, which leave her exhausted, spent, and basking in big jolts of opioids and oxytocin—bliss and fondness—bringing these in turn into her life and into her relationships.

But here is the catch: you can't *will* the ANS to do anything. You can't say to it: "Turn me on." This is true for other processes it regulates: you can't *will* the "letting-down" of your milk, as many new mothers know; you can't speed up or slow down digestion through your conscious intention, or give birth more efficiently. As many women (and men) know to their frustration, the more you try to *will* yourself to feel aroused and reach orgasm, the more elusive these states can become.

To enter the transcendental state that takes the female brain into "high" orgasm, *you absolutely need to feel safe;* safe from "bad stress," in the sense of knowing you are entering a trance state in the presence of someone who will protect you if necessary at the very least, and not endanger you or put you in circumstances out of your control. The trance state is very nice if you're in a modern suite at a hotel in the Caribbean, but what about when our foremothers were making furtive love in the brush of the savannah? Obviously, it would have been highly dangerous, and thus not evolutionarily valuable, to enter into this disinhibited trance state in the vicinity of wild animals or aggressors from another tribe, or any everyday natural threats. This biological, evolutionary connection for women of possible ecstasy to emotional security has implications that cannot be overstressed. *Relaxing allows for female arousal.*

Just as being valued and relaxed can heighten female sexual response, "bad stress" can dramatically interfere with all of women's sexual processes. I became interested in the role of stress in relation to the "performance" or "failure to perform" of the vagina—and breasts, and uterus—a decade ago, when I was working on my book about childbirth, *Misconceptions.* It became obvious from the research I did at that time that the uterus, cervix, birth canal, vagina, and perineum were all substantially supported by relaxation in "performing" their powerful ANS tasks in childbirth and lactation. A low-stress environment of soft lighting, soothing music, caring attendants, and the loving presence of family, all actually helped the female body birth a baby, and then feed a newborn, successfully, in clinically measurable ways. Many studies also confirmed that stressful hospital birthing environments, in which women in labor are hooked up to intravenous devices, or to fetal monitors that consistently show false-positive "fetal distress," cause so much "bad stress" in mothers that the stress itself biologically—not just psychologically—arrests labor contractions, and inhibits lactation.[4]

In the decade that has passed since I first explored this brain-uterus, brain-breast-tissue connection, these studies have multiplied. Stress can and often does stop the uterus from contracting in childbirth; it can stop the birth canal from drawing the baby toward the vaginal opening; it can stop the muscles from relaxing, that need to open in order to birth the baby without tearing the mother's perineum; it can stop the milk glands from filling. Ina May Gaskin, famed alternative childbirth educator and author of the enduring bestseller *Spiritual Midwifery,* has delivered more than five hundred babies at home or even in tents in the woods, with very low rates of complications. She often tells couples to lower lights, play music, have the man stroke the woman, and to kiss and make out during labor, because of how often she has seen that a soothing and even seductive environment supports effective contractions during birth, and supports milk "let-down" for breast-feeding.

"Farm midwives might give a couple instructions on how to kiss more effectively," she writes. "A loose mouth makes for a loose puss which makes the baby come out easier." She teaches her midwives to teach the husbands or partners of birthing women to stimulate women's nipples to aid contractions: "Our group of midwives had known this [about stimulating birthing women's nipples] and used it as a tool for two or three years before we heard that the medical community, in doing experiments, had discovered that there is a powerful endocrine hormone called oxytocin that is produced by the pituitary gland, which can be prompted to [bring about contractions of the uterus] by stimulation of the breasts. We had been using this in starting labor in the woman . . . or . . . in speeding it up. We prefer to do this by pleasanter means than an IV drip." As she puts it, the same sexual energy that got the baby in, is best at getting it out.[5]

If you look at the neurology and biochemistry of childbirth and lactation, you will see that it is not weird at all, really, to maintain that the vagina sends signals resulting in thoughts and emotions, because the uterus in labor and delivery—the breasts in lactation—send signals that result in thoughts and emotions, too.

When a baby passes through the birth canal, the contractions trigger oxytocin in the mother's brain. Affectionately called "the cuddle chemical," oxytocin is a hormone well known for its role in birth and lactation in the postpartum period, and in the establishment of mother-infant attachments. It is also released during orgasm in both sexes, and acts as a neurotransmitter in the brain, facilitating bonding and the formation of trust. Hormones such as oxytocin can reduce fear or behavioral inhibition, and promote the expression of social behaviors, such as pair bonding, and sexual and maternal behaviors. Female rats with no prior offspring show maternal behaviors within just thirty minutes of oxytocin administration, and these behaviors can be completely abolished by treating the same rats with oxytocin antagonists.[6] Female prairie voles treated with oxytocin pair-bonded faster, and they lost interest in pair-bonding when the hormone was blocked. Anecdotally, some women who have had cesarean sections have trouble bonding, at first, with their newborns. These new mothers were not allowed to labor long enough for "mother love" to be chemically established within them. When a newborn suckles, the sucking reflex also triggers the release of oxytocin in the mother's brain. The baby is biochemically *creating* its mother's love and feelings of attachment.

I experienced some of the "thoughts" of the uterus myself. In 2000, I wrote about how oxytocin had made me gentler, more conflict averse, and basically nicer, when I was pregnant.[7] My uterus was doing some of my thinking for me, in spite of my will, and mediating my consciously autonomous, consciously assertive, feminist brain. I also experienced the delayed attachment that cesarean sections can cause due to their interruption of oxytocin production that contractions are meant to generate. It is not a radical idea that biology can condition consciousness; it is well established that the uterus in labor, and the nipples in breast-feeding, can mediate female consciousness. So it should not be odd to say that the biology of the vagina, in the context of sex, can mediate female consciousness as well.

"Bad stress," researchers have now abundantly confirmed, has exactly the same kind of negative effect on female arousal and on the vagina itself. When a woman feels threatened or unsafe, the sympathetic nervous system—the parasympathetic nervous system's partner in the ANS—kicks in. This system regulates the "fight or flight" response: as adrenaline and catecholamines are released in the brain, nonessential systems such as digestion and, yes, sexual response, close down; circulation constricts, because the heart needs all the blood available to help the body run or fight; and the message to the body is "get me out of here." Based on the insights in Meston and Gorzalka's work, we now know that a threatening environment—which can include even vague verbal threats centered on the vagina or dismissive language about the vagina—can close down female sexual response. (We will explore "good" sexual stress later.)

Don't take my word for this powerful evidence of the mind-body connection in women's sexuality. If you have a lover or husband who is willing, try this simple experiment. Wait for a moment after he or she has said something really reassuring or admiring of you as a woman; then let him or her touch your nipple. Watch how quickly your nipple seems actively to seek out your lover's touch. If he or she keeps talking along those lines, watch how readily your vagina responds to the touch—as the Tantric masters say, it should literally yearn toward and open for the lover's hand, to draw it closer, or do the same for a lover's penis. (Again, a similar connection between verbal appreciation and pathways of arousal may well be true for men: researchers have found that men's physiological distress levels in relationship conflicts lower, in response to female words of respect and appreciation.)

Try the experiment another way at another time. If he or she has said something offensive or annoying or disrespectful to you, see what happens if your lover touches your nipple; it is unlikely that you will be able to tolerate his or her touch comfortably, let alone welcome it. Many people don't like being touched if they are angry, but women seem to have more trouble than men with arousal if they are upset.

The difference in our bodies' responses may make male-female connection especially tricky in such moments: this one simple difference in female reaction to different ways of being spoken to is one enormously significant reason that so many sexual approaches from men to women in long-term relationships become derailed, to the great sorrow and frustration of both men and women; the woman literally often *can't* take an intimate touch if her lover has recently been verbally disrespectful, or has failed verbally to soothe "the Goddess in her" at some point beforehand, priming the release of oxytocin and vasopressin in her body and preparing the parasympathetic nervous system to do its magical work.

In the first flush of courtship, men often treat their female lovers in ways that deeply relax the women, supporting the work of the SNS; that activate their pelvic neural networks; and that trigger delicious hormonal activity in the female brain. But once the relationship is secured, many men tend to scale back those seductive words and lingering, relaxing caresses, or drop them altogether. This is a mistake, but it is not surprising: the "lingering caresses" kind of sex requires a great deal more time than does briefer, more goal-oriented lovemaking. Some might say it requires a good deal more "effort" from men; the Tantric practitioners I spoke with in the course of this journey would certainly say that it asks of men a great deal more "focus." Our culture even calls these caresses and words a preamble to the real action—the idea is embedded in the very word *foreplay*—so they are seen as sexual "extras." A whole set of words, actions, and gestures that women cannot do without, and that I call "the Goddess Array," are, in our culture, seen as mere invitations to the feast, and not as the feast itself.

But when you understand the role of the ANS in women, which is where the effect of seemingly "nonsexual" touches, seductive or admiring words, and that crucial sense of safety and of being uniquely valued, register, you will see what a terrible error this is. The sympathetic nervous system doesn't transmit sensations as such. It is part of the ANS that produces effects opposite to "flight or fight." But it sends out responses to the gentle caresses, words, and so on that I am describing, which affect female arousal as a whole. When it comes to the female brain's connection to the female body, as the brain mediates the ANS and is mediated by it, it becomes clear that *these gestures, touches, kisses, and words aren't extras*. They are integral parts of the activation of the female ANS—and in turn these words and gestures tell the female brain that this is a safe sexual environment. The linear, goal-oriented model of sex that is conventional in our culture makes many women feel frustrated and existentially unhappy over time—*even if they are having orgasms.* Since orgasms are seen as the "goal" of sex in our culture, this can be confusing. Well-intentioned men might understandably feel baffled as they witness a wife or girlfriend grow irritable and dissatisfied over time, with this kind of culturally perfectly adequate lovemaking.

But men who really want to understand their wives and girlfriends and make them existentially happy will simply need to understand the female ANS, and seek out a deeper understanding of the life of the vagina. Such a man will need to become "more Tantric," more sensual and romantic in bed, but he will, just as importantly, need to be much more attentive to what the woman wants in her life at any given moment. He will need to totally forget whatever he thought "worked" with his last lover, and learn from the very beginning, following her individual response. He will have to be far more inventive, creative, and attentive than the conventional model of heterosexual sex "scripts" him to be. A male lover of a woman, in other words, has to be far more patient, tactile, and time invested than he has probably been raised to be (and probably much more than he is initially inclined to be, after a long day at work). He must become far more interested in her state of mind, her level of stress or of relaxation, the skin of her whole body, a breath in her ear, a heavier touch and a lighter touch; far more interested in really gazing into her eyes, in light kissing and deep kissing; far more interested in offering stroking and caresses to her that do not feel to the woman as if there is a goal-oriented "agenda." He must stimulate, sensitively and skillfully, whatever combination of the woman's clitoris, vagina, G-spot, labia, perineum, rectum, and mouth of her cervix really makes her happy. He needs to be highly attentive to whether she wants soft, lingering lovemaking at that moment or hard, powerful sex or some exciting combination, because at different times of the month—or depending on her mind-state, which affects her body—her wishes may vary. He will need to know the difference between "bad stress" and "good stress." Penetration may be part of the pleasure nexus, of course; orgasm is part of the pleasure nexus; but there is much, much more.

———————

How exactly does your sexual neural network function? You can see from the Netter image of the autonomic nervous system how the genitals connect to the lower spinal cord, which in turn connects to the brain.[8]

The Netter image shows a close-up of the spinal cord and the nerve roots that connect the spinal cord's impulses to the vagina and vice versa. These impulses end up in the female brain. All the neurotransmitters send signals from the clitoris, vagina, cervix, and so on up the spinal cord, and finally they reach the hypothalamus and the brain stem.

The pituitary gland is under the brain, and the hypothalamus right above it. The pituitary is called the "master gland" because it regulates all the hormones in your brain and body—the production, for instance, of oxytocin—the chemical "love factory" that generates feelings of bonding, trust, and attachment. The pituitary gland is where all the emotional action takes place. Here is one place where a dopamine system is regulated that will make you more or less aroused; another, midbrain dopamine system makes you incentivized and focused, before and during sex. Dopamine is associated with arousal and desire. Oxytocin and other emotion-generating hormones, which will make you think your lover's otherwise annoying habits are really cute, are processed in the hypothalamus. And prolactin, which will make you finally get up out of bed to get some laundry done, or to do some other work, is also processed in the hypothalamus. So it is right to say that the vagina is sending signals to the brain during lovemaking that mediate consciousness.

That skein of living threads in the female pelvis—so intimately in communication through the spinal cord to the brain, with its shifting bath of chemicals—triggers opioids and oxytocin release after orgasm, which, as we will see, makes us ache physically when we have started to fall in love with someone. It is why women go into that disinhibited, out-of-control trance state when they climax that involves different parts of the brain.

Though delicate, that network underlying our clitorises, vulvas, and vaginas is incredibly powerful: the orgasmic pleasure generated there sends our brains messages with power to help regulate our menstrual and hormonal cycles, make us more or less fertile, calm us down at the scent of a lover, or vaginally lubricate when we are praised. By the same token, the brain also sends signals to the clitoris, vulva, and vagina, indicating when it is the right time and situation in which to lubricate, flush with blood, climax, and bond. This network is so influential over all the relevant systems of our bodies that if we are neglected sexually—or if we sexually neglect ourselves if we are not partnered—the messages sent from these pathways up the spinal cord to the brain, and the hormonal reactions in the brain, can lead us into depression, or even heighten our risk of injury or heart disease. This network is continually sending moods, sensations, and emotions to our brains and from our brains to our inner and outer skin; it is not the vagina itself but that network underneath everything that leads us to feel much of what we feel; that leads each woman to shiver differently, in response to a different touch; that leads female consciousness itself to fluctuate, as these messages along these pathways fluctuate—a flux heightened by the cyclical nature of female sexual desire. If femininity resided anywhere, I would say it resides there, in that electric inward network extending from pelvis to brain.

This neural pathway, and other evidence we will look at, explains why our notions of female sexuality are so often wrong. Since Masters and Johnson wrote *Human Sexual Response* in 1966, which they based on their studies of men and women having orgasms in lab conditions, our culture has accepted the single model of human sexual response they described of excitement, plateau, orgasm, and resolution, which, they argued, is similar for women and men.[9] Their summary of the vagina asserts that "it should be stated parenthetically that vaginal (natural or artificial) response to sexual stimuli develops in a basic pattern" regardless of the stimuli's origin, a view that new science suggests is too simplistic. Even today, our culture tends to present male and female sexual response as analogous or parallel, while acknowledging that some women have more orgasms with less of a "refractory period" rest time in between than men need. That "one model" for human sexuality has even been seen as liberated—it does allow women sexual needs, since it allows men sexual needs—and it fit the Second Wave of feminism's, and the sexual revolution's, comfortable idea that women were, sexually at least, "just like men."

The Masters and Johnson model is being challenged as too reductive when it comes to women, on several fronts. The latest science—including from such researchers as Rosemary Basson, M.D., at the University of British Columbia, Irv Binick at McGill University in Montreal, Quebec, and Barry R. Komisaruk, at Rutgers University in New Jersey—is confirming that there are many variations, for women, on what now looks like a far too basic model.[10] It is more accurate to say, based on the newer science, that though female sexuality has *some* superficial analogues to male sexuality, additional levels of experience and sensation are also often involved.[11] Female sexuality is very far indeed from being merely a female version of what has traditionally been understood, often from a male perspective, as "just sex." They are finding that the vagina and brain cannot be fully considered separately: Basson found that women's subjective sense of arousal must be measured in mind, not just body; Komisaruk and his team found arousal and orgasms *only,* for injured female subjects, in the mind.[12]

My journey finally led me to conclude that, with the exception of a few healers, teachers, and practitioners, we are indeed, for all our "liberation," constraining the vagina in sexual ideologies that are actually much less than liberating and that are sometimes new, "hip," or "sexy" forms of old-style enslavement and control. Or else we are actively ignorant of the true role and dimensionality of the vagina. I came to conclude that the vagina is not nearly as free today in the West as we are led to believe—both because its full role is seriously misunderstood, and also because it is disrespected.

## Confidence, Creativity, and the
## Sense of Interconnectedness

*The sister didn't even get the watercolors—they puzzled her—
looked several times—always seeming to question—The man on
horseback she liked . . . I'll take it to school tomorrow—showing
it to folks that can't see hurts but I'll do it anyway— . . . Is it
because there is more animal in me than brain—that I want to
be near you to tell you how much I like it—No—it isn't animal at
all—it's touch—Touch may be God or the Devil with me—I don't
know which— . . .*

—Georgia O'Keeffe to Alfred Stieglitz

*A*round the same time that I was stuggling with my medical
situation, I went back to graduate school to work toward a
degree in Victorian and Edwardian women's literature.

I began to notice that many women writing between 1850 and
1920 articulated aspects of female sexual experience that did indeed often suggest a connection between a sexual awakening and
a creative awakening. These pre–sexual revolution, pre–Second
Wave feminist writers such as the British Victorian lyric poet Christina Rossetti, turn-of-the-twentieth-century American novelist Kate
Chopin, and Anaïs Nin, the memoirist writing in France in the

1930s, wrote about female sexual passion as if it were an overwhelming force that made short work of will and self-possession. They often seemed to connect sexual self-knowledge or sexual awakening in women with the growth or awakening of other aspects of female creativity and identity. Unlike those women writers and artists of the post-1960s era, they did not ever portray female sexuality as being "merely" about physical pleasure.

I found something else quite surprising: though misogynist commentators had often suggested that brilliant women could not be sexual—versions of the sexless, intelligent "bluestocking" have surfaced since the medieval period—and that highly sexual women had no brains, the biographies of creative artist after creative artist suggested the very opposite. In life after life of women writers, revolutionaries, and artists, a particularly liberating sexual relationship or affair—or hints of sexual self-discovery, even if the artist was unpartnered—would precede a luxuriant stretch of creative and intellectual expansion in their work. And, judging from their private letters, I saw that some of the most creative and most intellectually and psychologically "free" women of their eras—from Christina Rossetti to George Eliot, Edith Wharton, Emma Goldman, and Georgia O'Keeffe—were also, evidently, remarkably sexually passionate women.

George Eliot described her heroine Maggie Tulliver, in *The Mill on the Floss* (1860), "throwing herself under the seductive guidance of illimitable wants."[1] According to her annotator, novelist A. S. Byatt, Eliot herself "too had fears that she might because of her passionate nature become demonic. . . ." In a letter to friends, Eliot wrote of her own fear of becoming consumed with sensual desire: "I had a horrid vision of myself last night becoming earthly, sensual and devilish. . . ."[2]

Poet Christina Rossetti wrote exquisitely about the torments of female sensual temptation: the heroine of "Goblin Market" (1859), Laura, "sat up in a passionate yearning / And gnashed her teeth for baulked desire, and wept / As if her heart would break. . . ." Laura's sister Lizzie, who has eaten "goblin fruit," in contrast, is intoxicated and evidently addicted to wanting more: Lizzie cries, "Hug me, kiss me, suck my juices / Squeezed from goblin fruits for you / Goblin pulp and goblin dew. / Eat me, drink me, love me; / . . . make much of me. . . . / She kissed and kissed her with a hungry mouth." The "wicked, quaint fruit-merchant men" in "Goblin Market" pressed upon the two girls fruits that were "like honey to the throat / But poison in the blood."[3]

The young painter Georgia O'Keeffe wrote to her love object, Arthur Whittier McMahon, in 1915, "It seems so strange—not to give myself—when I want to. Love is great to give. . . ." To photographer Paul Strand, whose sexual relationship with the artist coincided with a period of tremendous artistic growth for her, she wrote— conflating the excitement of a new foray into abstraction with the excitement of thinking about kissing a man: "Then the work—Yes, I loved it—and I love you—I wanted to put my arms around you and kiss you hard. . . . It's so funny the way I didn't even touch you when I so much wanted to. Still am telling you that I wanted to. . . . Take me out on the Drive some nights with you—will you?" Her biographer notes that she concluded this letter "provocatively," referring to Riverside Drive, where lovers sought darkness in the evenings.[4]

For many of these creative artists, apparent sexual awakening and creative surges had at certain key times in their lives seemed to fuse together, and seemed to elicit a phase of work that reached a higher level of insight and energy than had the just-previous work in their *oeuvres*. These arcs of accomplishment—these creative "high points"—seemed as if they might help confirm further my growing conviction that women experience the vagina as integral to a core self, and that it can also serve as the trigger or entry point to an awakening of sensibility that can at fortunate moments fuse the creative and the sexual.

Women writers often describe such sexually awakened moments in terms of a kind of mist falling away, heightening a sense of the *female* self. In their private letters, they often describe a startling, intoxicating discovery of self through the catalyst of the sexual love they are experiencing. As the young Hannah Arendt wrote to her lover Ernst Blucher after their affair began—an affair that was described as intensely intellectually engaged and intensely erotic, for a young woman who had never been especially physical before—"I . . . finally know what happiness is. . . . It still seems to me unbelievable, that I could achieve both—a great love, and a sense of identity with my own person. And yet I achieve the one only since I have had the other."[5] Often, no matter what they suffer for their passion, these writers' heroines refuse to regret the sexual awakening that has brought them the suffering: in Kate Chopin's 1899 novel *The Awakening,* Edna Pontellier muses that "among the conflicting sensations that assailed her, there was neither shame nor remorse."[6]

Edith Wharton's letters and novels, in particular, made me eager to pursue this line of inquiry. For most of her adult life, Wharton was married to the conventional, upper-class dilettante Teddy Wharton, a man to whom she was not suited. By her own account, and others', their sexual life was almost nonexistent. But in 1908, she experienced a dramatic sexual awakening when she entered into an extramarital affair with the handsome, seductive, and provocative bisexual journalist Morton Fullerton. In her private love letters to him, published for the first time in the 1980s, she writes of this sexual awakening as threatening a dissolution of her self, a loss of her control. She writes—reverting to French, the language in which she addresses sexual pleasure—that his touch leaves her with "no more will": *"je n'ais plus de volonte."*[7] She speaks of Fullerton's sexual love as "a narcotic"—a metaphor echoed in the fiction by other women writers of this period. (Edna Pontellier, in *The Awakening* [1899], also describes her lover Robert's touch as "a narcotic"—a metaphor that would become more scarce after the Second Wave of the 1970s made such admissions of perceived dependency by omen on men politically incorrect.)[8]

In one letter, Wharton describes a conversation with Fullerton in which, after she conveyed to him the effect on her of her having become orgasmic, he responded that she would write better as a result of that experience. Fullerton, as it turned out, was right: Edith Wharton did indeed do some of her best work after her sexual awakening. Interestingly, in *The House of Mirth,* published in 1905, there is virtually no language of physical passion in relation to her women characters, so their attachments and motivations seem incomplete.[9] Suppression is well expressed, but not fulfillment. Female sexual passion, however, in many manifestations, suffuses her *Summer* (1917) and *The Age of Innocence* (1920).

After 1908–10, Wharton's prose becomes richer and more tactile; the world of pleasure and the senses enters into it more fully, as does a sense—a tragic sense, at that time, necessarily—of feminine longing for ecstasy, life, and sensation at all costs. The theme of a woman who is changed and awakened by her own sexuality—and who does not regret the consequences, though she suffers as a result—is consistent in Wharton's fiction after 1908–10.

I looked at biographies of these and other great women artists, writers, and revolutionaries from the eighteenth and nineteenth centuries, and into the early twentieth: Mary Wollstonecraft, Charlotte Brontë, Elizabeth Barrett Browning, George Sand, Christina Rossetti, George Eliot, Georgia O'Keeffe, Edith Wharton, Emma Goldman, Gertrude Stein—all women whose lives, letters, and choices, even at great risk or sacrifice to themselves, revealed their intense, often sexually passionate natures.[10]

In life after life of this now-expanded circle of women artists, writers, and revolutionaries, the same arc appeared: a flowing of creative insight and vision seemed to follow a sexual flowering. One can often see a shift in perspective chronologically for these writers, artists, and revolutionaries: their palettes suddenly broaden, or possibilities of another world swerve into view.

George Eliot, after she began her illicit relationship with her lover George Lewes, wrote her first important piece of fiction, *Scenes of Clerical Life* (1857). Soon after Georgia O'Keeffe began a highly erotic relationship with photographer Alfred Stieglitz, her daring experimentation with form and color, represented by her flower paintings, revolutionary for their era, began. As she wrote to him in 1917, conflating artistic and sexual excitement, "I feel as though I have lots to do—*lots*—and one thing to paint—It's the flag as I see it floating—A dark red flag—trembling in the wind like my lips when I'm about to cry— [. . .] There is a strong firm line in it too—teeth set—under the lips—

"Goodnight—My chest is very sore and I'm tired—couldn't sleep or eat for excitement down there—and hurt—and wonder—and realizing—"[11]

Emma Goldman's radical critique of existing social norms intensified sharply after the start of her passionate affair with Ben Reitman in 1908. She also took stands that led to her arrest. Typical of such a muse, Reitman did not just seduce Goldman, he also offered her his "hobo hall" for her lectures, when she could not secure another forum. When Gertrude Stein met and began living with Alice B. Toklas—which allowed her to explore her inner life as a lover of women—her work leaped forward in terms of the level of its experimentation, as well as in terms of its sensuality.

Even recent women writers sometimes seem to make this connection—and sometimes in surprising detail: in "A Conversation with Isabel Allende," which reporter Melissa Block conducted for National Public Radio on November 6, 2006, Block asked Allende about the genesis of the vividly realized seventeenth-century Spanish character Inés Suárez, heroine of Allende's novel *Inés of My Soul:* "The first sentence just popped out of my womb," Allende replied, to a perhaps startled interlocutor. "I wouldn't say my head—but my womb. It was, 'I am Inés Suárez, a townswoman of the loyal city of Santiago de Nueva Extremadura in the kingdom of Chile.' And that's how I felt. I felt that I was her and that the story could only be told in her voice."[12]

In the biographies I read, the lover is often a kind of muse figure—not always a staid partner, but often a man or woman who respects the creative artist or revolutionary intellectually, while stirring her erotically. For so many of the great women artists, writers, and revolutionaries, it seems, a sexual awakening coincided with risk-taking on other levels—social and artistic—and with other kinds of awakening: of mastery, expression, and creative powers.

I began to wonder: Was there, perhaps, some connection we

were missing between freedom and creativity, and an awakening to women's own most passionate natures?

Could something deeper, I wondered, be going on here?

## THE TINY RAT-PLEASURE BRUSH

After my spinal surgery and its attendant restoration to me of joy, color, confidence, creativity, and a sense of connection between things, there was no way for me to ignore the fact that the injury to my consciousness that I had suffered before my operation had to be related to some physical causation, as the changes in consciousness correlated so strongly to injury to and recovery of my pelvic nerve. What had happened to me? And what did it mean? Was this cause and effect a freak of my own weird subjective neurology and biochemistry—or was this an insight potentially generalizable to all women?

About four months after I had mostly recovered from spinal surgery, I was invited to speak to a group of brilliant young women at a university. To conceal identities, I will place this event in rural Canada, and locate it at a state university. Many were biology or neuroscience students, and they had decided to put together a conference. Their goal was to have some conversations about the issues they might face as women when they left the school setting and entered the "real" world.

It was a warm, breezy day as we gathered to talk in the living room of a cottage on an old farm. There were deep soft couches covered in scarlet fabric, faded crimson rugs, and baskets of dried flowers in the massive fireplaces. Through the windows, the honeyed sun poured in: we could see a deep-green river valley before us, and beyond it, the blue, mounded hills.

After a conversation about their projects and their future lives, we all decided to go for a walk in the warm bright air. One of the young women, who knew the area, led us on cow paths and through hedges, over muddy bends in the dirt road, and then up and over a hill. As we crested the hill, I saw that it was as if we were in another ecosystem. The domestic coziness was suddenly far away. Wild gray-green fields dropped away from all sides, and a strong, steady wind blew. I decided to put directly before them what my puzzle was.

"I think that there might be a connection between the vagina and the brain that most of us don't fully understand. I'm finding that there may be some relationship between female orgasm, and confidence and creativity. There may also be a relationship between the vagina— and orgasm—and the ability to see the connections between things."

The young women were silent for a moment. Then one young woman, an historian, spoke up. "That is absolutely true for me," she said definitively. "When I have really good sex. But I mean, *really* good sex"—everyone laughed, quite aware of the difference—"I feel like I can do anything. I feel great about myself. My confidence goes through the roof. And I am not always like that. But also it shows up in my work for a while afterward: I see things I did not see before, connections I might have missed. I do feel more of a sense of mastery about my perceptions."

Another young woman, a political scientist, agreed: "It makes me feel invincible. It makes me feel like running a marathon. Totally happy about myself." There was the silence again, the silence of intense thinking.

"I used to work in a lab where my job was to give female rats sexual pleasure," said a young scientist. She had a mischievous smile.

"What??" we all exclaimed.

"It's true!" she laughed. "I had a tiny brush." She made a gesture with her fingers, as if painting a tiny point in the air. "After a while it is just part of the job."

"I didn't even know female rats could experience sexual pleasure," I marveled, struck by my own ignorance.

"All female mammals have clitorises," she explained, in the calm tone of a scientist for whom this was interesting, but also just another data point. "They all have clitorises," she repeated. A cow tilted her head and glanced quizzically at the creature to her right. (Indeed, I was to learn that two-thirds of mammalian clitorises are on the anterior wall of the vagina—like the human G-spot; at that time I had no idea that mammals generally had clitorises.)

It was quite a remarkable moment. A fog had started to drift in over the rounded hills that extended away from us; the wind was softly blowing. The women were talking quietly about orgasm, insight, and energy. I was amazed that I had never known that fact, obvious though it should have been. *All female mammals* were designed by the process of evolution to experience great sexual pleasure.

"Female rats, when they want sex, go like this." She held up her hands like little paws and arched her back. We all laughed. It was a gesture I would learn later was called "lordosis." She described the lab and its results further, and I agreed to find out more about it.

We talked for a while longer, but the wind grew too strong for us. We drifted back at last to the cozy fire, the chintz, and the teapot, a little sorry to leave that slightly wild, slightly inexplicable moment— when the wind, the grass, and the animals had all seemed a part of what we were learning about ourselves: that we and our specific feminine pleasure had a firm place in the natural order of things.

I was sorry for the moment to end, but buoyed by the young women's curiosity, and their openness to discovering if what excited them in their intellectual work was part of other kinds of excitement that they had, until then, understood, in isolation, as physical.


## THE ONSTAGE ORGASM

In the next few months, other women, from many different backgrounds, confirmed to me that they, too, had experienced a connection between their sexual well-being and their confidence levels and creative lives.

One evening I attended a crowded premiere party in New York City, where I was surrounded by film and theater professionals. The noise was deafening. Standing at the crowded bar, I introduced myself to a statuesque woman in her early forties who was waiting next to me. She was radiantly elegant; she wore red lipstick, pearls, and a black cocktail dress that evoked the flapper era. She told me that she was an actress—she had had a role in the film we had just seen—and she asked me what I did for a living. I told her that I was a writer, at work on my next book. She asked what it was about. "It's a book about the vagina," I said. She smiled. Her pupils dilated.

By this point, it had happened often enough that I was aware that many people had immediate, probably measurable physical reactions when they asked me this question and heard the word *vagina* in my response. Some, both men and women, smiled immediately: beautiful, heartfelt smiles. Others looked frightened or disgusted, as if I had suddenly produced from my handbag a trout and placed it on the table before us, or had held it up for discussion. Still others, usually men, burst out laughing, angrily and inadvertently, usually to their own embarrassment.

Given the actress's dreamy smile, something suggested to me that I could go ahead. "Actually, right now," I confessed, "I am trying to figure out a possible link between female orgasm and creativity."

The actress turned pale and self-conscious. "I can't believe you said that," she said. "I want to tell you something. It's something I've never told anyone." She took a deep breath. "I'm a Method actor." I knew that Method actors use visualization to act "from the inside out"—that is, they invoke the consciousness of the character whose role they are playing, to experience and then express that character from within, rather than "acting" as if they are that person. "When I start to rehearse a role and go deeply into the character, my orgasms change. They start to become more, more . . ." She was gesturing with her wineglass, as if at an imagined cosmos, at a loss for words.

"Transcendental?" I asked.

"Exactly. Ask my boyfriend. And then"—she looked around, to make sure no one was listening—"I find it a heightened erotic state for me to be in character, performing." She looked around again, but soldiered on, wishing, it seemed, to get this insight on the record. "I have had an orgasm while I was onstage. Just from being in that heightened creative condition."

I clutched my wineglass. So it was not just that orgasm might heighten creativity in women; maybe creativity also heightened orgasm.

"Really!" I said.

"Really," she said.

"Wow. Do you think that has ever happened to anyone else?"

"I know it has. It has happened, I am certain, to other women in the creative arts. I know women who have had orgasms while painting. And I know the two feed each other: the sexuality fuels the creative work, and the work fuels the sex." She gave me her card and promised to introduce me to these female artists who had orgasms from their creative work.

I thanked her and walked out into the night, making my way gingerly past the actresses around me to the coat check, as if they were demurely dressed minefields of Eros that might erupt at any moment. But as I looked up at the starry New York winter night, I felt light-headed myself.

That night I began work on an informal survey. I put forth a set of questions to the women in my Facebook "community" of 16,800 people at that time. The questionnaire asked them if they had ever experienced any seeming connection between sex and creativity; if they had ever had a sexual experience boost their confidence levels and sense of self-love; if a sexual experience had ever led them to see better the connections between things; and if, on the other hand, periods of sexual loneliness, depression, or frustration had negatively affected their confidence, creativity, and energy. Their answers confirmed that the young scientists, the actress, and I were not so aberrant in our gender.

A typical question-and-answer e-mail went as follows:

NW: Has a really profound sexual experience ever affected your confidence levels?

RESPONDENT: Yes.

NW: Given you more energy?

RESPONDENT: Yes.

NW: Made you like yourself more?

RESPONDENT: Yes.

NW: Boosted your creativity? If so, please specify how.

RESPONDENT: I am a painter, and did an artist's residency in Vermont for a month about a year ago. I was away from my husband at the time. Because of the private space that I was provided, I ended up delving into [sexual] memories dealing specifically with past relationships. Having a good relationship—both sexually and otherwise—does boost my self-confidence, and my motivation to pursue my artwork . . . after visiting my husband mid-residency, I returned [to work] feeling more confident, and had more self-love. Someone at the residency commented, "You look really nice today," and I'm sure it was because seeing my husband had boosted my confidence.

Women from many different backgrounds e-mailed me in droves. Many women spoke of unusually profound orgasms—not the everyday kind—as experiences that were followed with a sense of unusual power, energy, and confidence; of self-love; and of the world sparkling.

"Laura," a British thirty-four-year-old administrative assistant, wrote to me. "I met someone at work," she confided, "and we developed a fast attraction. It was very quick for me and I suspect he was interested in me for a while. Anyway, we had a go, and a really good sexual experience that changed me deeply. My confidence level shift was immediate; I stood taller and walked stronger. More energy? Every day for two months I woke up and exercised, joyfully. I loved my self more too; started getting pedicures to express it. Creativity? I played guitar every night, and learned four new songs. Connections between things? This relationship restored a dormant psychic ability that has enhanced all of my thinking since. Conversely: that relationship has not continued. Lately I have begun to grieve and miss it; mostly I miss all of the above." She went on, "I am sad and feel the return of my old stories of negative self-image, of rejection. I find this to be strange, and unsettling to experience." She concluded poignantly, "I have also tried sleeping with other men and have not felt anywhere near this influx [of feelings]."

Laura wrote that she was orgasmic with the other men; indeed, even more so than with the one with whom intimacy caused such an awakening. Many other women echoed this idea, that what was transformative to them in those profound sexual experiences was not a simple matter of the quantity of orgasmic "fireworks." What was transformative for them was something subjective about the quality of the orgasm that merged the physical realm with the realm of emotions or perception: the intensity that it created, and in turn the confidence and creativity it unleashed.

I asked this same set of questions of an old friend "Patrice," a woman my own age who was now an accomplished businesswoman. We were sitting out in her back garden in a pretty suburb of what I will say, to conceal identities, was Ann Arbor, Michigan. She had a postage-stamp garden; her laundry was drying in the sun on a line just beyond us; and her six-year-old boy was playing with a friend in the glass conservatory that we could see from where we were sitting at an outdoor table by a plot of herbs. She looked like a perfectly "ordinary" wife and mother in her forties. Oddly enough, though we had talked frankly about our sex lives for twenty-three years, since we first met, we had never talked about the possible connection I had set before her, simply because it had never occurred to me. She looked at me, again, as other women had, with that abrupt expression of surprise and recognition.

"Oh my God," she said, and started laughing. "Ohhh . . . *Naomi.* Wow. Oh, definitely. I can have perfectly fine sex most of the time, fine orgasms, and what you are talking about does not happen. But then, once in a while, there are those amazing times just after sex like that, you feel—oh, things are electric! And you have insights about your work. It is like you get some kind of superpowers. And you just want to run a marathon, or write an opus. Climb the Alps!" She was laughing hard now. "But," she cautioned, "it is not every time, by no means every time. I mean, I wouldn't want it to happen every time, right? Because you would never want to do anything else if it did, or else you would be walking around in a creative mania all the time. If it happened every time, you would never get out of bed."

Does really special sex, sex that engages the vagina, emotions, and body in very specific ways—ways that involve very concrete kinds of activation of the parasympathetic nervous system—actually lead to female euphoria, creativity, and self-love?

"Laura," whom we met earlier, eloquently described this transformation of her whole self via sexual experience as "strange and unsettling" to go through. This sense of bafflement or mystification at our own reactions as women came up many times in the e-mail responses I received. If we don't understand our own neurology and biochemistry in sex and love, our own female selves can be very "unsettling" to us.

What had happened to us? What had happened to the actress who was transformed in an erotic ecstasy onstage? What had happened to the scientist who saw new connections in her lab, and to the entrepreneur who "wanted to write an opus"?

# Dopamine, Opioids, and Oxytocin

*I write like I love . . . the kisses we gave each other at ten o'clock that night of Saturday, October 12 . . . how many fields of wheat, how many vineyards, there are, between you and me! I hate the law . . . I want to feel—to make others feel . . .*

—Explorer Isabelle Eberhardt, 1902

What had happened to us was that dopamine—among other substances, including oxytocin and opioids—had hit our systems, before, during, and after lovemaking. Dopamine is the ultimate feminist chemical in the female brain.

When a woman's dopamine system is optimally activated—as it is in the anticipation of great sex, an effect heightened by a woman's knowing what turns her on, letting herself think about it, and letting herself go get it—it strengthens her sense of focus and motivation levels and energizes her in setting goals. All those effects are involved with dopamine activation. It is accurate to say that if you activate your dopamine system in seeking out great sex, as a woman, your brain can take those heightened capabilities of energy and focus into other areas of your life and into other endeavors.

But this heightened superpower, this self-potential, is dependent on reward: on getting what you want. If, as a woman, you are frustrated sexually, and, even worse, aroused but denied release, your dopamine system eventually diminishes in anticipation of sex; you eventually lose access to the positive energy that you might otherwise have had both in sex and also subsequently, to take elsewhere in your life.

You are less likely to get what scientists call "activation"—loosely translated as "excitement"—from anything; you could be depressed and be likely to experience "anhedonia"—the literal meaning of which is "no pleasure"—a state in which the "world looks colorless." With low dopamine activation, you will suffer from a lack of ambition or drive and your libido levels will be low.[1] But if your dopamine levels are just right, you are confident, creative, and talkative, and you trust your perceptions.

An illustrated chart (see insert) compiled by dopamine researcher Marnia Robinson shows how dopamine affects human behavior in relationships and in social settings.[2] Focused drive has been shown to be related to dopamine activity.

Opioid release, which is measurable in brain scans, and which meditators describe as states of "awe," "bliss," and "oneness," is boosted by orgasm. There have been suggestions that the "out-of-body" experiences some people have during surgery, and the "near-death" experiences that lead dying people to feel euphoria and bliss, are also probably related to dopamine and opioids.

By the same token, a female self's experience of freedom, and its impulse to seek more freedom, and to do so from a basis of self-love—the feminist quest and the feminist sensibility—are all strengthened in women by preorgasmic dopamine, and by the effect of orgasm on the brain. The brain's limbic system, as we saw, mediates the hormones the female brain receives in arousal and produces after orgasm (or lack of orgasm). So in this way, the vagina is the delivery system for the states of mind that we call confidence, liberation, self-realization, and even mysticism in women.

Just because these states are chemically mediated does not mean that they are not "real" self-love, "real" attachment to freedom, or "real" bliss. Those of us who are not scientists often forget that brain chemicals are vehicles for very profound human truths. Remember how, after my spinal injury, but before I was diagnosed and treated, I saw the world as flatter, less colorful, and less interesting than it had seemed to me before I was injured? That change in worldview was probably due to inactivated dopamine and opioids in my system, since one of the pelvic nerve branches that would have triggered dopamine activation was frozen. Because of the impairment to the nerves in one of the branches, there was lower than usual dopamine, oxytocin, and opioid activation in my brain. I was getting some level of the hormones from the clitoral orgasms, but missing the full activation of those same chemicals in the brain that I would have expected from a fully functioning pelvic neural network. As one of the few women in the world—as far as I know—to have, neurobiologically speaking, experienced the interruption of these circuits and their healing, I consider my experience a control with some important information: the world looked different, and I was different.

A woman with low dopamine will have low libido and depression, as we noted. On the other hand, if you are a woman, and your dopamine levels are optimally activated, you will be confident, creative, and sociable. You will have strong opinions, clear boundaries, and you will take pride in your own work. You will experience feelings of well-being and satisfaction; have a sense of directedness and persistence in accomplishing tasks; experience strong feelings toward others; make sound choices; and have realistic expectations. These are qualities that every CEO writes about as critical to accomplishing game-changing work and affecting the world in major ways.

Your life is more likely to feel meaningful—as long as you continue to get reward at the end of your experience of sexual arousal—and you will see the connections between people. Because of the role of dopamine, you will also see the connections between your own body and actions and reactions from others. As Dr. Jim Pfaus of Concordia University, Montreal, Quebec, put it, "You could call dopamine the 'cause-effect' chemical."[3] You activate dopamine's release in various ways: aerobic exercise, taking drugs like cocaine, socializing, shopping, gambling—and having good orgasmic sex.

The feminist echo of the consequence of a woman's regularly strengthening her brain's perception of a direct link between cause and effect—between one's agency and a desired outcome—is obvious. "Dopamine's optimal work in your brain is about flexibility in decision making: it helps you make the right decision at the right time for *you* in an ever-changing world," notes Dr. Pfaus. It is the "decider" chemical, the chemical involved in leadership and confidence building.[4]

Experts such as David J. Linden, whose book *The Compass of Pleasure: How Our Brains Make Fatty Foods, Orgasm, Exercise, Marijuana, Generosity, Vodka, Learning, and Gambling Feel So Good* explores dopamine's effects, point out that dopamine makes you feel good about yourself, makes you feel as if you have a strong ego, and makes you feel open to new challenges.[5]

Dr. Helen Fisher, anthropologist and author of *Anatomy of Love*, found that romantic love is not an emotion—it is an overwhelmingly powerful part of the "motivation system" of the brain—a drive, part of the reward system of the brain.[6] Dr. Fisher found that romantic love has three different chemical components: lust, composed of androgens and estrogens; attraction, driven by high dopamine and norepinephrine levels and low serotonin (this accounts for mood swings in early courtship); and finally, attachment, made up of oxytocin and vasopressin. And all these mood-altering chemicals can possibly become higher, because of their multiorgasmic potential, in some women than in most men.[7] Researchers Cindy M. Meston and K. M. McCall, in their 2005 essay "Dopamine and Norepinephrine Response to Film-Induced Sexual Arousal in Sexually Functional and Dysfunctional Women," also reported finding a link between well-functioning dopamine (and norepinephrine) systems and strong female sexual response. Regarding dopamine and norepinephrine, the authors wrote, "these transmitters play a prosexual role in female sexuality."[8]

French neuroscientist Claude de Contrecoeur, who looked (by using different drugs) at the effect of serotonin and of dopamine on behavior and on feelings, finds that dopamine has an opposite effect to serotonin. If you stimulate the neurotransmission of dopamine in the brain, what happens? Your mind becomes more active and you want to move around. "Dopamine stimulates motivations and lifts indecisiveness," he finds. It raises self-confidence, he maintains. "Dopamine alleviates depression by stimulating action and lifting indecision," he writes. "Dopamine activates blood flow which may be an important factor in its anti-depressive action." If dopamine is overactivated, he warns, then self-confidence can even increase to self-delusional levels.[9]

But it is important to understand serotonin, too.

Millions of women and men are prescribed selective serotonin reuptake inhibitors (SSRIs), which are the modern form of anti-depressants. Women far outnumber men in being prescribed SSRIs. Are these same millions of men and women warned that SSRIs may well send their libido and ability to experience orgasm plummeting? SSRIs produce a state of satiety, due to raised serotonin levels; raised serotonin levels make you feel satiated—which is pleasant—but the same situation reduces your motivation. SSRIs inhibit serotonin uptake: de Contrecoeur found that raised serotonin anesthetizes emotion, suppresses or blocks sexual desire, and makes people sleepier and less aggressive—they even move around less.

On the other hand, lowered serotonin levels raise dopamine activity, de Contrecoeur believes, which in contrast leads people to experience "stimulation of sociability and mood, aggressivity and sexuality."[10]

The political implications of these two mood, or mind, states are obvious.

Patriarchal societies, even without the benefit of what current science is now documenting, have, I contend, noticed the link between sexually assertive, sexually self-aware women—and focused, motivated, energized, biologically empowered women.

This is why I call dopamine the ultimate feminist chemical. If a woman has optimal levels of dopamine, she is difficult to direct against herself. She is hard to drive to self-destruction, to manipulate and control.

Other neuroscientists and evolutionary biologists are also confirming that something significant to mood happens in the brain when a dopamine rush prepares the way for orgasm. After orgasm, gender differences emerge. For men, dopamine drops drastically after orgasm, and men lose interest in sex, for a time. They have a refractory period during which they can't get aroused. But does dopamine drop as far in the female brain—and does prolactin step up the "enough already" response for a woman in the same way, especially if she is multiorgasmic? Not necessarily. If a woman goes on to have another orgasm and then another, she will continue to mainline boosts of dopamine. And new research shows that virtually all women are able to have orgasms fairly easily under the right circumstances.

Why does this matter? Because it suggests that all women who are orgasmic (and especially women who are able to be very orgasmic) have the capability to receive much more dopamine, and more opioid boosts, over the course of a really good day than the men they have just slept with, and more than other women who lack knowledge about their own sexual pleasure.

I asked Dr. Pfaus, "Wouldn't more female orgasms trigger more opioid release?"

"It might well do that," he said. "For women who have multiple big ones, you would expect them to have more opioids." [11]

Female orgasm also, surprisingly, boosts the levels of testosterone in women. That is one more reason that great sex makes women hard to push around easily. Science writer Mary Roach points out that testosterone "more than any other hormone . . . influences a woman's libido" and also makes women want to have more sex. [12] So sex raises women's testosterone, which in turn raises their libido further, which in turn makes them more assertive and more interested in having even more sex. (This connection is well documented; testosterone therapy, for instance, a controversial menopause treatment for women, raises women's assertiveness levels as well as their libido.) [13] So the fear that patriarchy always had—that if you let women have sex and know how to like it, it will make them both increasingly libidinous and increasingly ungovernable—is actually biologically true!

I don't like any kind of feminism that sets one gender above another, so I do not mean this in any way as a value judgment. Neither gender is "better." But one gender is theoretically able to get more of a certain kind of dopaminic and opioid activation during sex, which has a very specific effect on the brain and even the personality. We cannot escape what this math implies for female sexuality, in its unmediated, un-messed-up state: nature constructed a profound difference between the sexes, which places women in, potentially, a position of greater biochemical empowerment than men, through the medium of satisfying sexual activity. (Of course, it is not a zero-sum game: men have other ways of getting extra dopamine hits.)

The good news is that all this dopamine will—if women and their vaginas are not hurt, suppressed, injured, or demeaned—make women more confident, more euphoric, more creative, and more assertive—possibly more than a male-dominated society is comfortable with. Feminists are continually seeking to elicit the suppressed female "voice." Serotonin literally subdues the female voice, and dopamine literally raises it.

Dopamine causes focus and initiative, according to science's latest model. Opioids cause bliss, the "oceanic feeling," the sense of the sublime. Have you ever seen a group of people who have just snorted cocaine *talk*? You can't shut them up. Cocaine causes these effects by stimulating dopamine release in the brain; indeed, cocaine was first abused by Dr. William Halsted at Johns Hopkins Hospital because it made him feel invincible, filled him with energy and confidence, and fought his fatigue.

How many heterosexual women reading this can remember a time when you made love and found yourself afterward mysteriously suffused with chattiness, just at the moment your male lover was crashing into sleep? *You just wanted to talk.* You had so much to say! Studies show that an embarrassing number of women confess to having woken up a sleeping male partner to speak with him. If you have done that, you know who you are—though you may not have known why you had that intense drive to do so. That is the unstoppable sociability of dopamine, in the anticipation of one more orgasm.

To restate what by now should be obvious: the healthy, sexually well-treated vagina *regularly* delivers a strong activation of dopamine to the female reward system, as well as surges of oxytocin for connection, and opioids that drive the sensations of joy. So the vagina delivers to women the feelings that lead them to want to create, explore, communicate, conquer, and transcend. And since women can potentially have more orgasms than men, theoretically, and can theoretically release more oxytocin in lovemaking, they risk also feeling more: more love, more attachment, and more affection afterward.

Let's look at oxytocin—"the cuddle hormone"—on its own. Oxytocin's function in humans is to bond people to each other so they are better able to survive. Oxytocin also allows people to see the relationships between things and between people more clearly. David J. Linden reports that nasal oxytocin sprays that were designed to help new mothers release milk for lactation—the brand is called Liquid Trust—have been put to other uses. Those who inhaled the spray became more trusting of strangers, even after they had been betrayed in a game. They were more willing to take greater social risks. They were also more likely to see "the connections between things," meaning, in this case, they were better able to infer others' emotional states. In a famous experiment, oxytocin helped subjects correctly intuit another person's emotional state—when the subjects were given photos of human faces in which only the eyes were visible.[14]

Oxytocin is women's emotional superpower. Oxytocin induces labor contractions and helps release breast milk, as we saw; its evolutionary role is to bond us to our children and to our mate long enough to maximize the chances that a child will have two caregivers during its long dependency.[15] In experiments, when scientists block either oxytocin or dopamine, mother mammals will ignore their offspring. It reduces cravings.[16] When scientists administered it to rodents who were addicted to cocaine, morphine, or heroin, the rats opted for a lower level of the drugs and showed fewer symptoms of withdrawal.[17] "Oxytocin and its receptors appear to hold the leading position among the candidates for the substance of 'happiness,' " assert Navneet Magon and Sanjay Kalra in "The Orgasmic History of Oxytocin: Love, Lust and Labor."[18] Oxytocin also calms—one rat injected with oxytocin will calm down a whole cage full of anxious rats.[19] It increases sexual receptivity.[20] It is not so surprising that when the neural pathways from brain to vagina are damaged, one feels that life has less meaning; truly, the well-treated vagina is a medium that releases, in the female brain, what can be called without exaggeration the chemical components of the meaning of life itself.

## IS THE VAGINA AN ADDICT?

*During that month I have been completely happy. . . . What joy, dear, to find your letter. . . . I won't say I need it desperately, because that is my chronic state. . . . Before that [happy hour with you] I had no personal life: since then you have given me all imaginable joy. Nothing can take it from me now, or diminish it in my eyes . . . [it] has set my whole being free. . . . I can't say this to you because when I do you take me in your arms et alors je n'ais plus de volonte. . . .*

—Edith Wharton to Morton Fullerton[21]

So dopamine makes you confident and gives you faith in rewards; opioids provide addictive boosts of happiness and good feeling; oxytocin, which studies have shown is increased upon orgasm, and so women who are multiorgasmic can theoretically produce more of than men, makes you bond, feel affection and trust, and leads you to want to make love some more.

Could this explain why, even though most actual sex addicts are men, so many women feel at times that they are "addicted to love"? Our highs are potentially higher; but the downside is that when that dopamine and opioids leave our systems, we are potentially in a lower low than most men experience—a withdrawal state that is exactly like opiate withdrawal. The biochemistry of addiction means that if we have *more* of a dopamine burst to start with, our fall will be that much harder. So women have more of a tendency to be mystics than men—because of all this potential dopamine production—and more of a risk of being sexual love addicts (to distinguish from straight sexual addiction, which men are more often treated for). The higher rates of oxytocin and dopamine that we can potentially produce—and potentially painfully lose—potentially make us dependent on our love/sex object in ways that may not always be mutual.

---

I turned once again to the scientists.

I interviewed Dr. Jim Pfaus in his lab at Concordia University in Canada. Dr. Pfaus is a pioneer in the study of new frontiers of female sexuality. He noted that it was reasonable to see a connection between female orgasm, dopamine activation, and heightened focus and confidence.

I was lucky to witness an extraordinary experiment in this lab, as Dr. Pfaus and his team of graduate students demonstrated the role of female sexual pleasure in mate selection. This jaw-dropping experiment would be published in March of 2012 in the *Archives of Sexual Behavior* as "Who, What, Where, When (and Maybe Even Why)? How the Experience of Sexual Reward Connects Sexual Desire, Preference, and Performance."[22]

Dr. Pfaus himself is a youthful-looking scientist with an energetic demeanor, who wore, in his off hours, a casual T-shirt, boots, and a black leather jacket. Dr. Pfaus's lab was in a pleasant modern quadrangle on the Concordia campus, which is in a handsome red-brick suburb on the outskirts of the relaxed and intellectually curious city of Montreal. In a brightly lit, cheery lab with stacks of well-tended male and female rats in clean plastic cages lined up against the walls, Dr. Pfaus introduced me to his even more youthful, highly focused team of researchers, at least half of whom were women.

Then, before my eyes, Dr. Pfaus and his team proved the role of female sexual pleasure in mate preference among lower mammals—the role of the pleasure-seeking vagina, clitoris, and cervix in the evolutionary dance.

One female scientist gently lifted up a "naive" (that is, virgin) black-and-white female rat and showed me, while stroking her, how she would be injecting the animal with naloxone to prepare her to not have a good time for the first sexual experience of her life. I could have imagined it, but as we both watched the adolescent virgin rat scramble about curiously after her injection, a hint of melancholy, from me and from the young scientist watching her subject, was in the air.

While one group of sexually naive female rats was injected with naloxone, which blocks the experience of pleasure, a control group of virgin female rats was injected with saline, which does nothing. All the rats were injected, too, with hormones that made them ovulate, ensuring that they would, under ordinary circumstances, very much want sex.

The female rats were then placed into cages designed by a female scientist: the cages had four little openings in a Plexiglas divider. These allowed the female rats to scamper in and out of the area where the male rats were waiting for them (since the males are bigger, the males could not follow the females through the little doors). The doors gave the females control over the contact.

The female rats injected with the saline—that is, those who could feel pleasure—were—there is no other way to say it—wildly flirtatious; they scampered in and out of the males' space; they "solicited" the males repeatedly (I learned that female rats solicit males by making a "headwise orientation"—gazing directly into the males' eyes—then running away); they hopped around the males, another sign of female rat sexual desire; they presented their genitals to the males to lick and sniff. One feisty female kept trying to mount the male in her cage—finally reaching a point at which she simply resorted to hopping onto his shoulders and mounting his *head*. What was unmistakable about the activity was that it was being reinforced—the "saline" females were getting something they wanted from the males that made them more and more interactive with them, and more and more excited. For the saline group, it was prom night. Excitement, activity, interaction!

For the naloxone females, in contrast—they all soon looked like characters in an Ibsen play. There was some initial sniffing and palpating from the males, but soon the females just gave up responding to, or initiating, contact. You could see the moment at which they did, almost perceptibly. After a few forays, they stopped interacting with their partners; stopped scampering over to the male's sides of the cages; stopped "headwise soliciting"; stopped trying to climb onto the males. Soon each female was gazing bleakly into the middle distance in her own area in the cage that the male could not get to— though one male, I will never forget, was desperately trying to get himself through the too-small doorway and, in a begging posture, tried to drag his mate through the tiny door by her tail with his teeth. Finally the females were permanently on "their own side of the bed." They stopped moving much at all—wouldn't look at the males—and appeared listless. They were not being reinforced by sexual pleasure. What struck me about that scene was not just that *sex* wasn't being reinforced for these females—but that *nothing*, really, was being reinforced; they weren't interacting with their own environments.

The experiment in its later stage showed an even more dramatic outcome: at this point, the scientists ran the naloxone experiment with a scent—such as lemon or almond—associated with the male rat: the scent was placed into the male rat's fur. Later, when the young, naive female rats who had had naloxone were put in a "ménage à trois" situation with two male rats as potential sexual partners—that is, in a situation in which the females could choose— they avoided the male rat that was scented with an aroma, even if it was a new male rat—and even though these females now could experience pleasure. In other words, the females were showing proof of *memories* of a bad sexual experience, and making decisions accordingly. Dr. Pfaus noted that they showed a lot of activity in the prefrontal cortex during that experiment: it proved that even lower female mammals have sexual memories and think about avoiding bad—pleasureless—sexual experiences. In strikingly poetic language for a scientific journal, he writes that his experiment proved "that a critical period exists during an individual's early sexual experience that creates a 'love map' or gestalt of features, movements, feelings, and interpersonal interactions associated with sexual reward."[23]

I left the lab that day feeling strangely validated and elated by what I had seen (though glad that the naloxone rats would get a chance to have the saline in the future). Nature had spoken. Those females in the first experiment—the saline group, so eager for sexual pleasure that they were mounting the *heads* of the happy males— were, as Dr. Pfaus points out only partly joking, making decisions in an environment in which no one had ever called them sluts, or unladylike. I felt strangely freed by seeing how directly nature or evolution had placed that intense female sexual desire firmly inside every little female mammal on earth.

## A THIRD SEXUAL CENTER FOR WOMEN?

Sexuality is under observation in many labs, and experiments are producing much new information about female arousal, desire, and emotions.

I was interested to note that Dr. Pfaus's other recent experiments show that female rats, given the option, prefer penetration (that is, penetration that they can control)—with clitoral, vaginal, and cervical stimulation—to the "brush" that stimulates the clitoris alone.

The latest MRI experiments from Dr. Barry Komisaruk's lab at Rutgers University in 2012 confirm a possibly related finding in human females, too. The vagina and the mouth of the cervix seem to be evolutionarily rigged to need an "other."

Dr. Komisaruk's MRI study showed that genital stimulation (clitoral, vaginal, and cervical) in women activated different but adjacent parts of the cortex, and that these areas also relate to different functions and emotional centers. This experiment confirmed in a vivid new way—among other amazing hypotheticals—the existence of a third sexual center for women, this one at the mouth of the cervix.[24] (Beverly Whipple's experiments had provisionally identified it in the 1980s.)

The idea of another sexual center in women made perfect sense to me. I had experienced it myself, even though, according to our until-recent understanding of the anatomy of female orgasm, it was not supposed to exist. It makes evolutionary sense, of course; while it is handy from an evolutionary point of view for women to have clitoral pleasure, it is superefficient, for reproductive reasons, for women to experience additional extreme pleasure from pressure at the very mouth of the cervix, as that kind of pleasure encourages penetration and thus pregnancy. I was also aware that for many women, when there is sexual pressure against the cervix, orgasms can feel far more emotional—women can burst into tears after orgasms that strike the mouth of the cervix. Many women have described to me becoming emotionally "addicted" to this sensation from a lover.

A Komisaruk team experiment asking women to rank orgasms subjectively confirmed heightened emotional subjectivity as well, in relation to some sexual areas more than others.

These experiments should, I believe, help to radically change our notion of what the "self" consists of. Since the eighteenth century, the self has been defined in the West as autonomous. But the vagina and cervix of even the most empowered woman cannot choose autonomy so simply. The vagina and the mouth of the cervix seem to be evolutionarily rigged to need "others" and to place the female brain in an unchosen but demanding connection to others.

The vagina and cervix, with their built-in craving for "the other," seem to be evolution's guarantee that heterosexual women will always interdepend with men and be willing to have intercourse with them, even with its many dangers, emotional as well as physical. This arrangement seems to guarantee that women will be driven by strong desires from within to attend to building complex bonds with others, even at the risk of their personal autonomy. And it comes as no surprise, then, to discover that many women find that vibrators alone or masturbation alone do not do exactly what lovemaking does for them emotionally. Dr. Pfaus believes that maybe we are "hard-wired to associate that kind of stimulation with another individual that we have to work on in a relationship; and having the stimulation disembodied—though pleasurable—is not the same degree of pleasure that we experience with another individual living entity." [25]

What if there is nothing wrong with this? Dr. Helen Fisher argues that male and female biologies and drives arose, for evolutionary purposes, to be interdependent with one another: to maximize each person's success if the two genders work as a team. What if sexuality and satisfaction actually require both perspectives—the more autonomous male and the more interdependent female? What if the vagina's longing is nature's way of correcting the potential imbalance of a worldview based on male biology alone?

"A woman without a man is like a fish without a bicycle," the Second Wave feminist slogan assured us, but maybe the fact is, well, no. I now think that denial of this need for men for sexual pleasure in straight women's lives was not actually feminist and did not actually help heterosexual women. Obviously, straight women do not need just any man. It is an insult to these women to dismiss their longing for the one they feel is *the* man, or to deride their mourning if he is gone. Nor does this denial of the paradox of our feminine autonomy, coexisting unsettledly with our feminine need for interdependence, help lesbians or bisexual women understand why, so often, the need for the lover is so intense. This ideology does nothing to help women of any sexuality understand why, often, the vibrator and a pint of Häagen-Dazs are pleasurable but that other longings for connections can remain strong.

To respect the central paradox of the female condition—the sexual/emotional need of the vagina and cervix—might mean that we need to face the fact that women are, in a sense, more easily addicted to love and to good sex with the person who triggers that heady chemical bath, than men are. The work of Dr. Daniel G. Amen, in *The Brain in Love,* along with that of many other neurobiologists whose work has not yet been "translated" into mainstream culture, suggests that some of women's behaviors currently seen as needy or masochistic are in fact better understood as natural and probably evolutionary responses to the brain changes caused by female orgasm. Good sex is, in other words, *actually* addictive for women biochemically in certain ways that are different from the experience of men—meaning that one experiences discomfort when this stimulus is removed and a craving to secure it again. Bad sex—inattentive sex with a selfish or distracted partner—is *actually* chemically dispiriting and damaging psychologically to women in a way that is different from men's experience. We will see why.

Neuroscientist Simon LeVay, in *The Sexual Brain,* points out that orgasm triggers, for both genders, the same mechanism as addiction, and he notes that all addictive mechanisms share a basis in dopamine. "Porn, accumulating money, gaining power over others, gambling, compulsive shopping, video games . . . if something really boosts your dopamine, then it's potentially addictive for you." Addiction highs can "hijack" our wiring, leaving us with little choice about seeking that high again and again, even if we suffer for the need in other ways. Of thousands of different chemicals, just a few— alcohol, cocaine, and other opiates and narcotics—boost dopamine. Highly stimulating versions of ordinary behaviors also boost dopamine, which is why exercise and pornography can be addictive.[26]

But we are living in a postfeminist world that tells women to just "fuck like men"—that doing so is a sign of liberation—and encourages young women to engage in "friends with benefits" relationships as an act of self-confidence, to roll out of bed with the same casual carelessness that men have traditionally demonstrated.

That male-model ideal of not-caring, take-it-or-leave-it sexuality is, I argue, setting up yet another impossible ideal into which women are supposed to shoehorn their actual needs, at some violence to themselves. Because sexually addictive behavior—or I should say, addictedness to a lover who is "right" for the autonomic nervous system—in women is hardwired. This is possibly the not so well-kept secret of women and love: we talk about great personalities or impressive résumés, similar backgrounds or common interests in prospective mates or new lovers. But though this dimension of our courtship experience is critical, certainly at first, the truth is that if he or she didn't make you feel that great in your body—if he or she didn't smell that good to you, taste that satisfying, touch you in ways that suited your unique needs to be touched, or make you come satisfyingly—you wouldn't care *that* much if he or she never called again. If he or she is the one who turns the ANS on high alert, who delivers the dopamine high from anticipation, who leaves you with the world aglow from opioid release—that is the same man or woman who makes you ache with anxiety for the follow-up call. If this is the person with the right touch to activate your unique neural network, *you will go into withdrawal* if he or she is not around to do this again, and fairly soon. Actual, painful, real withdrawal.

So when women have good, satisfying sex—what I call "high" orgasm: caring, attentive sex that activates the entire pelvic neural network and also intensely engages the ANS—they experience a major brain high.

This bath, of what are essentially drugs, primes women's neural systems to overcome huge obstacles to getting to the loved one; to engage in extreme behavior in pursuit of love and sexual pleasure; and to be physiologically unable to compartmentalize, to pull themselves up by their bootstraps, or just to "get a grip" or "get over" him or her. If they manage to "snap out of it," it is with superhuman effort and at a cost. This major brain high can also involve the hormones that elicit obsessive thinking about a loved one, and that elicit nurturing and even self-sacrificing behaviors. This major brain high is a factor for both genders. Both genders, of course, experience passionate attachment and suffer from unrequited love. And yes, the issue of the way intercourse differs emotionally and physically from masturbation for men, the role of male attachment, and the relationship of male sexuality to consciousness, deserves its own book.

But: women are potentially multiorgasmic, which changes, to some extent, one aspect of the "major brain high" equation.

Sappho wrote of jealousy "underneath my breast, all the heart is shaken . . . underneath my skin the tenuous flame suffuses . . . fever shakes my body." [27] The author of the Song of Songs (whom many scholars presume to have been a woman) wrote, "Strengthen me with raisins, / refresh me with apples, / for I am faint with love. . . . All night long on my bed / I looked for the one my heart loves; / I looked for him but did not find him. / I will get up now and go about the city. / Through its streets and squares; / I will search for the one my heart loves. / . . . I . . . would not let him go . . . / Blow on my garden, / that its fragrance may spread abroad." [28]

The grieving Dido, abandoned by her lover Aeneas; Charlotte Brontë's small, impoverished governess, who nearly died in a blazing bedroom trying to rescue her love in *Jane Eyre;* George Eliot's Maggie Tulliver, in *The Mill on the Floss,* who witnessed her reputation, her role in society, and her obligations to convention, all wash away from her as she allowed herself to be swept down a soon-to-be-fatal river with a man to whom she was powerfully sexually attracted; and you, my dear reader, who have probably—likely much to your own mortification—obsessively checked for a response to an unanswered e-mail or sat by an unringing phone, as have I; are we masochists, are we pathetic, or trivial-minded? No, to the contrary. Rather, we are subject to a force that is extremely powerful—one that perhaps no man can truly understand. I think that what drives us is rather noble.

An essential paradox of the female condition is that for women to really be free, we have to understand the ways in which nature designed us to be attached to and dependent upon love, connection, intimacy, and the right kind of Eros in the hands of the right kind of man or woman.

I believe we should respect the potential for "enslavement" to sexual love in women; to our place with Eros and love. Because only by making room for it, rather than suppressing or mocking it, can we strive to understand it. When a woman is engaged in this struggle with love and need, she is not "subject" to the person in question; she is actually engaged in a struggle with herself, to find a way to reclaim her autonomy while somehow not cutting herself off from the part of herself that was awakened by the beloved in the longing for connection.

A woman struggling with attachment and loss of self is engaged in a struggle for the self as demanding and rigorous as that of any man on any quest narrative. Of course, the biological responses I am talking about here have long been identified in psychoanalysis and in literature; only recently has science added new dimensions to and explanations of these mind-states elucidated by poets, novelists, and students of the psyche.

One of my favorite slang terms for the vagina in the United States is "the force." This is what we should be talking about. Women indeed take love, sex, and intimacy seriously, not because women, intimacy, and Eros are trivial but because nature in its clever and transcendental wiring of women's genitals and their brains has forced women to face the fact, which is simply more obscured to men (though actually ultimately no less true for them), that the need for connection, love, intimacy, and Eros is indeed bigger and stronger than anything else in the world.

A culture that does not respect women tends to deride and mock women's preoccupation with love and Eros. But often we are preoccupied with the beloved not because we have no selves of our own, but because the beloved has physiologically awakened aspects of our own selves.

Should we not, rather, be proud of who we are?

We should be proud.

## What We "Know" About Female Sexuality Is Out of Date

*They had laughed and made love and laughed again . . .*

—Nancy Mitford, *The Pursuit of Love*

This journey showed me, to my surprise, that even though we talk about sex all the time, the information we have about female sexuality is generally out of date. If women had easy—or at least easier—access to and could draw on the new scientific discoveries about female sexuality, which have not been widely reported, they would have a much deeper understanding of their own sexual and emotional responses—and could feel far more sexually alive and connected. Many of these new discoveries illuminate our conflicted feelings vis-à-vis our drive to be loved, and speak directly to the need for men and women to engage with what I will call "the Goddess Array," the set of behaviors that activate the autonomic nervous system in women.

Sex educator Liz Topp, author of *Vaginas: An Owner's Manual*, in an eye-opening interview with me (in which she reported that senior girls in high school, even in our enlightened age, and even in excellent schools, have no idea where on the chart of the vulva the clitoris is—and neither do senior boys), referred to some of these behaviors, only half jokingly, as "the things that women need that men don't need."[1] The latest science confirms that these "little" gestures and flourishes, which are so often relegated to the category of "things that people do in courtship and stop doing in a long-term relationship"—those sexual or romantic "extras" that are sort of nice to dole out to women but are not deemed essential—are in fact physically and emotionally fundamental to women's vibrancy. These practices radically boost a woman's orgasmic potential. But at least as importantly, they help support her relationships, and are even essential to her mental health and peace of mind. They all add up to gestures and attentions that compose "the Goddess Array."

Why, one might ask, don't more people know about this information? There are several reasons for this reticence. One reason is that it is still often taboo to write and talk substantively in public forums about the actual vagina and its actual needs and experiences, as opposed to talking about female sexuality from a more conventional women's magazine "sex advice" angle.

Another reason this new information has not "crossed over" into mainstream conversation is that much of it can risk, at first, sounding terribly politically incorrect. It is not easy to address the biology of women's sexuality without sounding reductive or running afoul of gender politics. If we try to address women's basic animal nature, we run the risk of sounding as if we are casting women as *only* animal-like, or as more animal-like than men.

The tricky part is, if you look at the new science, that women *are* indeed, in sex, in some ways more like animals than men are; the new science also reveals that, in sex, women can be more like mystics than men are. These are controversial statements, but as a feminist I believe that a frank exploration of the potential animal and mystical aspects of female sexuality does not in any way undermine women's rational, intellectual, and professional capabilities.

Finally, these important new discoveries are not widely discussed in mass media yet because the "solution" to many of the sexual problems that women report is not a lucrative new drug, but rather a change in human interaction. Specifically, the solution is often that

least easy goal to reach—a sweeping change in how most straight
men behave in bed with most straight women. Major pharmaceuti-
cal companies—which are the major funders of ads for newspapers,
magazines, and websites that address female sexuality—will not
realize any profit from millions of men simply learning how to touch
their women better, gaze at them longer, hold them more skillfully, or
bring them to more transformative orgasms.

But it is important to get this new information out into the world
nonetheless, because our conventional wisdom about female sexuality is badly out of date. The last broadly reported investigation that
still informs our notion of female sexuality was the survey of ten
thousand cycles of orgasms surveyed in the William H. Masters
and Virginia Johnson classics, *Human Sexual Response* (1966) and
*Human Sexual Inadequacy* (1970), and the survey of 3,500 women
by Shere Hite, *The Hite Report on Female Sexuality* (1976). As mentioned earlier, Masters and Johnson concluded that women and men
were essentially similar in their sexual responses. They also concluded that there was no physiological difference between a "vaginal
orgasm" and a "clitoral orgasm."

Masters and Johnson also annoyed feminists by maintaining that
penile thrusting alone should give women enough stimulation to
have orgasms. Shere Hite contested this conclusion in her own survey. She cited data that about two-thirds of women could not have
orgasms during coitus but often could while masturbating, but that
only about a third had orgasms through intercourse alone.[2] Masters
and Johnson's conclusions that the sexes' responses are essentially
the same, along with Hite's interest in highlighting the importance
of the clitoris and diminishing the importance of the vagina—joined
as she was by a wave of feminist commentary also supporting the
importance of the clitoris and downgrading the vagina, in such essays as Anne Koedt's "The Myth of the Vaginal Orgasm" (1970)—all
served to leave us where we are today: with a general impression that
female sexuality is a lot like male sexuality, except that some women
can have multiple orgasms; the general belief that the vagina is not
as important as the clitoris (women's advice columns still, wrongly,

echoing Anne Koedt's vastly influential essay, misinform woman that the vagina "has very few nerve endings"); and a consensus that it is good etiquette for men to give women, chivalrously, a bit of advance help in the stimulation department (these gestures, cast as gildings on the lily of intercourse, are still infuriatingly called "foreplay") but that the pacing of "sex" is essentially that of the male sex response cycle.

These assumptions are not accurate. It turns out that male sexuality and female sexuality are *very* different. It turns out that, for women, the clitoris is sexually important, the vagina is sexually important, the G-spot is sexually important, the mouth of the cervix is sexually important, the perineum is sexually important, and the anus is sexually important. Recent research has found that what Masters and Johnson argued—that all female orgasm goes through the clitoris—is incorrect. According to the newest data, the G-spot and the clitoris are both aspects of a single neural structure; and women have, as we saw and as Dr. Komisaruk's MRI findings confirm, at least *three* sexual centers: clitoris, vagina, and the third at the mouth of the cervix. (He adds a fourth, the nipples.)

When I first learned that new science had confirmed the sexual responsiveness of the cervix, I was shocked that I had heard nothing about it from science reporting (though I had from literature: "At the back of the womb there lay flesh that demanded to be penetrated. It curved inwards, opening to suck. The flesh walls moved like sea anemones, seeking by suction to draw his sex in. . . . She opened her mouth as if to reveal the openness of the womb, its hunger, and only then did he plunge to the very bottom and felt her contractions . . . ," writes Anaïs Nin, who was not waiting for scientific confirmation, in *Delta of Venus*[3]). That elision of information was one of many weird omissions I would find on this journey as I stumbled upon hugely important scientific discovery after hugely important scientific discovery that had received virtually zero mainstream ink. If a sixth unknown sense were confirmed by science, if they had found that every man had, tucked away, somewhere about his person, an extra sexual organ, for God's sake—*would that not make the evening news?*

Another recent study has found that the whole "clitoris versus vagina"—Masters and Johnson versus Shere Hite—debate is itself wrongly framed: the G-spot, in the anterior wall of the vagina, is now being understood by many researchers to be *part* of the anterior root of the clitoris. The female sexual organ, which includes all these areas, is being proved by new science to be far more complex and far more magical than the utilitarian thrusting totted up by Masters and Johnson can account for, or the goal-oriented, male-identified model of female sexuality mistakenly popularized to this very day in sex advice columns in magazines from *Good Housekeeping* to *Cosmo*.

It turns out that women are designed to have many different kinds of orgasms; that women have the potential to have orgasms without any end except physical exhaustion; that if you understand female sexuality, you pace all the action around her; that while this is a high bar to set, you still want to set it, because properly treated, some women can ejaculate, and because all women in orgasm can go into a unique trance state; that women's orgasms last longer than men's; that memory plays a role in female arousal in a way that is not the case with male arousal; and that women's response to arousal and orgasm is biochemically very different from men's. We're like guys sexually in superficial ways, but in many ways we are, sexually, profoundly *not* like guys.

Maybe one reason this new information has been underreported has to do with anxieties about the male ego, even if the censorship involved is unconscious. Why wouldn't every newspaper be reporting new data that suggest that women are potentially sexually insatiable? Or that many of them are unhappy with the current sexual status quo? Or that certain kinds of seductive behavior and attention from their partners doubles or even quadruples the "microvolts" in the climaxing cervix and vagina? What's not to like about this information? Perhaps the lack of attention to this new information is the fear of implying a new "task"—that of sexual muse and sexual artist—to be put upon male shoulders, even as most men are already overtired and overworked.

I believe, though, that this hesitancy underestimates most heterosexual men's interest in making the women in their lives truly happy—not to mention these men's own vested interest in having sexually vibrant and joyful lovers, which in turn can help make heterosexual men themselves happy.

## AN EPIDEMIC OF FEMALE SEXUAL UNHAPPINESS

I now had reached the point in my journey at which I had begun to believe that our misunderstanding of what women really need sexually—as well as how sex affects them—has led to a great deal of sexual suffering among women today. The numbers show that we have an epidemic in the West of women—"free," presumably sexually literate women—who are suffering from a terrible and preventable sexual malaise. One American woman in three reports that she is suffering from too low levels of sexual desire, and for one woman in ten the absence of desire is so severe it is clinically diagnosable. Indeed, a low sexual desire level—medically defined as "hypoactive sexual desire disorder"—is the most common form of "female sexual dysfunction" reported in the United States.

J. A. Simon's 2010 article in *Postgraduate Medicine,* "Low Sexual Desire—Is It All in Her Head? Pathophysiology, Diagnosis, and Treatment of Hypoactive Sexual Desire Disorder," points out that

> *The Diagnostic and Statistical Manual of Mental Disorders, Fourth Edition, Text Revision (DSM-IV-TR)* defines female hypo [low] sexual desire syndrome as "persistent or recurrent deficiency or absence of sexual fantasies and thoughts, and/or desire for, or receptivity to, sexual activity, which causes personal distress or interpersonal difficulties and is not caused by a medical condition or drug." . . . Sexual function requires the complex interaction of multiple neurotransmitters and hormones, both centrally and peripherally, and sexual desire is considered the result of a complex balance between inhibitory and excitatory pathways in the brain. For example, dopamine,

estrogen, progesterone, and testosterone play an excitatory role, whereas serotonin and prolactin are inhibitory. Thus, decreased sexual desire could be due to a reduced level of excitatory activity, an increased level of inhibitory activity, or both.[4]

These few sentences are a model of scientific understatement, in the sense that the neutral language of science—which is basically saying that a woman's low sexual desire is a result of neurotransmitter and hormonal disconnects or imbalances—is not addressing, or is disregarding, the fact that while menopause, medication, and other immovable factors that the authors name can play a role in low sexual desire, a thousand other psychosexual, interpersonal, and even mood-lighting influences that *can* easily be changed and made better, can also play a major role in lowering many women's levels of sexual desire.

I learned on my journey that women's sexual desire can often fairly easily be turned way back *up*—but they can't do this easily by themselves, or alone with their doctors. Their lovers and husbands have to pay attention to what will, in Tantric terms, "stoke the fire."

The data on low female libido present an even more striking set of facts than they seem to at first glance. A substantial number of women report sexual dissatisfaction, even as "sex" is everywhere and sexual "information" has never been easier to access.

According to an American Psychiatric Association symposium, "Sex, Sexuality And Serotonin," 27 percent to 34 percent of women—more than double the 13 to 17 percent of men—reported experiencing low sexual desire. An extraordinary 15 to 28 percent of women—from one woman in six to one woman in three—reports that she suffers from "orgasmic disorders." This percentage has *risen* in the four decades since the height of the sexual revolution—1976— when about 25 percent of women complained of problems with desire.[5]

A 2009 study, the National Health and Social Life Survey, based at the University of Chicago under the direction of Edward O. Laumann, reported that 43 percent of women—as opposed to 31 percent of men—suffered from what was identified as a "sexual dysfunction."[6]

J. J. Warnock, in "Female Hypoactive Sexual Desire Disorder: Epidemiology, Diagnosis and Treatment," writes that "Female hypoactive sexual desire disorder (HSDD) may occur in up to one-third of adult women in the US. The essential feature of female HSDD is a deficiency or absence of sexual fantasies and desire for sexual activity that causes marked distress or interpersonal difficulty."[7]

An even newer report, released by Indiana University in 2010, reveals that only 64 percent of women participants reported reaching orgasm the last time they had had sex (which means that 36 percent, almost four in ten, didn't), but that 85 percent of the male participants in the same study *told* researchers that their most recent female sex partner had reached orgasm: the data were adjusted for men having sex with men—and the adjustment did not account for the gap between the number of women whom the men *thought* were climaxing during sex with them, and the much smaller number of women who were actually *doing* so.[8]

Whether so many women having such disappointing sexual experiences is leading to many couples having very little sexual intimacy, or whether so little sexual intimacy leads to so many women reporting their low libido, sexual sadness, and frustration, the data show that one heterosexual couple in five is scarcely making love at all.

We have to conclude from this and other studies with similar numbers that the Western sexual revolution sucks. It *has not worked well enough for women.*

In this liberated, postsexual revolution, postfeminist era, when women can do "whatever" they wish sexually and be "bad girls" with little stigma—when any fantasy is available at the touch of a remote control and any sex appliance available rush delivery at the click of a mouse—an astonishingly high percentage of ordinary women, from one in five to one in three, still report feeling little desire, or have trouble regularly reaching orgasm, or report being angry about something involving sexual intimacy. Now that I know more completely how connected the vagina is to female mood and consciousness, I will coin a phrase and say that between one woman in five and one woman in three seems to be suffering from something very like sexual, or even like vaginal, depression.

Oddly enough, our ostensibly pro-sex culture seems very comfortable with this incredibly high rate of female sexual unhappiness. There are no campaigns calling urgent attention to this epidemic of female sexual absence and sorrow. Australian sex therapist Bettina Arndt's book *The Sex Diaries* (2009) sold widely in part because it addresses directly many women's startlingly low levels of desire. Arndt reported that it is quite common, in her clinical experience, for women to want sex less often than their husbands do, and that this is the unacknowledged secret behind many divorces, and even behind many male infidelities.

We will see that new studies show that when circumstances are supportive, virtually every woman can reach orgasm. What if so many women are suffering from low levels of desire, from frustration, and from sexual withdrawal, because—there is no way to say this but honestly—*many men are taught about women in such a way that they don't really know what they are doing?* These numbers must mean, too, that even in this post-sexual-revolution era, many women don't know how to identify, and then ask for, what they need and want.

If a man follows this culture's sexual "script" about what the vagina is, what female sexuality is, and how in general to relate to a woman—he is very likely, against all of his dearest wishes and best intentions, to miss, over time, knowing what is necessary to keep her aroused. The most destructive thing that men are being taught about women is that the vagina is just a sexual organ, and that sex for women is a sexual act in the same way it is for men. But neither gender is being taught about the delicate mind-heart-body connection that, it turns out, *is* female sexual response.

From what I was learning about an optimal state of female sexual and emotional health, which leads women to be passionate and orgasmic to a high degree, this terribly low level of female sexual happiness and desire is a clear marker that something has gone widely amiss. The low levels of female libido that all the recent studies report should be read as signs of a raging disease: signs of *something being very wrong for millions of women in terms of what is happening to them sexually.*

The next part of this book shows how this disconnect took place over the course of a couple of millennia—and what to do about it now.

*two*

*History:*

*Conquest and Control*

# The Traumatized Vagina

*Scapegoating the victim—saying that she brought the situation
on herself—is necessary . . . just as the efficacy of ritual sacrifice
once depended on the delusion that the victim was responsible for
the sins of the world.*

—Peggy Reeves Sanday, *Fraternity Gang Rape*

*J*ust as good sexual experience in the vagina drives joy and creativity into the female brain, the obverse is also true, due to the
same neural pathways: the traumatized vagina, the abused vagina,
the vagina that is part of a neural network that is being neglected by
a withholding or sexually selfish mate—literally *cannot* effectively
condition the female brain with the chemicals that constitute the
emotions of confidence, courage, connection, and joy.

So if you are to subdue and suppress women, and in such a way
that you don't need to actually pen them in or lock them up—in
such a way that they come to "do it to themselves," to suppress
themselves, to lose joy and self-direction, to have no pleasure, to
distrust the strength of love, to think human connection frail and
unreliable—*you must target the vagina.*

As I learned about the incredible connection of the pelvic neural
network to women's minds and emotions, I could not help thinking

about women I had met, from all walks of life, who had been terribly injured in just the ways that would harm or interfere with that mind-body circuitry. I could not get their faces out of my mind. I could not forget certain things they said, certain aspects of their affect, which so many of them had shared. I wondered if there were connections that we were blind to, in the way in which we were currently interpreting this kind of suffering. I realized that women I had met who had suffered vaginal illness, trauma, or injury, across many cultures and of many different ages, often shared in common certain ways of holding themselves; of standing and moving; and a certain expression in their eyes. I kept hearing how the phrase "I feel like I am dirty—like damaged goods" echoed in the words of so many women I had met: from women at a refugee camp in Sierra Leone, many of whom had suffered vaginal fistulas as a result of having been raped as an act of war, to women calling in to a rape crisis center in Edinburgh, Scotland, to the woman I met at a crowded café in Chelsea, Manhattan, who suffered from vulvodynia.

Were we missing the significance of vaginal trauma—just as we were missing the significance of female sexual pleasure—by reading vaginal trauma as "just" physical, or by misunderstanding the trauma of rape as "just" a PTSD-type reaction to a violent act? Were we missing what could be a much more profound and delicate understanding of just *what was being harmed* when a woman's vagina was harmed?

I knew that for women, a fully functioning pelvic nerve is crucial for producing the dopamine, oxytocin, and other chemicals that raise levels of perception, confidence, and feistiness. Would injury or trauma to the vagina and the pelvic nerves materially interfere with the neural pathway's delivery of those intoxicating chemicals to the female brain? And then, another vista swung open: *Could that be why women's vaginas were targeted with violence millennium after millennium?* I could not argue that this was consciously tactical. But could it have been established, subconsciously, over the millennia, because it is *effectively* tactical? It is hard to repress and control a majority of the human population. What if this targeting had been discovered as an efficient tool?

In other words, just as men over the course of generations, in our earliest history, would have noticed what we can now understand as a biologically-based link between a sexually empowered woman and her high levels of happiness, hopefulness, and confidence—would they have noticed the effect of a corresponding biologically-based link between a sexually traumatized woman and a lowered ability to muster happiness, hopefulness, and confidence?

When you spend time in a rape crisis center, as I have done, it is hard to avoid wondering if men are monsters. Why is rape a constant in every society?

Why does war always include mass rape of the enemy's women? Why do so many men rape in a context of war? Feminists such as Kate Millett in *Sexual Politics* (1970), who argues that "rape is generally the result of male sadism and hatred of women," and Susan Brownmiller, in *Against Our Will: Men, Women and Rape* (1975), who argues that war turns men into perverts in order to turn them into rapists, tend to follow the individualized reading of sexuality posited by Freud. Thus they tend to psychologize all rape, which leads to the alarming possible conclusion that all men as individuals are potential sadists. But what if some rape is not personal, but instrumental and systemic?

In 2004, I went to Sierra Leone to report on the mass sexual violence that had been part of the brutal civil war that tore the country apart. The International Rescue Committee took me and several other supporters and journalists to recently rebel-held territory; there, we encountered hundreds of women who had been raped in the war, and in separate visits we met with dozens of rapists from the conflict. It was this trip that persuaded me that the Western model of rape—in which rape results from individual dysfunction, hostility, or perversion—could not account for the instrumentality of rape in the context of war.

We met the women in various settings, but on one visit we went to a refugee center, a walled compound—set in the midst of an open, barren plain—that housed what seemed like thousands of women who had been violently raped in the recent conflict. A single tree provided a little shade, and low, simple concrete structures that housed the women surrounded an unpaved courtyard. It was a haunting, Purgatorial setting: for as far as the eye could see, women drifted slowly, aimlessly around the compound, and except for one or two aid workers and the security guards stationed at the compound entrance, there was not a single adult man.

The women showed tremendous courage. They performed a theater piece for us, which used elements of tribal dance to dramatize their emotions. One woman, playing a rapist, "attacked" another woman. The raw violence in the scene was startling.

After the performance, a female doctor introduced us to several of the women. One woman sat in painful silence as the doctor explained that the woman suffered from a vaginal fistula resulting from her attack. "A vaginal fistula," the doctor explained, "is a tear or puncture in the wall of the vagina, which connects it to another organ, such as the bladder, colon, or rectum." It was a very common injury in the region. Since there had not been enough antibiotic medication in the woman's village to treat the woman, the infection in the wound had led to an odor that had driven her husband to repudiate her. That, too, was a fate that had befallen many of the other women at the compound who also suffered from vaginal fistulas.

At another point, we met a woman—a child really, fifteen years old—who had been kidnapped in Liberia (fifteen thousand teenage girls suffered a similar fate in the conflict), held as a sex slave, and raped repeatedly. She had managed to trick her kidnapper, take her year-old baby (whose father had been her captor), and escape. She had walked through the bush, eating wild yams, until she had made it across the border to an IRC compound, and relative safety.

These women were different from the women we met who were traumatized by amputations, or by gunfire, or by being forced to work in the diamond mines. There was something about what had happened to the rape victims that had efficiently switched a light off in them. These women, rejected by their tribes and families, moved in great groups together over the dusty mounds of earth as if they were adrift together. In spite of their individual courage, what was unmistakable was that aspects of their very souls, in some profound way, had been hollowed out of them. In any one woman, this dimming of vitality was notable; but when you saw this nation of drifting women, it was impossible to ignore. Something systemic had been done to them that had somehow, in a way unique to *this* trauma, blunted them at the level of engagement, curiosity, and will.

The doctor explained exactly how these women had sustained their injuries. The women had been shredded internally; deliberately. By the points of bayonets; by sharpened sticks; by broken bottles; by knives. Tens of thousands of women had been injured in exactly these ways. The doctor spoke about these injuries not as resulting from deviant acts perpetrated by random perverts, but as a common outcome in the conflict.

Why would thousands and thousands of soldiers, in a conflict situation, have used sharp objects to destroy the vaginas of thousands and thousands of women? There was nothing about the rapes, with these injuries, that seemed sexual to me or even psychodynamic. I now believe, given my understanding of the pelvic nerve and its relationship to female confidence, creativity, and will, that these tens of thousands of men were not "getting off" on damaging the internal pelvic structures of these tens of thousands of women.

Women are brutalized in conflicts in Africa and around the world in this way decade after decade. It was the commanders in Sierra Leone and in the Democratic Republic of the Congo who ordered this kind of atrocity, and who ordered their troops to rape. Individual soldiers the IRC has interviewed have explained that they had no choice but to follow these orders—lest they be shot themselves. Why would such an order go out from a commander in an armed conflict? Could these commanders be giving these orders on the basis of something that is a kind of folk wisdom? In other words, could these commanders be ordering their troops to engage in atrocities that damage the female pelvic nerve, because centuries of experience have shown that a consequence of this kind of violence is that the women who experience it will be easier to subjugate?

I later interviewed others who work with women who have been violently raped in war. Jimmie Briggs, founder of the global antirape and antiviolence organization Man Up (Briggs was named a GQ Man of the Year in 2011 for his work on behalf of women traumatized by rape in war), travels frequently to the Democratic Republic of the Congo, which is one of the Ground Zeros of this practice: the United Nations estimates that four hundred thousand women have been raped during the recent civil war in that country.[1] Briggs has written a book on the subject of rape in war: "There is something different about victims of violent rape," he said. "I will go on the record about this. I have interviewed people who have been traumatized just as severely in other ways and there is not this same outcome. I have seen the difference of the result of this kind of trauma from other kinds of trauma. It is indeed as if a light has gone out of these women's eyes."[2]

In another very different refugee camp, in a room with concrete walls painted blue-green, where white light slanted in from high unglassed windows and a few English sentences had been scratched onto a makeshift blackboard, I was introduced to some of Sierra Leone's most brutal rapists: they were twelve-, thirteen-, and fourteen-year-old boys—child soldiers. They were being rehabilitated by the IRC, which was working to educate them and provide them with a safe harbor. Their eyes were overcast with pain; their polo shirts were ragged; drugs and terror had stunted their growth. These were simply children, who had themselves been kidnapped and traumatized, forced at gunpoint to rape. These children, who played soccer in a dusty courtyard after we had spoken with them, obviously did not do what they had done to the women in the other camp out of perverse pathology. The Freudian model that violent rape is the result of individual sexual deviancy simply does not account for the systemic use of violent rape in war.

Radical feminism sees rape as simply a demonstration of unequal power relations and takes as its motto the assertion that rape is about power, not sex. This is closer to what I now believe to be the truth, but it still misses the ultimate insight: If it is just about power, why involve the sex? Why not just beat, threaten, starve, or imprison a woman? You can get plenty of power over women in ways that are nonsexual.

But if your goal is to break a woman psychologically, *it is efficient to do violence to her vagina.* You will break her faster and more thoroughly than if you simply beat her—because of the vulnerability of the vagina as a mediator of consciousness. Trauma to the vagina imprints deeply on the female brain, conditioning and influencing the rest of her body and mind.

Rape is part of the standard tool kit in the deployment of genocidal army tactics. This insight allows us to understand that many men who rape—and perhaps most men who rape in war—are not doing this as a function of personal perversion. Understood in this way, rape is instrumental. Rape is a strategy of *actual physical and psychological control of women,* traumatizing via the vagina as a way to imprint the consequences of trauma on the female brain.

If we understand this, we understand that what happens to a woman's vagina is far more important, for better and for worse, than we have realized. We can see that rape is a far more serious crime than the model of rape as a "sex crime" or a form of "violence" that lasts for the duration of the crime, and then perhaps posttraumatically. We should understand that while healing is possible, one never fully "recovers" from rape; one is never just the same after as before. Rape, properly understood, is more like an injury to the brain than a violent variation on sex. Rape, properly understood, is always aimed not just at the female sex organ but at the female brain.

## RAPE STAYS IN THE FEMALE BRAIN

According to aid workers, body workers, and doctors I've interviewed, as well as according to some pioneering new research on trauma, rape can change the female brain and female body systems in complex and long-lasting ways. But do you have to suffer a dramatically violent rape like the women in Sierra Leone for trauma to the vagina to affect the brain? Dr. Burke Richmond's research suggests not.

Dr. Richmond is a neurologist at the University of Wisconsin,

Madison, Wisconsin, specializing in otolaryngology. He studies neurological problems such as chronic dizziness, vertigo (the feeling of being off-balance), and tinnitus (chronic ringing in the ears). He also runs a clinical practice for patients, mostly women, who suffer from these and related conditions. His research in perception disorders has demonstrated that there are various ways in which rape or child sexual abuse imprint the female brain and body.

I met Dr. Richmond in the summer of 2010, on a mutual friend's boat. His three lively children scrambled about on the deck. A witty but serious physician in his forties, with dark hair and a focused expression, he told me that a disproportionate number of his female patients who suffered problems with balance had histories of rape or sexual assault. Their problems with balance often remained for years after the attacks. He had concluded that, while the causation was not yet proved—his evidence was at that point anecdotal—there was a high enough incidence of correlation between patients with balance problems and patients who had a past history of rape or sexual assault that it was statistically significant and bore additional investigation. I was so gripped by his descriptions of rape apparently literally affecting some of his female patients' abilities to "stand their ground" that I spoke to him for two hours, oblivious to the bright sunshine and the yellow-gray cliffs falling away in the distance.

His findings confirmed something I had noticed in my ten years of teaching voice—public speaking and presentation—at the Wood-hull Institute, a leadership academy for young women, which I had cofounded. Part of my training involved teaching young women how to stand tall, to "stand their ground" when speaking—that is, how to occupy a four-foot space on an imagined stage. I noticed again and again, over the course of many years, that a minority of young women literally couldn't stand their ground—they could not stand still, straight, and tall, no matter how much they wished to do so; they kept imperceptibly swaying from side to side.

These same young women's shoulders also seemed energetically to yield, somehow, under my hands, without the natural resistance that other young women's shoulders presented as I adjusted their posture.

Finally, this same subset of young women tended to have constricted voices: tension in the larynx often made their voices sound high and childlike. When we practiced voice exercises to open their throats and diaphragms, two things happened almost universally: their voices deepened to a more natural and more authoritative register, and following shortly thereafter, they would burst into convulsive sobs.

Often these young women, after they had wept deeply, and after they had made it through the public speaking exercise successfully with their "new" voices and open throats and chests, showed an amazing transformation—a glow, a radiance, a new authenticity and vitality, as if they had just now come "into focus." I learned again and again that the young women who presented this constellation of "symptoms" had suffered childhood or adolescent sexual assault, or had been raped. I noticed that this cluster of symptoms was very different from the presentation of the many other young women we had in the program who had suffered just as severe, but other, nonsexual forms of trauma.

So when Dr. Richmond shared with me his findings that revealed that patients of his who were literally not able to resist being "pushed over" had also had high rates of sexual assault or rape in their backgrounds, I was riveted.

Some of his patients, Dr. Richmond told me, come to him with a symptom called "phobic postural sway"—which means they sway under stress, or can be pushed over easily. Others have "conversion gait disorders"—their gait swerves, even though there is nothing apparently physically wrong with them. Still others experience "visual vertigo," meaning that they feel dizzy for no obvious reason. Other symptom clusters he found that appeared along with histories of rape included the feeling of falling continually, or morning nausea. "In a group of women that I've seen who fall over easily, in a test in which I push them, I will ask about sexual abuse history—and frequently I will find it. That is a bias: I don't ask all my patients this question. That is, I don't ask those who don't demonstrate these symptoms if they've been sexually abused. But it is useful to ask about sexual abuse when these symptoms do appear, because that can lead to the right diagnostic test."

"So you can literally push rape and sexual abuse survivors over more easily?" I asked.

"Yes," Dr. Richmond confirmed. "If I ask these women to close their eyes and stand, there may be a slight sway. Most people do not have a perceptible amount of sway. If you lightly push most people, they will resist. They won't sidestep or fall over, or be grossly off balance. But these women will. If you push them, they will keep falling over; you have to catch them. It is a disproportionate physical response not congruent with their physical functioning. They have normal strength, normal reflexes, normal physical functioning; they have no objective neurological deficits—no vestibular lesions or other brain injuries, which can cause a similar finding, for instance. These women have no physical evidence of a neurological problem, but their bodies are reacting as if they *do* have a neurological problem.

"Once I instruct them to resist," Dr. Richmond said, of his sexually traumatized patients, "I can push with all of my strength and they will be solid as a rock."

That astonished me: when a rape survivor is told to resist, her body reacts differently. "So that's a mind-body thing."

"Exactly—for what it is worth. I imagine my role as a physician and an authority 'allows' them to resist. The stability is there—once they have been 'given permission' to resist. These are the same patients who, without the instruction, fall over when pushed."

To restate what Dr. Richmond is saying: rape victims are sometimes *literally* "destabilized" by the rape.

I wondered about the relationship of this information to the brain-vagina connection: Had trauma to the vagina also affected the brain, or was it an unrelated but just as intriguing imprint on the brain from sexual abuse?

"There is no doubt that when you have extreme levels of trauma, you can see that in the body. I don't ask everybody about sexual abuse but when I see this pattern and ask about it, it is amazing how often

I will find it. I say it is an interacting variable. They may have other things going on, but this question of sexual abuse needs to be incorporated into the treatment if you want an explanation for why these symptoms are happening to this person now. They have multiple layers of medical problems that accumulate over time, from obesity to migraines to mental health disorders."

"Because of the sexual abuse?" I asked. "Yes," he answered. "I get that you are saying we can't say one thing is the cause. But it sounds like you are saying that the effect of sexual abuse on the female body should be a field of study."

Dr. Richmond agreed. "Nobody fully understands 'conversion disorders,' " he explained. "The term refers to a physical abnormality generated by a mental state." The popular expression for conversion disorders is *hypochondria,* or the phrase "it's all in your mind." With a conversion disorder, someone suffers a real symptom, but the cause is not apparently physical. "Though there is nothing apparently 'physically wrong' with these patients," said Dr. Richmond, "we need to take what is happening to these women seriously. Their symptoms may be caused by an abnormality in the brain generated by abnormal memory traces or abnormal neural circuitry.

"If you've been attacked by somebody repeatedly, you develop a whole behavioral motor response to that attack. You may later passively dissociate and feel, 'Somebody's doing something to someone's body, but it is not my body.' " Dr. Richmond said that one's learned response to that attack could be carried through life.

I told him about how I was looking at pelvic nerve mutilation in women who had been violently raped in Sierra Leone, and at the interruption in dopamine delivery to the brain that the injury involved. I explained that I wanted to understand if, and if so how, sexual assault to the vagina might have a physical effect on the female brain.

"I would argue," he said, "that it is the brain that affects the body after trauma. You get direct nerve injury from vaginal assaults such as the ones in Sierra Leone, but it is the brain affecting the entire system after that, or apart from that gross trauma. In the West you can see these effects on women from sexual trauma of less obvious kinds.

Behavior is a global response: if someone is traumatizing you, your visual system is affected, your auditory system is affected; these are all integrated, and your brain is continually learning new reactions from the trauma."

I restated: "So it is accurate for me to say that if you traumatize a woman sexually, even if there is no 'violence,' you are physically traumatizing her brain."

"Yes," he repeated. "I think that is something that is fair to say." He thought some more. "I had this one patient who had a history of sexual abuse in childhood. As an adult, she presented with an aversion to certain sounds: this is a condition called misophonia, a spontaneous emotional response to certain sounds. Imagine how you feel about fingers against a chalkboard; for people with this disorder, clicking or chewing or other sounds can become intolerably emotionally abrasive. The adult disorder may have some original link to early sexual abuse from her father. She remembers him in the corner, making these noises, and it was a linked memory to the abuse."

I told him, in response to this, about the puzzle that had bothered me for so long about women's recovery from rape—that so many women who had, through therapy, dealt intensively with the psychological effects of their rape, who had had good sexual responses before their rape, and were with safe, supportive, loving partners, simply could not enjoy sex again the way they had done before the rape.

"So," I asked Dr. Richmond, "does this dysregulation of the autonomic nervous system after sexual trauma possibly help explain what I observed about rape survivors—that they may be having trouble with sexual arousal and pleasure after the assault in part because of actual physical changes to their autonomic nervous system, due to that trauma?"

"Can rape or sexual assault induce a permanent shift or change in the autonomic nervous system? Arguably it could; a growing literature confirms this. Some people's systems may make them more vulnerable to this. It may be that some women are more resilient than others, some men more resilient than others, against PTSD, in terms of the question of possible damage to the autonomic nervous system from sexual trauma. But wherever your emphasis, it is clear that when people have extreme experiences outside the norm, those experiences will have an effect on vulnerable populations and will affect the autonomic nervous system." Indeed, other recent studies confirm that women who have been raped or sexually abused, especially in childhood, show striking physically measurable brain differences from women who have not been raped through changes in the size and activation of the hippocampus, and differences in cortisol levels.[3]

In other words, when you rape a woman (and perhaps also when you rape a man, though the data here are based on female victims), or if you sexually abuse her in childhood, you may be repatterning her body, possibly *for the rest of her life,* in ways that embed fear, more easily triggered stress responses, and attendant risk aversion, into the very neural fabric of her responses to the world, and that, as we will see, in the case of the changes in the hippocampus, may even interrupt her ability to process recent memory in a way that might strengthen her ongoing sense of self.

For at least one of Dr. Richmond's patients, there was a vocal symptom related to sexual trauma. "I have a very interesting case," he told me. "It appeared that this patient had episodes of 'expressive aphasias': for long periods of time, she had a complete inability to talk. She had suffered horrendous abuse before the age of two—when she was preverbal. This person's physical behavioral response when she was an adult under stress was to regress to a preverbal state."[4]

A broad study has confirmed that many health problems, seemingly unrelated to the original rape, follow a sex crime: Roni Caryn Rabin, who wrote "Nearly 1 in 5 Women in U.S. Survey Say They Have Been Sexually Assaulted" in the *New York Times,* reports on the many health problems that can follow rape: The National Intimate Partner and Sexual Violence Survey supported by the National Institute of Justice and the Department of Defense, she wrote, looked at 16,507 adults. A third of women said they had been victims of a rape, beating, or stalking, or a combination of assaults. *Rape* was defined in this study as "completed forced penetration, forced penetration facilitated by drugs or alcohol, or attempted forced penetration." By that definition, "1.3 million American women annually may be victims of rape or attempted rape." (One in 71 men has been raped, according to the same study.) "A vast majority of women who said they had been victims of sexual violence, rape or stalking reported symptoms of post-traumatic stress disorder."

Other surprising, and seemingly unrelated, health problems also correlated with the sexual assaults. The women who had been sexually assaulted had higher rates than the nonassaulted women did of asthma, diabetes, irritable bowel syndrome, headaches, chronic pain, sleep difficulties, limitations on mobility, and poor physical health in general, as well as higher rates of mental health problems. This link between sexual assault and other chronic health problems in other body systems seemingly unrelated to the assault, confirms findings in smaller studies reported by Lisa James, director of health for the nonprofit Futures Without Violence: her data, too, suggest that even a one-time act of sexual violence can chronically affect the victim with seemingly unrelated health issues.[5]

So is all rape about sexual aggression or male neurosis? Or can the sustained cultural presence of rape also or even instead, at times, be about reprogramming women at a core physical level to be less brave, less secure, less robust in other ways, and to go through the rest of their lives, potentially, with a less stable sense of self?

I would soon speak with a Tantric guru named Mike Lousada, and an osteopath named Katrine Cakuls, read a book by an energy worker named Tami Lynn Kent,[6] and interview my own gynecologist, Dr. Coady; all of them would describe a constriction in the musculature of the vagina as a response to trauma as well. Dr. Coady would identify it as vaginismus; Lousada would describe "knots" in the vaginal musculature of rape survivors; Kent would note that muscle constriction in the vagina can cause other kinds of imbalances in the rest of the body; and would describe as constricted the vaginas of women who believe they are "uptight" emotionally—women who often turn out to have had sexual shaming, or worse experiences, in their pasts.

Katrine Cakuls is a highly trained Manhattan cranial osteopath at Cranial Osteopathic Approach, who heals women by, among other treatments, doing internal nonsexual vaginal work. She is also sure that emotion affects women's vaginal sensitivity and muscle tone and can even exacerbate vaginal and other kinds of pathology. She, too, believes from her experience in her own practice, that when she "frees" tensions in the vagina, she can free other emotional issues in the female mind that may have gotten stuck, releasing areas of a woman's creativity and sexual health that had been suffering from low vitality. Tami Lynn Kent, author of the cult bestseller *Wild Feminine: Finding Power, Spirit & Joy in the Female Body,* is a body worker who does nonsexual vaginal massage. She has a national following of body workers who hold similar beliefs and who work on the same area. Her view is that different quadrants of the vagina hold different kinds of blocked emotion, and that these can be released through internal manipulaion.

I interviewed the clients of body workers who specialized in nonsexual vaginal massage, or osteopathic adjustment, and many of them said that the intimate and unconventional treatment had effected remarkable emotional healings. All this, of course, would until recently have been considered fringe in the formal medical establishment. But medicine and science are in some places catching up with the anecdotal evidence of the cranial osteopaths and body workers. Researchers Yoon et al., as we will see, have recently found that stress and trauma actually do affect the very functioning of the vagina.

I remarked to Dr. Richmond, "It seems that women who present with symptoms that may result from sexual abuse are dismissed by medical professionals as hysterical if there is no physical cause—or else pathologized as nuts by psychiatrists."

"Many women would say that," he responded. "Women do not want to hear from doctors that 'it is all in their head' and, by the same token, many are scared of going to psychiatrists because they fear being labeled crazy due to their symptoms, when they know they are not crazy.

"As the growing field of neuropsychoimmunology shows, the mind-body connection is very real. Science is now developing tools to objectively demonstrate these changes, and reflect our greater understanding of the complex responses between brain and body: the functional ways in which memory is laid down and physical responses follow.

"It is easy for me to say, 'It is all in your head,' " he concluded. "That is, everything neurological is real, and it can also be all in your head."

What Dr. Richmond was seeing anecdotally has been documented in recent studies. There is growing, if still preliminary, evidence that rape and early sexual trauma can indeed "stay in the body"—even stay in the vagina—and change the body on the most intimate, systemic level. Recovery is possible, but treatment should be specialized. Rape and early sex abuse can indeed permanently change the working of the sympathetic nervous system (SNS)—so crucial for female arousal; and, if she is not supported by the right treatment, it can permanently alter the way a woman breathes, the rate of her heart, her blood pressure, and her startle reaction, in a manner that is not under any conscious control.

At least one major 2006 study confirms that the trauma of a history of sexual abuse not only can dysregulate the SNS—creating, as Dr. Richmond saw, a permanent higher "baseline" SNS activation in sexually traumatized women—but also can lead the vagina to respond differently—less effectively, with less engorgement—to exercise, and even to the subjects' viewing of erotic material.

Researchers Alessandra Rellini and Cindy Meston, when both were in the psychology department at the University of Texas, confirmed that sexual trauma in childhood really can affect and damage not just the psychology but the physiology of the vagina—and of female sexual arousal—years after the trauma took place.[7] They checked the cortisol levels from the women's saliva, heightened their SNS reactions through exercise, and then showed them erotic videos. They measured the women's "vaginal pulse"—the ease of their vaginal engorgement—via the strength of the blood's beating through that area.

Rellini and Meston found significant differences in "vaginal pulse" measures for women with traumatic sexual abuse in their histories, compared with those who had never experienced sexual abuse.

Rellini and Meston, like Dr. Richmond, found excessive baseline SNS activity in women who had been traumatically sexually abused.

This dysregulated SNS, they confirmed, affects the women's later sex lives, since a balanced (not an excessively heightened) SNS is critical to female arousal. Women with a history of sex abuse show higher "baseline" or resting SNS activity, the authors found—confirming the work of other researchers.

In other words, women can get aroused most easily when the SNS is in good working order; and the trauma of rape or child sexual abuse seems to mess with the good balance of the SNS in many women. (It is also interesting to look at this data for many reasons: raped women's bodies don't respond the same way to exercise as do nontraumatized women's bodies. There is a notable weight difference in the subjects of the experiment who did and did not have abuse in their backgrounds; the sexual abuse/PTSD women were on average about thirty pounds heavier than the control group. This difference could certainly be explainable by many factors, but it bears more investigation.)

The authors note that there is not much research on the effect of sexual trauma on women's relationships, and that what research there is tends to focus on cognitive treatments, rather than looking at the biology of trauma. "Despite the detrimental impact of PTSD on women's relationships, few treatments have been developed specifically for couples' issues experienced by CSA survivors with PTSD . . ."[8] "[E]ven fewer therapies address sexual dysfunction experienced by this population."[9]

The researchers explain their finding further: "Studies conducted on women with a history of [child sexual abuse and posttraumatic stress disorder] show increased sympathetic nervous system . . . at baseline levels. During a stressful experience, the [SNS] becomes activated and releases catecholamines, such as norepinephrine, which increase glucose availability, heart rate, and blood pressure. . . ." [10] "After a nontraumatic stressor, the body returns to its original state. However, after a trauma, the homeostasis of the individual is often altered, and this is associated with the development of PTSD. The literature on veterans and adult survivors of childhood maltreatment shows that baseline levels of SNS activity are higher in trauma survivors with PTSD than in healthy control women." [11]

We have all seen movies about war veterans who are startled into a state of pounding heart rate and hyperventilation by a car's backfiring. Traumatized rape and child sexual abuse survivors appear, according to this study, to show the same kind of overall, chronic dysregulation of the system responsible for breathing, heart rate, and blood pressure:

"Impairments in the hypothalamic-pituitary-adrenal (HPA) axis also are found in women with PTSD; these include higher levels of adrenocorticotropic hormone (ACTH), lower levels of cortisol, and a down regulation of glucocorticoid receptors. . . . Lower levels of cortisol may lead to excessive SNS activity, which may cause an over-expenditure of energy and a maladaptive adjustment to subsequent stressors." [12] This may be the same dysregulation and overactivation of the stress response to which Dr. Richmond was referring; he and others have linked that elevated SNS activation to many health problems that are seemingly unrelated to the original sexual trauma, from vertigo to motor control issues to visual processing problems to high blood pressure and an elevated startle response. Translation: women who have been sexually traumatized experience brain changes that damage the body system that regulates the reaction to stress.

How does this relate to impaired female sexual response over time, resulting from sexual trauma? "The [SNS] is also thought to play an important role in the early stages of female sexual arousal," the authors emphasize.

"An additional study by Meston and Gorzalka (1996a) found support for the idea that there may be an optimal level of SNS activity for facilitation of sexual [arousal] and that too much or too little SNS activity may have a detrimental impact on physiological sexual responding," they point out. In other words, women have to have balanced levels of SNS activity to become aroused well; being freaked out or terrified, or feeling threatened, often impairs female sexual response. Since levels of SNS activity increase in a natural way during lovemaking, the hypothesis in this study is that for traumatized women, whose baseline SNS is so elevated, lovemaking unbalances the SNS's workings and impairs their arousal. The authors suggest this in scientific language: "It is conceivable that when women with [posttraumatic stress disorder] engage in sexual behaviors, their [SNS] baseline levels become excessively activated due to their high [SNS] baseline levels. . . . This may have a negative impact on their physiological sexual responses. Hypothetically, this could explain the high incidence of sexual arousal difficulties noted in women with a history of [child sexual abuse and posttraumatic stress disorder.]"[13] The study sought to investigate this hypothesis—and the authors concluded that their findings confirmed that it was true.

So the trauma of rape or childhood sexual abuse can lead to dysregulation of the sympathetic nervous system, a dysregulation that leads in turn to the vagina's *physical inability* or impaired physical ability to engorge with blood upon a woman's seeing erotic material—even if this arousal is taking place many years later in life than the original attack. In other words, rape and sex abuse trauma can actually damage the vagina's functionality. It can damage the vagina's engorgement capabilities much later in life. It can affect the system that, in the male body, would allow a man to achieve erections, or affects the system that in a man would affect, in turn, the hardness or softness of his erection.

Rape and sexual assault can break, in other words, the delicate physical balance that underpins the female body's *physical* mechanism for getting turned on. It seems that the aftereffect of sexual trauma can dysregulate the *physiology* of female sexual arousal—leaving entirely aside the *psychology* of the event and its many emotional aftereffects.

Rape tends to be understood and even prosecuted—if there is no weapon involved, and no additional physical assault, no visible bruising and no blood—as if it is "just" forced sex, rather than a highly violent act resulting in potentially lasting physical damage. But this new science shows that "mere" fear and "mere" violation, when imposed on a victim through a "nonviolent" sex assault, even a date rape, can imprint and harm the female brain and body in measurable, long-lasting ways. Indeed, Dr. Coady believes that sexual assault and abuse can affect women's experience of physical pain later in life, and new data do relate sexual trauma to some women's later seemingly unrelated perception of chronic pain—that is, if you are raped or suffer child sexual abuse, and you have a much later "unrelated" health condition, it can feel as if it hurts you more than it would women in a control group without that history. She believes in this potential result to the point that Dr. Coady says that "for 'rape' you can substitute 'pain.' "

Surely this new science should lead us to support rape victims to heal in ways that involve more than just verbal, emotionally-based counseling. Perhaps it will lead to the development of standard practice for treating a victim of "nonviolent" rape to include counseling by those who are more specifically trained in the science of PTSD and in behaviorally/neurologically based treatments, such as those in use at New York City's Bellevue Hospital Center's Post-Traumatic Stress Treatment facility, to help the brain and the impaired SNS physically to recover. Perhaps, too, civil suits by victims can draw on evidence of later health issues, or even tests of stress reactions, to get civil damages from rapists where the courts have not gone far enough. This trauma and its physical consequences can be treated— but it takes treatment that incorporates the science of PTSD.

Understood in this way, and with this significant evidence, rape and sexual assault, with their attendant trauma, should be understood not just as a form of forced sex; they should also be understood as a form of injury to the brain and body, and even as a variant of castration.

## VULVODYNIA AND EXISTENTIAL DESPAIR

My thesis, to be sound, needed a control group. Obviously, it would be unethical to harm the female pelvic nerve or interfere with orgasm deliberately to see what happens to the female brain when those chemicals are not being delivered to it from the pelvic neural network. Such studies do not exist. So one must explore what happens to women who have suffered damage to this mind-body system through a medical condition, or who have suffered the trauma of rape. Would we see the changes in these women's confidence, creativity, sense of connectedness, and hopefulness, which I was investigating? It made sense for me to talk to Nancy Fish. Fish knows all about trauma to the vagina, both as a patient herself and as a counselor to sufferers of vulvodynia—which means "vaginal pain"—and pelvic nerve damage. She is a therapist at SoHo Obstetrics and Gynecology, Dr. Deborah Coady's practice, the foremost vulvodynia practice in the United States. Fish runs SoHo OB/GYN's support group for sufferers of vulvodynia, and she is the coauthor, along with Dr. Coady, of the book *Healing Painful Sex*.

Vulvodynia is, generally, a poorly understood condition that affects, at some point in their lives, a shockingly high number of women—16 percent of all women, according to Dr. Coady and Nancy Fish's research. (A *Newsweek* survey showed women self-reporting sexual pain at the rate of 8 percent to 23 percent, so Coady and Fish's numbers, which seemed improbably high to me when I first heard them, are a confirmed median.)

When a woman suffers from vulvodynia, it means that something is inflaming or irritating some part of the pelvic neural network, causing pain in the vulva, vagina, or even the clitoris, which leads to painful sex. I knew from having interviewed several vulvodynia sufferers that they had a "light gone out of them" quality about them when their condition worsened, and that their radiance shone brighter when their condition improved. Of course, that is an anecdotal and not a scientific observation, and of course they were depressed for obvious reasons when they were suffering; but I needed to know—was their depression due primarily to the pain itself, and to the related misery of not being able to have normal sexual intimacy; or did it also, possibly, involve this larger neural disarray of the brain/vagina feedback loop?

On a budding day in May 2011, I sat on the screened porch of my house and interviewed Ms. Fish. When we spoke, her voice was faint—she was recovering from surgery to release her own trapped pelvic nerve—but she pushed herself quite admirably to raise her voice above the murmur her energy level could comfortably muster, to help me get these questions answered.

A Columbia University–trained therapist, Fish runs a private practice in Bergen County, New Jersey, counseling women with vulvodynia, in addition to her work at SoHo OB/GYN. "I see young women, older women, single, married, lesbian, straight, bisexual, from all backgrounds," she explained. "There is such a diversity in my practice that that is one way I know this is a medical condition and not psychologically generated." Fish is also very open about having suffered from the condition herself for many years.

Fish explained that vulvodynia is another outcome of a trapped pelvic nerve, but that instead of an absence of sensation, a woman with vulvodynia experiences pain. I spelled out to her my theory that the pudendal nerve helps deliver feelings of well-being to the female brain, and thus the vagina mediates a woman's sense of her core self.

"Does this make sense, in your experience? Or is this crazy?" I asked.

"Oh no," she said. "That's totally normal. Any time there is any kind of problem in the vulvovaginal region, it affects your whole sense of self. A lot of women *feel* crazy for feeling that their whole sense of self is involved with the vagina, but I tell them they are not. Having pain or discomfort in that part of your body is not like having pain in another part of your body. People talk about 'sciatic pain' or 'migraine pain,' and they are very comfortable talking about it. But most women are ashamed to talk about pain in that area of their bodies. So not only do you walk around with horrible pain, but you can't even talk about it."

"Vulvovaginal pain has been 'read' as psychologically caused, for the last few decades, I gather," I said.

Fish agreed. "Women are often told it's all in their heads." She continued, "Anxiety and depression can certainly make the pain worse. But we have never met a woman for whom this pain has psychological roots. It is physically based.[14]

"The majority of doctors have no clue as to what is wrong with these women. A patient sees an average of seven doctors before she gets an accurate diagnosis, and is often told the most outlandish things. I went to one crazy doctor who works in this field, who calls herself a real expert. She told me I had a severe vitamin D deficiency—she never did an internal exam with me! She never mentioned the pelvic floor! She is still practicing—though I brought charges against her with the State Board."

I wondered if that core sense of self in relation to the vagina's well-being could be evolutionary or neurobiological. I heard so many women from so many different cultures and economic backgrounds say that they felt like "damaged goods" when there had been an insult to or trauma to the vagina.

I pushed further. "How often do you hear that expression 'I feel like damaged goods' from your patients?"

"Almost with every person I see," she replied. "It is almost impossible not to say that, it seems, at a certain point."

"I feel," I speculated, "that there is something about a sense of an intact, healthy vagina that goes to a core sense of the female self. Is *that* crazy?"

"No," she assured me. "When your foot hurts, you may feel depressed; it doesn't affect your core sense of self as when the vagina is injured or in pain."

"Do many of your patients feel depressed?" I asked. I was wondering if vaginas that were not working well neurologically were not delivering dopamine to the patients' brains, which would stand to reason.

"*All* of them feel depressed. *All* of them have depression," she stressed.

"Do you think that the nerve damage in the vagina may be a physiological cause of the depression?" I continued.

"When there is pain to the vagina, your whole central nervous system gets affected. I am sure there are biological things going on."

"How does this depression manifest in your patients?"

"It is like: 'Why me? I've been a good person.' "

"It is existential depression," I remarked.

"Yes. I see young women whose lives are shattered. It can happen from one moment to the next. They go from normalcy to severe pain.

"I had one patient," she continued, "a businesswoman. The day before she was supposed to go on a business trip to India, she was struck with horrible clitoral pain. Her pudendal nerve became inflamed. She went on this trip to India nonetheless, and she was dying the entire time. She tried to put herself through the meetings. At the hotel she would put an ice pack between her legs and start to drink. She said that if she had spent the rest of her life like that, she would have killed herself. Most of my patients have had suicidal ideation."

"You are saying," I confirmed, "that this is different from patients of yours with equally severe pain elsewhere in the body. Is there anything else specifically about pain in the vagina that would make women especially want to kill themselves?"

"The inability to have normal intimacy makes it all the more desperate, though I have met really terrific men who are incredibly supportive."

"What does it feel like for women to never be able to use their vaginas in a healthy way?"

"They don't feel like they are whole."

"In a different way than an amputee?" I kept restating the question because I wanted to be sure I was isolating "vaginal grief" from general physical grief.

"Yes," she affirmed. "While I was going through my journey with vulvodynia, I also had a lateral mastectomy. That was a piece of cake compared to this. You feel unattractive, like your partner is not going to want to touch you. I have said at certain points [to my husband],

'Why don't you just go have an affair?'; I feel so bad that he cannot have typical intercourse. My clients have told me they said the same things to their partners. People worry about their partners leaving them. They don't feel like whole women."

I asked her whether there was any message regarding their vaginas she wanted women reading to know.

"Women have so little understanding of their own bodies—because the science is missing, I am finding," she said. "The science is missing. If people had a better understanding of the biology of women, this area would be so destigmatized."

"You are saying that modern science doesn't distribute widely enough an understanding of women's vulvas, vaginas, and pelvises, and so women do not understand themselves either?"

"Yes," said Fish.

"So science is in the Dark Ages regarding the vagina, and so are women?"

"Yes. We are *so* in the Dark Ages when it comes to medical care and understanding in the area of the vagina."

"I didn't even know I had a pudendal nerve," I commented.

"Oh my God! When I say 'pudendal nerve,' no one knows what I am talking about. People in the *medical profession* don't know what I'm talking about! Women need to become more comfortable with their vaginas. When women first come to see Dr. Coady, no one has ever heard of the pudendal nerve, and they don't know what pelvic floor muscles are, or that these are also connected to their vagina and can affect their sex lives. . . . Some women don't know exactly where their labia are, or their clitorises. Deb always gives them a mirror."

"What happens when women heal and can use their vaginas normally again?" I asked.

"It takes time," she replied. "Some women will always have cautiousness there." Fish explained that some of her clients said that even after they had recovered, they felt that their "sexuality was amputated." "They have anxiety," she went on. "They have hypervigilance there about everything they do."

"So the experience of pain or trauma in the vagina, *even after it is over,* leaves women with some psychological scars—anxiety, hypervigilance, a sense of 'amputation' of an aspect of the core self—that are hard to just ignore even after the vagina is 'better'?" I asked. I thought again of all those women in Sierra Leone moving like ghosts in a settlement of ghosts; I thought of all the women I had met in Western Europe or North America who had been raped, and who were still moving through life with "the light," as Jimmie Briggs had put it, having "gone out of their eyes."

Did her patients, I asked her, report any general flattening of excitement, enthusiasm, or creativity when their vaginas were so—for lack of a better term—despairing?

"Oh yeah," she confirmed with certainty in her voice. "Everything—*everything* becomes flattened: their feelings about work, their feelings about their friends, about their partners, about family members. Their perception changes because of the way they feel about themselves. They start to feel damaged, so they project it onto everyone else. It is indeed despair that they report: despondency and hopelessness."

"Does anyone talk about a loss of creativity with vaginal injury? Did you yourself experience a loss of creativity?" I asked.

"When I am in really bad shape . . . yes, everything becomes hampered," she said sadly. "I feel less creative about everything: about interactions with children, with friends."

"Do people find when they get better their creativity and hope come back?" I pressed on.

"Yes . . . they do," she mused. "Like any loss, the trauma stays with you on some level even after you get better. But hope, confidence, creativity—yes. When women start to heal, they do start once again to be able to appreciate things on a deeper level." She was silent, thinking. "Hope, creativity, confidence . . . ," she said, almost to herself, as she pondered again. "Their affect *is* much different," she confirmed at last. "They begin to feel like a whole person again, not like damaged goods. Do they seem more excited, more hopeful?" she asked herself again, connecting my questions, which were new to her—as they were new to me—to her clinical experience. "Yes, *definitely,*" she said, after a long pause. "They can have intercourse again. Their confidence comes back. Once they do recover their sense of being intact human beings . . . they do get back a deeper sense of meaning. The things that seemed insignificant before, while they were suffering, can indeed become significant again: good things—the sense of connection to family and friends."

"And that sense of connection to family and friends gets lost or damaged when they are suffering vaginally?" I repeated.

"Yes, it does."

"What I am really teasing out is whether your clinical experience confirms what is right now just an intuition for me, with some science to hint in that direction."

"I definitely think based on my clinical experience that what you are saying is very, very valid," she said. "One treatment for chronic pain is SSRIs [selective serotonin reuptake inhibitors]. Of course your norepinephrine and serotonin are affected by pain. If those chemicals aren't functioning properly—that is bound to affect your mood. Psychologically, chemically—definitely: there is a chemical alteration when there is any kind of vaginal or vulval-region problem; there has to be a chemical alteration in the female brain. Everything is connected; you can have pain there, then you can have peripheral nerve pain, then it can affect central nervous system pain. There is a whole mind-body connection—like a vicious cycle."

"Your brain is connected to your vagina," I restated, glad that she had confirmed, from her much deeper background, the possible link I was investigating.

"It definitely is," she said.

"So let me take a giant leap now," I said. "There are countries where all the women are put into vulvovaginal pain systematically through female genital mutilation, which includes cliterodectomy and infibulation. Would you say from your clinical experience that this would be putting most of these women into a state of permanent lack of affect, anhedonia (low ability to experience pleasure in general), and depression?"

"I don't see how they can't be. There has to be permanent damage to the pelvic nerve. There has to be psychological damage when somebody amputates that part of their body [Fish is using a metaphor; the pelvic nerve would be, rather, severely scarred]: the same things I am seeing, I imagine. Despair and hopelessness."

"It is a reasonable hypothetical?" I asked.

"Oh yeah, it is reasonable."[15]

"If I can show the implications of a brain-vagina link," I mused, "well, it seems to explain so many otherwise weird things that are done to the vagina in history."

The pelvic nerve of the vagina—which I am using interchangeably with "pudendal nerve"—in contrast to the pelvic nerve that terminates in the male prostrate, rectum, and penis, is terribly vulnerable, physically. It can be injured or irritated in childbirth, in episiotomy, and in many other less dramatic ways. The pelvic neural system in women is so delicately exposed to the environment, so lightly shielded by thin vaginal membranes, that in some cases a woman's having merely sat for too long in the wrong position, placing pressure upon it, can injure the female pelvic nerve permanently. Dr. Coady made an important discovery that many women are suffering permanent or severe injuries to their pelvic nerves merely from yoga leg stretches, or from dance classes.

Because of the differences in male and female pelvic anatomy, the female pelvic nerve is of course far easier to attack and injure intentionally than is the male pelvic nerve. You would literally have to pierce a man through the perineum to do the same kind of damage to the male pelvic nerve that a violent rape or sexual injury can do to a woman.

Men would suffer from disruptions of delivery of opiate-type hormones to the brain, if they suffered injuries to their own pelvic nerves, obviously. And such injuries do happen—notably, in prison populations, where, it is well worth noting, violent male rape is widespread and accepted by authorities in a de facto way, and where inmates' passivity is also valued. But these kinds of injuries to men, because of their more defended pelvic anatomy, are far more rare.

Does this insight about how damage to the pelvic nerve affects the female brain completely change our understanding of what rape is? It certainly should. In war, time after time after time, women suffer the insertion into their vaginas of blunt objects, of bottles, of bayonets. Gang rape rips them up at the site of the vagina and where the prostate would be, between vagina and anus—two of the three termini of the female pelvic nerve. In culture after culture, cliterodectomy is also practiced—cutting off and traumatizing the final terminus of the female pelvic nerve.

This has long been misunderstood as a sex crime. It is actually a technique.

### RAPE STAYS IN THE VAGINA

Mike Lousada is the world's nicest former investment banker turned male sexual healer. His mission, as he describes it, is the sexual healing of women, and he is highly trained both as a therapist and as a Tantric practitioner. He has a well-regarded practice in Chalk Farm, London, where he has sexually healed or sexually enhanced the responses of hundreds of women through a combination of Tantric gaze and touch, and orgasmic "yoni massage." (*Yoni* is the Hindi word for "vagina"—it means "sacred space.") Lousada is one of a growing number of practitioners from various disciplines who are certain that the vagina mediates female emotions and thoughts. His success rate has been so consistent that he has begun to address mainstream British and international medical panels of physicians who treat low sexual desire and sexual dysfunction in women, and Dr. Barry Komisaruk, the MRI/female orgasm researcher at Rutgers, has contacted him to study his practice with MRI machines.

Outside a small library at a medieval college, I Skyped with the man whom I was starting to think of as a resident adviser for all things yoni.

I had met Lousada a year earlier, when I had interviewed him for a London newspaper about his yoni massage work, and I wanted to ask him now about his views on what Dr. Richmond had reported to me, and about the questions raised by the recent scientific reports on the effect of rape on the female body. Does sexual trauma stay in the vagina in a physical way, in his experience? He had worked intimately with the vaginas of so many women, many of whom had experienced some kind of sexual trauma. What would he say?

I sat on a low ledge that was part of an ancient wall at the edge of the green in the center of the college. It was early June: heavy pink heirloom roses scented the air, shedding petals along the path to the small stone library. Clusters of pale cherries, not yet ripe, hung from the boughs of a massive tree at the corner of the green. These were not the dark-crimson American cherries I was used to, but Shakespeare's buttery-rosy English cherries—a common metaphor in Elizabethan poetry for lovely cheeks or lips, or for the general deliciousness of women.

I was on my second vagina guru of the day, and it wasn't even lunchtime.

Earlier that morning I had been studying in another library. At the university where I had been working, scores of students had been silently focused on reviewing their Swinburne or Lawrence. While trying to open a document on my laptop, I had inadvertently pressed "play" on an audio file of an interview I'd conducted with Charles Muir, the American Tantric guru. Muir was the man who claimed to have brought awareness of women's internal "sacred spot" to America in the 1970s. Suddenly, in the silence of the library, a Queens-accented, resonant voice had rung out clearly from my computer: "There are *trillions* of cells in one ejaculate. A typical man ejaculates with so much force that . . ." Rows of curious faces had swiveled toward me simultaneously. I'd frantically tried to press "stop," tapping the trackpad over and over, but Muir's confident cadences grew only louder. "And *every* time he ejaculates . . ." Finally I seized my computer and, red-faced, carried Charles Muir's voice at a run out of the double doors.

Now it was Lousada's voice, softer and London-accented, that my computer broadcast, as I asked him whether, in his experience, he had seen any physical markers of sexual trauma in his clients. Dr. Richmond and others had shown how trauma to the vagina can leave a mark on the brain and nervous system. Now I wondered if, in the feedback loop that characterized the brain/vagina connection, memory of trauma might leave a physical imprint on the vagina.

"From my own experience," he said, "that theory makes perfect sense."

Before he went on, though, he cautioned me: "When I am seeing a client for sexual healing, I am seeing them on two levels: physical and spiritual." I assured him that I understood that.

He confirmed that what I wondered about was indeed true: that there were in fact physical differences between women with no experience of sexual violence and those with a history that included rape or sexual abuse. "How could that be?" I asked. "What was the mechanism?" Lousada answered, "The vagina is designed partly for pleasure. Then our life experiences come along. It is as if the tissues of the vagina receive emotion that is poured into them. With more experiences, the emotion becomes compacted, especially if you have had pain. Pain eventually turns into vaginal numbness; which is, actually, desensitization, which is very common."

I asked him to put this process into more basic terms. "When I am doing yoni work, if the vaginal tissues have reached some level of numbness, in order to help my client with her own healing process, I must take her back from numbness, to pain, to emotion, to pleasure." He also spoke about something that he acknowledged was hard to describe: an "energetic disconnect" in the bodies of women with rape or sex abuse in their pasts—their vaginas seemed "energetically" disconnected from the rest of their bodies, even if they were orgasmic. (A male physician, who reviewed for me Lousada's perspective on the "desensitized" vagina, pointed out that while there's no "single cell" of the tissues of the vagina, "rather, there are a multitude of different cells arranged into the various tissues that form the organ as a whole—exactly analogous to the pharynx. Mucus-secreting and highly sensitive cells line the 'cavity,' underlain by the powerful 'constrictor muscles' that are in constant communication with the mucosal surface, the spinal cord, and the brain. Blood flow, cell membrane permeability, fluid and pheromone secretion, and a host of other 'local' biological processes all interact with one another and with the central nervous system. It is no surprise to me that Lousada, with his wealth of experience, should be sensitive to changes in this symphony, to dissonant notes, or to sections of the orchestra that have gone silent.")

I asked Lousada how common a state of relative desensitization of the vagina is in our culture. Very common, he repeated. "For some women, the lightest touch from a feather can be orgasmic. But most women in this culture need a lot of friction-based stimulation, which suggests that there is a loss of sensitivity for them." I reminded him about women's varying neural wiring, but he clarified that this diminution of sensitivity he referred to can take place when there is nothing unusually challenging about a woman's neural wiring. He also said that vaginal sensation in these women improves after the work he does with them (which involves healing-oriented vaginal and vulval massage, often to orgasm, and other practices such as meditation and visualization). Lousada noted that studies have shown that virtually every woman can, theoretically, be orgasmic; because of this, he believes that the relative numbness or desensitization of many of the vaginas that he encounters in his work is the result of a woman's lifetime accumulation of negative experiences, ranging from ridicule of her sexuality in childhood, to sexual abuse itself.

How do these women describe their situation? I wondered. Did they think their somewhat dulled sensations were normal? Or did they show up in his living room describing this desensitization as a problem?

"They don't generally say, 'I don't have a lot of sensation,' " he emphasized. "They may say, 'Do you know what: I've never had an orgasm.' They might say, 'I have vaginismus [painful, involuntary tightening of the vaginal muscles before or during sex].' Or they may often say, 'I just don't enjoy sex.' "

I pushed Lousada to be more specific about the differences he had observed in the emotionally traumatized vagina. "Some lack lubrication," he said. "Some feel physically tight—not 'tight' like before having a baby, but rather, the quality of the tissue itself feels denser and tighter than other women's vaginas. If you massage these women's vaginal walls, there are knots of muscles there, in their vaginas," he repeated. "Vaginismus, in my experience, is almost always the result of sexual trauma."

I struggled to process Lousada's narrative—that many, maybe even most, women in our culture just didn't feel as much, vaginally, as they might, because of awful things that had happened to them emotionally.

I knew from having worked with rape and sexual abuse survivors that many such women had difficulties with even loving, consensual sex they wished to have with caring partners. They found themselves, again and again, up against an implacable, enduring wall between their intentional selves and their own sexual pleasure.

They were in loving, safe, supportive relationships. But they *still* struggled with their bodies' sexual resistance and refusal, which often lasted for years—or even a lifetime. Was this emotional "wall" possibly, for some women, also a physical wall—of tightened or knotted muscle?

If some of these effects of emotional trauma in the vagina were actually physical, and they were left untreated, then of course these life-damaging, relationship-damaging physical aftereffects in the vagina would persist and persist. Asking him to restrict himself to defining *sexual trauma* in the more commonly understood narrower sense, I asked him to estimate the frequency of this phenomenon: loss of vaginal and clitoral sensation due to sex assault, rape, or childhood molestation. "Look," he said sadly. "Twenty-five to thirty-five percent of women have had acknowledged sexual trauma." I knew that several studies confirmed that those numbers were correct. "How they often respond is through loss of sensitivity in the vagina: vaginismus, disconnection, due to the trauma.

"Or else they can go completely the other way: women can become totally orgasmic, though with a history of clear trauma. The attitude is: 'Hey, I'm cool with sex. . . .' But when we really get into yoni work, and I stimulate the vagina, she has one or two orgasms, and then huge bursts of grief or rage come up. So the body is using orgasm to mask the grief and pain."

I still did not get the biological mechanism, beyond the obvious point that we tighten our muscles when we are frightened. How could these effects be so physically long-lasting?

Lousada explained his theory for this, which he said was based on the work of Dr. Stephen Porges. "Porges came up with the scientific basis for the phenomenon," said Lousada. Dr. Porges, who is a professor of psychology and bioengineering at the University of Illinois and director of the Brain-Body Center there, developed a trauma analysis that is widely used called "polyvagal theory." I looked up Dr. Porges's theory.

Dr. Porges's "polyvagal theory" sees a connection between the evolution of the autonomic nervous system and emotional expression, including facial gestures, communication, and social behavior. He argues that through evolution the brain experiences a connection between the nerves that control the heart and the face; this connection links physical feelings with facial expression, voice, and even gesture. His practice teaches therapists to understand how "faulty neuroception" can have an impact on autonomic regulation, and how "the features that trigger different neuroceptive states (safety, danger, and life threat)" can actually be used, as Lousada uses them, within the context of treatment: the therapist's goal is to trigger in the patient's brain the "neuroceptive states of safety." [16]

If Dr. Porges is correct, and his treatment method has a reputable following in the trauma treatment community, it would mean that many of the 17 percent to 23 percent of women who have experienced sexual abuse or assault in their formative years would have the personality reactions that are so common to women in our culture— living in a state of continual anxiety, experiencing an inability to "just be," struggling with various kinds of defendedness and issues of control, with a trapped voice—all of which are states that are not conducive to women experiencing their full sexuality or power.

Briefly, Lousada went on, we have a "triune brain": a reptile brain, the amygdala, to deal with issues of survival; a mammalian, or emotional brain; and a neomammalian brain—the frontal cortex, where sophisticated social functions, among other processes, take place. When we feel threatened, he said, the oldest part of the brain, the amygdala, takes over. Most of us are familiar with "flight or fight," which is one amygdala response to threat. But Porges identified two others: "freeze"—sometimes when prey freezes, it can survive, because a predator might assume it is dead already; and "tend and befriend"— "If I do something to make you like me, you may not kill me."

Lousada adds to this set of responses to trauma one that he calls "the detach response." "If a tiger has his teeth in us, and there is nothing we can do, we go up out of the body into the mind," he said.

This "detach" reaction is well established from research on trauma. I knew from my own work with trauma survivors, especially survivors of childhood sexual abuse, how common that "out of the body" experience is during an assault. Many survivors of sexual assault I had worked with when I volunteered at a rape crisis center had described watching the assault dispassionately, especially if it was an episode of abuse during childhood, from a disembodied state, as if from somewhere else in the room. After a while, the child simply knows how to leave her body if an assault is on its way.

The vagina "freezes," I almost understood him to be saying, as in the common expression "freezes in terror," and the traumatized woman will also "detach" psychologically from "the crime scene"— from that part of her body. "Doctors will tell you then that a symptom like vaginismus is in the body. But it is the brain that tells the body what to do. The brain sends messages to the vagina, saying: 'It is not safe,' " said Lousada. This echoed what Dr. Richmond had said, though in a way more specific to vaginal tension.

"So I work with the client through these stages of trauma. If the traumatized client is detached from her body—she is in her mind— she may have numbness or vaginal tension. We move through that with touch. Then I'll move into working with her pressure points in the vagina. In vaginismus, there can be a spasming. 'Oh f—, that hurts!' a client might feel at that point in the healing. Then there is an energetic pulse that returns. And at that point something unblocks in the vagina. Once they feel safe enough to move from 'freeze' to 'fight or flight' they are likely to be moving also from numbness to pain or masking orgasms, to absolute rage—they may start yelling at that point, or revisit the trauma—but this time with a different outcome. They might shout, this time, 'Get your f—ing hands off me!' Memories may surface. They move into 'flight': sometimes the legs will involuntarily start kicking. Then they move into a social response: eventually they are able to engage with someone in a different way. Eventually intimacy doesn't retraumatize them. Porges says that the traumatized nervous system can profoundly affect relationships. In a fear-based response, people actually experience, for instance, a neutral response as threatening; this has been scientifically demonstrated. So I continue to heal them, through an empathic, gentle, loving touch."

I asked if in his experience a traumatized vagina correlated to a risk of depression for the woman in question.

"Yes," he said, since, in his view, "depression is repressed anger," and "in sexually traumatized women, the fight response has been repressed," which would lead to suppressed rage. He said that about 10 percent of his clients had been or were on medication to treat depression. (For contrast, the Centers for Disease Control reported in 2005–2006 that the percentage of noninstitutionalized people with depression is 5.4 percent.)

"So what happens to them sexually afterward, when they are healed?" I asked. "Do their vaginas actually change?"

"When they are healed, there is definitely a change in that area," he said. "Their vaginas do feel different: less rigid, more responsive. They do become more orgasmic, or they may allow orgasms for the first time. They can experience intimacy in relationships."

I thanked Lousada for his time. We had been talking about so much human grief and pain. But even though we had been discussing incredible sorrow, somehow the world seemed shot through with hope, and with a glimmer of something like illumination, something coming alive with light, like a cloud weighted with late sun.

"In Tantra," he concluded, closing the interview by bringing my attention back to what is a spiritual focus for him in this work, "this is spiritual work: a man can become enlightened just by gazing at the yoni. There are Tantric rituals in which a man gazes at but does not touch the yoni. I've done that ritual many times. And I actually had an experience of seeing the Divine within the vagina—an image came to me of the Virgin Mary." He explained that he had not been raised Catholic, or particularly religious, but that the image had suggested to him an "archetypal mother energy." "In Tantra, the yoni is not just a sacred place, but a 'seat of the divine.' " [17]

The image he described was indeed archetypal. I had a brief but striking memory: the previous morning, Dr. James Willoughby, a research fellow at Oxford University, who was archiving New College Library's ancient treasures, had kindly shown me an extraordinary illuminated volume, an Anglo-Norman version of St. John's *Apocalypse,* which had belonged to British noblewoman Joan de Bohun.[18] It had been created in the fourteenth century. It was worth about a million pounds. It was so lovely it nearly brought tears to my eyes. I could see the follicles of the vellum on the inner binding. Elsewhere, as I later investigated, on several parchment pages, a sacred lamb was framed in what Willoughby had called a "mandorla." Mary is shown also framed, throned in glory. Her cheeks are rosily tinted, her skin white, and her beautifully modeled hands open in compassion. She, too, is often framed in what Dr. Willoughby had called an "almond mandorla." This mandorla, curving around her on either side, and pointed at the top and bottom, had infinitely delicately rendered gradations of rainbow colors.

I had bitten my lip at the time in order not to ask further about the origin of the "almond mandorla," since it was so obviously an archetypal feminine shape. This was the archetypal mother energy, I thought, from which all colors emerge.

I had seen that shape in other works of art, including the double-pointed, double-curved, almond-shaped frames, also painted in rainbow shades, around Buddhist saints in classical Tangkas. The famous image of the sixteenth-century Mexican apparition of Mary,

Our Lady of Guadalupe—which, as two contemporary accounts maintained, manifested to Nahuatl peasant Juan Diego—also shows the Virgin Mother appearing within a similar, but not identical, radiant mandorla shape.

When I looked up the origin of the almond mandorla, I found that it was indeed a vaginal symbol that antedated Christianity—going back to the Pythagoreans—but that it was also used by early Christians. Early depictions of Jesus portrayed him as an infant within the vesica, or mandorla, which represented the womb of Mary. The mandorla also symbolized the coming together of heaven and earth in the form of Jesus—part man, part god. It represents a doorway or portal between worlds. By the Middle Ages, it was part of the church's sacred geometry. Other cultures also adapted the mandorla. In Hindu culture, the yoni is also a mandorla symbol: "the yoni is the gateway, or the zone of interpenetration, wherein two circles intersect." [19]

You can still see this symbol, now placed horizontally, in Piscean form, in stickers on cars of Christians asserting their religious identies; no doubt few realize that it was originally a schematic depiction of the archetypal womb, and related to early depictions of the archetypal divine feminine.

As Lousada and I continued talking, the afternoon had waned. By the time I disconnected from our Skype session, the light was lower, and high white clouds towered over the darker line of the medieval college's chapel roof. They looked like castles upon castles, like the mighty white clouds I had seen, painted with tiny brushes on vellum, through which a sacred lamb—or a beautiful, ancient Mary—had ridden in from heaven, as if explaining heaven to earth, while sheltered in the perfect double inward curves of a rainbow.

# The Vagina Began as Sacred

*At the summit of the world, give birth to the father; my womb is in the midst of the waters, in the ocean. Thence I extend through all the worlds and reach up to yonder sky with my greatness. . . . the Devi's womb (Yoni), sometimes translated as "origin" or "home," is her creative power . . . from this emanates the whole of the universe.*

—Deva Datta Kā Lī, *In Praise of the Goddess: The Devimahatmaya and Its Meaning*

*I*t would take many volumes to account comprehensively for the history of the vagina in the West alone; so this is necessarily an overview, concentrating on dramatic shifts in its cultural meaning and representation.

The vagina began as sacred. There are vagina symbols carved into cave walls in the earliest historic settlements. The earliest artifacts of human prehistory featured vaginas. Figurines such as the Venuses of central Europe, which probably represented fertility, often exhibited exaggerated pudenda. We can't know for certain exactly what these sacred vaginas represented, but feminist historians such as Riane Eisler, in *The Chalice and the Blade,* and others, are sure they represented a primordial state of matriarchy.[1] But the prominence given to representations of the vagina when human beings first made art certainly suggests that female sexuality and fertility were seen as sacred. From 25,000 to 15,000 BCE, "Venus figurines"—fertility images with pronounced vulvas—made of stone or ivory were abundant in Europe, and similar images crafted from the mud of the Nile were common in Egypt. Sir Arthur Evans, who discovered the Minoan civilization at the turn of the twentieth century, pointed out that the multitude of such fertility figurines in so many diverse parts of the world suggested that "The same Great Mother . . . whose worship under various names and titles extended over a large part of Asia Minor and the regions beyond" was "a worldwide fact."[2] As a number of historians, such as Rosalind Miles in *The Women's History of the World*, see it, "From the beginning, as humankind emerged from the darkness of prehistory, God was a woman."[3]

And from the beginning of recorded history, every early culture that has been studied had a version of a sex goddess, from the Sumerian creation epic *Gilgamesh*'s Inanna to the many versions of Ashtaroth worshipped in ancient Mesopotamia, to the sixth-century-BCE Egyptian goddess Astarte who grew out of Ashtaroth worship, and onward to the cultures of classical antiquity, Greece and Rome.

Five thousand years ago in what is now Iraq, Inanna's vulva was worshipped as a sacred site; Sumerian hymns praised the goddess's "lap of honey," compared her vulva to "a boat of heaven," and celebrated the bounty that "pours forth from her womb." The connection of her sexuality to the earth's fertility was so direct that even lettuces were described as the pubic hair of the Goddess.[4] Inanna's vagina was magical, a locus of pure holiness: "Inanna . . . leaned against the apple tree / When she leaned against the apple tree, her vulva was wondrous to behold / Rejoicing at her wondrous vulva, the young woman Inanna applauded herself / She said, I, the Queen of Heaven, shall visit the God of Wisdom. . . ."[5]

The core of the Sumerian religion was a "Sacred Marriage" between the shepherd god Tammuz and Inanna: coins from this era show Inanna spreading her legs wide apart in sacred congress with Tammuz.[6] Women worshippers dedicated vases symbolizing the uterus to Inanna. A sacred text of the period notes that "Once the Holy Inanna had washed / Then was she sprinkled with cedar oil. / The King then proudly approached her sacred lap. / He proudly joined with the glorious triangle of Inanna. / And Tammuz, the bridegroom, lay with her / Tenderly pressing her beautiful breasts!" Inanna's "wondrous vagina" is connected with the search for wisdom. Eventually all the early major Goddess religions included a male consort, with whom the Goddess would copulate in sacred marriage.

Qadesh, a variant on the Astarte archetype, the Egyptian goddess of nature, beauty, and sexual pleasure, was portrayed as a naked woman standing on the back of a lion, adorned with a crescent moon headdress. She was often shown holding snakes or papyrus plants in her right hand, which represented the penis; and in her left hand, lotus flowers, which stood for the vagina. Serpent symbology often accompanied representations of sex goddesses. Minoan goddess figures also depicted the Goddess bare-breasted, holding a snake in each hand. The story of Eve, tempted by the serpent into the original sin of her shameful female sexuality, is a later, Hebraic negative transposition of the sacred symbolism of the Goddess with her serpent.

Throughout the Fertile Crescent, worship of the sex goddess Astarte/Ashtharoth was universal in the period before the rise of the Hebrew patriarchal God. Goddess worship in this period identified Astarte with sexual generation, but also with the wisdom of the cosmos itself. But, as Judaism grew away from its Sumerian antecedents, all aspects of Goddess worship were gradually transformed into negatives, as the younger religion sought to focus its followers on a masculine version of the One God.[7] When the Hebrews developed monotheism, they did so in a context in which the Goddess religions had developed a system of sacred priestesses. At certain points in the calendar, these priestesses would copulate with male worshippers, a practice seen as bringing into the community the order and goodness of the Divine Feminine. Worshippers regarded sacred prostitutes reverentially, and in no way as degraded sex workers. There are many steles that depict these sexual priestesses having what was considered to be sacred intercourse with male worshippers.

The Hebrews' aversion to this form of worship—which again and again tempted the tribes of Israel—their political struggle to compete with such a religion, and the consequent hostility to the tradition of the sacred prostitute, are all evident in the horror with which the Five Books of Moses speak about unconstrained female sexuality, and especially about "harlotry." The Hebrews recast what had been seen as divine unions as abominations.

The worship of the sacred vagina and of female sexuality as metaphors for a larger divinity extended, before the arrival of Christianity, to Europe. In pre-Christian Ireland, and even into the Christian era, stoneworkers carved many Sheela-na-Gig figures on the outer walls of buildings. In these carvings, naked women—representing the "sacred hags" of Celtic mythology, and, as we saw, symbolizing liminality—are portrayed with their legs apart, hands holding open their labia.[8] Some architectural historians believe that even the dimensional, peaked stone folds that form the entrances of medieval European cathedrals incorporate vaginal imagery from this pre-Christian tradition. (Indeed, I was startled once as I wandered about the peaceful, and traditionally sacred, island of Iona, in the Scottish Hebrides, when I looked up onto the outer wall of an ancient nunnery and saw large and elegant labia carved, with nothing else around them, into the convent's stone wall.)

But sex goddesses were not all sweetness and light: in every culture that worshipped the Goddess, though she had a majestic and alluring aspect, she also had another aspect that was dark and potentially destructive. Many cultures have a version of what anthropologists call "the vagina dentata." This means, literally, "the vagina with teeth." In his *Theogony,* for instance, the Greek poet Hesiod described the unborn god Kronos reaching out from his mother's womb to castrate his father, Ouranos. In Hindu mythology, the demon Adi, in the form of the goddess Parvati, has teeth in the vagina. Author Erich Neumann, in his account of Goddess worship, *The Great Mother,* identifies the vagina dentata motif also in North American Indian mythology, in which "a meat-eating fish inhabits the vagina of the Terrible Mother."[9] Inuit myths also describe women with dog heads where the vagina should be. The archetypal and universal association (usually by men) of the vagina with the mouth make the vagina dentata a universal and timeless symbol of male anxiety about engulfment and annihilation by a threatening Mother—so universal that Sigmund Freud would explore this symbol in his *Three Essays on the Theory of Sexuality*.[10] These universal vagina dentata images are not about personal aversion to the human vagina, I believe; rather, they are archetypal images that are a necessary balance to the reverence for women's life-giving powers. They address the inevitable dark side of the Goddess by acknowledging that destruction is the other side of generation, that incarnation—the womb, the birth canal—is a gateway into being, but that incarnation also inevitably leads to death.

## THE VAGINA BECOMES PROFANE

While some of the power and seductiveness associated with the earlier goddesses still appeared in Greek narratives of female Eros and desire, women's subordinated status was complete with the establishment of the first Greek city-states. Some ancient Goddess symbolism survived into the classical period; in Ovid's *Metamorphoses,* for instance, in the story of Cadmus and Arethusa, Arethusa is converted into a serpent—which represents, counterintuitively, the vulva—and the man into a fountain, representing the penis. Another figure who echoes the powerful vagina symbolism in Goddess-worshipping antiquity is that of Baubo, who lifts her skirt to show her vulva, and who makes Demeter—who has lost her daughter, Persephone—laugh once again. Demeter's laughter helps restore fertility to a world threatened with barrenness by her grief.

No historian has conclusively explained how women lost status in the transition from the earliest civilizations to those of classical antiquity. By Plato's time (427–347 BCE), sexual perfection was seen as the union between a man and a boy; Greek wives were strictly for reproduction. Pleasure for women was restricted to the class of *hetairae,* or the courtesan class; wives were well contained behind the walls of private homes and immured in legally subordinated marriage. An exception was the poetess Sappho of Lesbos, who celebrated female eroticism, giving us the first vibrant metaphors in the Western poetic tradition for female arousal and orgasm.

Even the nature of female desire became hypothetical and contested in the classical period. Hippocrates (c. 460–c. 370 BCE) believed that both women and men needed to climax—both "bursting forth seed"—in order for conception to occur, but Aristotle (384–322 BCE) noted, in contrast, that women did not need to be aroused in order to conceive.

The Roman physician Galen (129–c. 200 CE) believed that the vagina was an inside-out penis: as Thomas Laqueur expresses the Galenic paradigm, "Women . . . are inverted, and hence less perfect, men. They have exactly the same organs but in exactly the wrong places."[11] Galen's influence extended for centuries after he was rediscovered in the Middle Ages. (He also recommended that single women masturbate for the sake of their health.) The Greeks maintained a concept of the floating uterus—they believed that the uterus traveled throughout a woman's body, and they developed the notion that women's nervous aspect and other diseases were caused by these agitations of the uterus, a belief the Romans adopted (the root of the term *hysteria—hyster—*comes from the Greek word for "womb").

## THE JUDEO-CHRISTIAN VAGINA:
### THE EVOLUTION OF SHAME

*Woman is defective and misbegotten.*

—Thomas Aquinas, *Summa Theologica*

While the Hebrew Bible was intent on condemning the "harlotry" of the sacred prostitutes of the polytheistic religions that dominated in the Fertile Crescent, as we saw, it almost never mentions the vagina directly, except euphemistically. But it does contain passages that eloquently express female sexual desire. The Song of Songs contains many subtle metaphors for female arousal and orgasm. The Hebrew tradition had not promoted a mind-body split, and sex was still sacred within the confines of marriage: rabbinical exigesis in the post-Exilic period insisted that a devout man must satisfy his wife sexually at least weekly, depending on his profession.

But Paul, a Hellenized Jew, introduced to the first-century-CE Jewish-Christian and pagan-Christian communities around the Mediterranean the Hellenic concept that the mind and the body are at war with each other. His letters codified the notion—so influential in the next two millennia—that sexuality is shameful and wrong, and that unbridled female sexuality, even within marriage, is particularly shameful and wrong. With the rise of the church in Europe and the spread of the Holy Roman Empire, Paul's teachings become synonymous with Christianity, and Christianity, with Western culture itself.

## THE CHURCH FATHERS:
## THE HATEFUL VAGINA

The rise of a Western ideology that cast the vagina as being especially hateful, and that portrayed female sexuality in general as a toxic lure to perdition, reached its formative point with Paul then with the Church Fathers of the subsequent four centuries. The Hebrew Bible certainly excoriates female sexuality that circumvents the boundaries of marriage—you can stone your daughter to death for fornication, for instance—but it also has harsh words condemning male infidelity and excess. Within marriage, both male and female sexuality are seen as blessings. The vagina is addressed, in Leviticus and in the Mishnah, in terms of menstrual uncleanness: women must abstain from sex, take ritual baths, and, the Mishnah maintains, use "testing-rags" in the "depressions and folds" of the vagina to ensure they are free of blood after the menses, and before sex.[12,13]

But the vagina that is hateful even within marriage, and the ideal of female virginity as a sexual status, arose only in the four post-Pauline centuries, especially around North Africa. The Church Fathers, who were practicing very extreme forms of asceticism in all-male environments and abasing the flesh in various ways, sought to outdo one another in reviling the flesh of women as sexual beings in particular. Paul had written, "It is good for a man not to touch a woman . . . [I]f they have not constancy, let them marry, for it is better to marry than to burn" (1 Corinthians 7:9). But Tertullian took this Pauline idea much further: now, intercourse was only for the begetting of children; and he cast women as seductresses luring men into a Satanic abyss of sexuality.[14] To him the vagina was "a temple built over a sewer," "the Devil's gateway": "And do you know that you are [each] an Eve? The sentence of God on this sex of yours lives in this age: the guilt must of necessity live too. *You* are the devil's gateway; *you* are the unsealer of that [forbidden] tree: you are the first deserter of the Divine law . . . on account of *your* desert—that is, death—even the Son of Man had to die. And do you think about adorning yourself?"[15]

The imprint of the equation of a female "virgin" with someone who is "good" and "pure" is so deep we scarcely think about whether those terms have any actual relationship; we assume the equation is an ancient notion, but the idea of the "pure" Christian virgin is fairly recent. Biblical scholars generally agree that the ideology of Mary's sacred virginity was a much belated construct of the Church, and that it cannot be confirmed in the original texts of the New Testament, which suggest that Mary had several children. The complex creed about Mary's virginity that we inherit was accepted, indeed, only five centuries after the events described or narrated in the New Testament—officially only in 451 CE, at the Council of Chalcedon.[16]

Little evidence survives of how the vagina was portrayed or understood in the Dark Ages, and the little there is comes from medical texts. In spite of the Church Fathers, for the first fifteen hundred years CE, Western women were still seen as needing sexual satisfaction if reproduction was to take place. Sexual frustration in women was understood for a millennium and a half as causing disease and mental suffering; in Hippocrates' era, doctors used genital massage on their female patients, or tasked a midwife with the therapy. The practice of prescribing medicinal genital massage to orgasm, as a remedy for "hysteria," lasted until the Tudor and Stuart periods in England.

As noted earlier, Galen, whose influence resurfaced in the Middle Ages, had developed a model of the female genitals' being an outside-in version of the male. The ancient Greeks had also maintained that women ejected semen, which contributed to conception. Since the uterus was understood to migrate around the body, women who had no sexual outlet were seen as being at risk of suffering from the unexpelled semen in their wombs corrupting their bodies, and sending "filthy vapors to the brain." [17]

Well into the Middle Ages, informal affection alternated with official condemnation of the vagina. A fair amount of folklore and bawdry in the late Middle Ages treat the vagina with a kind of colloquial affection—as in the play on the word *queynte* in Geoffrey Chaucer's "The Wife of Bath's Tale" and "The Miller's Tale" in *The Canterbury Tales,* which dates to the end of the fourteenth century. In "The Miller's Tale," at line 90, we read, "Pryvely he caughte hire by the queynte." [18] (In 1380, *queynte* was pronounced "cunt.") In *The Canterbury Tales,* Chaucer uses the word *cunt* not as an obscenity, but as it was used commonly in that era—in a simply lusty, descriptive manner.

This era, in spite of ideals of courtly love, also saw the beginnings of practices aimed at harming or constraining the vagina in new ways. The chastity belt, for instance, was invented in the early Middle Ages. Its use continued into the high Middle Ages. These were not delicate garments, but actual body locks made of metal. The device surrounded the wearer's hips with two iron bands, and a third iron band went between her legs. That band was closed with a lock. A woman's husband, if he wished to travel or was departing for a war, would literally lock up his wife's vagina, and take the key with him. The device did not simply prevent intercourse; it also made hygiene difficult, caused severe abrasions, and is best seen as a domestic instrument of torture.

In the fourteenth and fifteenth centuries, the "witch craze" swept through Europe. Its effect was to target female sexuality in multiple and terrifying new ways. In community after community, the women identified by inquisitors or by their fellow villagers as "witches" were often those who were seen as too sexual, or too free. And forms of torture focused on their sexuality. The "Pear of Anguish" was a torture device used on victims of all genders. It was a pear-shaped object made of iron that expanded inside the victim as the torturer turned screws. When it was inflicted on men, it was introduced into the mouth. But when it was used on women accused of witchcraft, or of inducing abortion, it was inserted into the vagina and expanded. During the witch craze in Europe in the fifteenth through seventeenth centuries, women's vaginas were targeted in searches for the "witches' mark" or "devil's mark" sought in their body cavities. Inquisitors also had suspected heretical women's vaginas mutilated.[19]

The Renaissance period in Europe saw the rise of the study of anatomy and, once again, the rediscovery of the clitoris. In this period, women were seen as sexually inexhaustible, and female sexuality was viewed as more overpowering than male sexual response—it was still taken for granted that women had to reach orgasm in order to conceive.

Dr. Emma Rees, a British literary scholar at the University of Chester who has written about the vagina in Elizabethan and Victorian literature, argues that Elizabethans intentionally elided the meanings of "lips" and "labia." She shows the similarities between two technologies of control from that era—chastity belts and "scold's bridles"—and she argues that Elizabethan audiences saw verbal and sexual license in women in similar ways. The chastity belt rigidly locked around the female pudenda, she argues, forcing a woman to be sexually inactive or "silent"; and, in the same way, the "scold's bridle" was a similarly constructed device, made of iron and leather, that locked around a talkative or argumentative woman's head, and gagged her mouth.[20]

Shakespeare, ever the neologist, innovated dozens of slang terms for the vagina, from "blackness" in *Othello* to "boat" in *King Lear*. Dr. Rees looks at all the vaginas in Shakespeare: she cites, for instance, the "detested, dark, blood-drinking pit" of *Titus Andronicus*. In this play, the heroine, Lavinia, is raped, and her rapists cut out her tongue. Dr. Rees argues that in this mutilation images of lips and labia collide: Lavinia's mouth and vagina are both assaulted in repeated acts of silencing and control.[21]

The idea of the female body as topography, and the vagina as either a sulfurous pit in that landscape, or else a bucolic spring, also became a standard part of Renaissance rhetoric. For a more pleasing version of the vagina/landscape analogy, see Shakespeare's "Venus and Adonis," as Venus offers herself to Adonis:

> *I'll be a park, and thou shalt be my deer.*
> *Feed where thou wilt, on mountain or in dale;*
> *Graze on my lips, and if those hills be dry,*
> *Stray lower, where the pleasant fountains lie.*[22]

With *King Lear*, Dr. Rees interprets Cordelia's resistance to doing as her father insists, in the context of the Elizabethan word *nothing* as slang for the vagina. Dr. Rees's theory is that, in Shakespeare, the vagina is often punned upon and used as a metaphor for the "otherness" of femininity, the unruliness of female sexuality, and the "diseased" and "contaminating" natures of both the female body and female speech, as they were understood at the time.

> CORDELIA: *What shall Cordelia speak? Love, and be silent.*
> (Aside) . . . *Nothing, my lord.*
> LEAR: *Nothing?*
> CORDELIA: *Nothing.*
> LEAR: *How, nothing will come of nothing. Speak again.*
> CORDELIA: *Unhappy that I am, I cannot heave my heart into*
> *my mouth. I love your majesty according to my bond, no more*
> *nor less.*[23]

"The vagina," Dr. Rees writes, "is emblematic of the chaos, of the 'can't' "—this is a Midlands pronunciation of *cunt;* Dr. Rees is punning—"that gapes at the play's heart." She writes, *"Nothing* is forced to take on the form of *something* through Lear's insistence upon it and his fascination with it prior to his agonies on the heath: 'nothing can be made out of nothing' (I.iv.130). But what remains the play's preoccupation is the fact that something *can* be made of nothing: if the vagina is the cipher, the absence, then what about when it brings forth a child? . . . When the Fool tells Lear that 'thou art an O without a figure' (I.iv.183–84), the 'O' could be read as emblematic of the vagina, and may suggest the increasing sense of emasculation Lear experiences."[24] Lear's emasculation, she writes, led to his curse of one of his two daughters' organs of reproduction:

> *Into her womb convey sterility,*
> *Dry up in her the organs of increase,*
> *And from her derogate [degenerate] body never spring*
> *A babe to honour her.* (I.iv. 270–73)

In this speech, the vagina and hell become one place: "Beneath is all the fiend's / There's hell, there's darkness . . . stench. . . ."

> *Behold yon simp'ring dame,*
> *Whose face between her forks presages snow,*
> *That minces virtue and does shake the head*
> *To hear of pleasure's name.* [IV.vi.116–19] . . .
> *Down from the waist they are centaurs, though women all above.*
> *But to the girdle do the gods inherit, beneath is all the fiend's:*
> *there's hell, there's darkness, there is the sulphurous pit, burn-*
>    *ing, scalding, stench, consumption!*
> *Fie, fie, fie! Pah, pah! Give me an ounce of civet, good apothecary*
>    *to sweeten my imagination.*[25]

The special ability of the vagina to serve as a cultural Rorschach— reflecting others' attractions to it and anxieties about it that were often contradictory—debuted with the early modern period. The ability of the vagina to signify heaven, hell, and "nothing" at all—the presumed female existential absence—was established in the West around this time.

In *King Lear,* the tropes around the vagina reveal that by the Elizabethan period, the Pauline Christian perspective on the hideousness and hellishness of the female sex organ and female sexuality were strongly embedded in the culture, just as other lyricists' work shows that at the same time, another stream of more classical references identified the same organ with pastoral delight and natural charm. "The symbolic power of the vagina is fundamental to understanding not only Shakespeare's but also Renaissance concerns more widely," writes Dr. Rees. By Shakespeare's time, *cunt* and *twat* were both considered obscene; which led the playwrights of the time to use punning and allusion to communicate their meanings directly enough—yet seemingly indirectly. In this punning passage from act 3, scene 2 of *Hamlet,* the subtext is Ophelia's vagina. Dr. Rees points out that "In Elizabethan English, the word lap could mean 'lap' as we now use the word, or it could mean, codedly, 'vagina.' And remember, 'nothing' also was understood at the time to mean 'vagina.' "

HAMLET: *Lady, shall I lie in your lap?* [Lying down at
   Ophelia's feet.]
OPHELIA: *No, my lord.*
HAMLET: *I mean, my head upon your lap?*
OPHELIA: *Ay, my lord.*
HAMLET: *Do you think I meant country matters?*
OPHELIA: *I think nothing, my lord.*
HAMLET: *That's a fair thought to lie between maids' legs.*
OPHELIA: *What is, my lord?*
HAMLET: *Nothing.*
OPHELIA: *You are merry, my lord.*
HAMLET: *Who, I?*
OPHELIA: *Ay, my lord.*[26]

"Country matters" meant, to an Elizabethan audience, sexual, that is, animal matters. When Hamlet asks Ophelia what she is thinking and she replies, "Nothing"—meaning that she is actually not thinking about anything, that she is intellectually submissive or neutral—Hamlet responds, tellingly, "That's a fair thought to lie between a maiden's legs." The pudenda—the "nothing"—is attractive in itself, but it is also attractive when there is neither a thought in the female brain nor experience in, or wisdom in, the female pudenda. When Ophelia replies, "What is, my lord?"—that is, what is a fair thought to lie between a maiden's legs? what is an appropriate way to be sexually female?—and when Hamlet replies, "Nothing," he is saying that a vagina—implicitly, an inexperienced or untried or ignorant vagina—is the right thing, an attractive thing, to find between a maiden's (virgin's) legs. Shakespeare has brilliantly managed a double mirroring of the connection between the female brain and the vagina, and he's reflected the Elizabethan understanding of the connections between the two—playing with his underscoring of the culturally understood fact that nothing is more attractive than "nothing" on the mind of a young women and that "nothing" in terms of sexual experience was the right evidence to find in the "nothing," the vagina, that lies between young or virginal women's legs. Ophelia's seeming ignorance of the double meanings of all the wordplay just heightens the culturally understood message about the attractiveness of sexual and intellectual ignorance in women "at both ends."

To King Lear, the vagina was a sulfurous pit; to Poet John Donne, who also used a subterranean metaphor, it was a blessed, and blessing, New World natural treasury, a "mine of precious stones": at a time of great discovery of new landscapes and valuable minerals and gems overseas, Donne, in his poem "Elegy XIX: To His Mistress Going to Bed," compares his beloved's lower body, and her vagina, to the treasures of a newly discovered empire:

> *License my roving hands, and let them go*
> *Before, behind, between, above, below.*
> *O my America, my new found land,*
> *My kingdom, safeliest when with one man mann'd,*
> *My mine of precious stones, my empery,*

*How blest am I in this discovering thee!*
*To enter in these bonds, is to be free;*
*Then where my hand is set, my seal shall be.*[27]

The sexual meaning of the vagina as a "kingdom, safeliest when with one man mann'd" is clear. "Then where my hand is set, my seal shall be" is another very tender metaphorization of the vagina: though it is true that the female body is conquered, as new lands at the time were being conquered and consecrated to England or Spain with the phallic planting of imperial banners, nonetheless the conquest in this case is celebratory and loving. The poet is caressing his lover's vagina with his hand, and if you understand what "my seal" meant to an Elizabethan reader—a signet ring at the time would be pressed into wax, to create a personal mark—Donne's erotic regard for the vagina is overt. Though Donne is claiming the vagina as "his" by metaphorically impressing a "seal" against it, it is also true that wax must be gently warmed and melted to receive and retain the impress of the signet ring.

This tension about whether the vagina was heaven or hell was reflected in the fact that, just as anatomy began to be firmly established as a Renaissance discipline, so the clitoris as an organ began a centuries-long process—which historian Thomas Laqueur identified, and which I referenced in my book *Promiscuities: The Secret Struggle for Womanhood*—of being lost and found and lost and found by anatomists. The cultural history of Western anatomy does not reveal any parallel continual misplacement and "forgetting" of the location, role, or function of other organs on the human body. The pancreas, let alone the scrotum, once identified on the body and their function once understood, *remain* located and understood—indeed the understanding of other organs' functions has only improved over the past four centuries, while the understanding of the role of the clitoris continually reeffaces and redegrades.

This "Where did it go?" "What was it for again?" intellectual journey regarding the clitoris should also reflect to us Western culture's ambivalence about the role of the clitoris not just as a trigger to female sexual excitement, but as the gateway or catalyst to female courage and confidence. Ambivalence about identifying, once and for all, the clitoris—where it is and how it works—can surely, we now see, given the brain-vagina connection, reflect ambivalence about handing to women, once and for all, the keys to the kingdom of personal assertiveness, and of the desire for freedom.

The clitoris has been discovered, "lost," and rediscovered consistently since 1559. That year, Renaldus Columbus identified the site he called "preeminently the seat of women's delight." "If you touch it," he noted, "you will find it rendered a little harder and oblong to such a degree that it shows itself as a sort of male member [. . .] since no one has discerned these projections and their workings, if it is permissible to give names to things discovered by me, it should be called the love or sweetness of Venus." He added that "if you rub it vigorously with a penis, or touch it even with a little finger, semen swifter than air flies this way and that on account of the pleasure [. . .] without these protuberances, women would neither experience delight in venereal embraces nor conceive any fetuses." In 1671, midwife Jane Sharp identified it yet again, noting that it "will stand and fall as the yard [penis] doth and makes women lustful and take delight in copulation."[28] *The Anatomy of Humane Bodies,* a medical textbook written by William Cowper in 1697, showed it for the first time as a distinct organ. And Laqueur cites another seventeenth-century textbook, this one French, which points out that the clitoris is "where the Author of Nature has placed the seat of voluptuousness—as He has in the glans penis—where the most exquisite sensibility is located, and where he placed the origins of lasciviousness in women."[29]

But these "forgettings" and rediscoveries merely foreshadow the greatest "forgetting" yet, which lay still ahead.

# The Victorian Vagina:
# Medicalization and Subjugation

*The state of arousal, which had occurred very frequently...*
*leased entirely after the surgery... on January 6, 1865, the*
*wound was totally healed, the condition of the patient good...*
*nor was she troubled by sexual excitement.*

—Gynecologist Gustav Braun, "The Amputation of the Clitoris and
Labia Minora: A Contribution to the Treatment of Vaginismus," 1865

The "modern" Western conception of the vagina, the one we
inherit today—shamed, sexualized in a narrow and functional way, desacralized and scientifically scrutinized—developed
in the nineteenth century. As Michel Foucault points out in *The
History of Sexuality*, this was the century of medicalized control of
sexuality in general.[1] The vagina was medicalized and controlled
in highly specific ways in this era that were unprecedented at the
time, but that have endured since—and that descend to us, often
intact.

As industrialization and increased education created an expanding class of increasingly restless and enfranchised women, new
sources of sexual subjugation worked to repress those women.
Growing cultural forces sought to keep women ignorant of their

anatomy and sexual responses and to develop a state of sexual "passionlessness." Many new sources generated these repressive pressures: newspaper commentators, doctors' manuals, marriage guides, and the rise of gynecology as a medical specialization.

This era saw the dissemination of the theory that the clitoris was a cause of moral turpitude, that reading novels could drive young girls wild with unconstrained desire, and that "good" women had no sexual (especially clitoral) feelings whatsoever, but that "bad" women could be ruined by their sexual appetites.[2] Paradoxically, this period also saw the explosion of treatments that let women have orgasms without losing social standing, because they did so at the hands of physicians. Some doctors simply advertised "uterine massage" for nervous conditions—and made fortunes masturbating their high-status, ladylike female clients on their treatment couches. Some doctors, no doubt exhausted from the demand, even developed electrical masturbation machines to bring about female "nervous release." Many kinds of electric dildos were developed at this time, too, all advertised for euphemistic purposes.[3]

The deeply ingrained idea that we inherit "good" and "bad" vaginas—the former, that will be protected by society and the state, and the latter, fair game for punishment and violence—descends from this moment. It was in this period that our uniquely modern anxiety—that "good," or respectable, vagina, which through its respectability lays claim to some social protection, not "degrade" itself through our own wantonness, inviting all the punishments that accrue to "bad" vaginas—became codified. By the mid-Victorian period, medical discourses about "respectable" women's vaginas, and pornography or punitive legislation aimed at "bad" women's vaginas, were virtually the only two discourses in which the vagina appeared in public or private commentary at all.

I cannot stress enough how many of our current anxieties about the vagina and about female sexual pleasure were introduced to society at this time and descend to us even now in forms recognizably dating to this period.

Until the mid-nineteenth century, women's devilishness—or, less judgmentally, their lust—was seen as integrated in women, if not as laudable. That unified, if not especially admiring, view of female sexuality changed for good by about 1857, and it was a dramatic change. Before 1857, the year of the first Obscene Publications Act in Britain, a wave of erotic lithographs, as well as slang and bawdry, treated the vagina in ways that descended from the raunchy but amused tradition of depicting the vagina—the lustful, active vagina—in such eighteenth-century erotic classics as John Cleland's 1748 *Fanny Hill*. But the Victorian era created our duality: a medicalized "good" woman's vagina, and a harlotized, pornographic "bad" woman's vagina. The Victorian ideologues of gender rejected the bawdy, sometimes adoring, more integrated middle ground in relation to the vagina and clitoris that the previous century had taken for granted. The new discipline of gynecology recast female masturbation, which had to that point been scarcely noticed and hardly commented upon, as an obsessed-over sinkhole of shame and degradation, and also recast female sexual pleasure in intercourse, which to that point had been taken for granted, if sometimes inveighed against, as a chimera, a blazing stigma, or a degrading grotesquerie.

It may also have been an unconscious cultural expression of an innate recognition of the dopamine-vagina-brain connection: in this period, middle-class women were successfully pushing for greater access to rights and influence of all kinds. They lobbied for the right to divorce from abusive husbands (the Married Women's Property Act, 1857); opposed the rounding up of women accused of prostitution, who were then forced into brutal pelvic exams (the Contagious Diseases Acts of 1864, 1866, 1869); fought for greater control over their own earnings and inheritances in marriage (the Married Women's Property Act, 1870); and sought the right to leave a marriage with their own property and retain custody of their own children (the Married Women's Property Act, 1882). By the end of the century, they were establishing women's colleges at Oxford and Cambridge and fighting to get into the professions. Given the dopamine-vagina-brain nexus, it is not unreasonable in retrospect to understand that an ideology would arise—however subconsciously—

that would increasingly rigorously keep these same newly educated, middle-class Western women, who were seeking and gaining so many new rights, from understanding how their own vaginas even worked, and that would indeed punish them in many ways for even considering touching their vaginas and clitorises in ways that would activate more unruly dopamine.

By the 1850s, Victorian medical and social commentators were asserting that masturbation for both sexes led dangerously to "a spectrum of physically horrible diseases" that finally brought the self-abuser to a state of madness. But the preoccupation with the dangers of female masturbation led to violence. The Victorian obsession with stamping out female masturbation was often tied to fears about women's education, and often connected to images of girls or women seduced by reading. (The seventeenth and eighteenth centuries had virtually no such preoccupation with a potential link between female reading and female masturbation.) In the pre-Victorian world in which even elite women were generally uneducated and propertyless, it really didn't matter much to anyone if they masturbated. This nineteenth-century obsession with the dangers of female masturbation, which emerged in a century in which women secured legislative victory after legislative victory involving access to rights, must be understood as a reaction against the dangers of female emancipation from the patriarchal home.

Gynecologist William Acton asserted, in his influential 1875 treatise, *Functions and Disorders of the Reproductive Organs,* that "masturbation may be best described as an habitual incontinence eminently productive of disease." He noted, though, that "the majority of women (happily for them) are not very much troubled with sexual feeling of any kind." Acton also believed that "As a general rule a modest woman seldom desires any sexual gratification for herself. She submits to her husband's embraces, but principally to gratify him . . . the married woman has no wish to be placed on the footing of a mistress."[4]

Many women today feel that their sexuality is something distinct from the rest of their character and is cut off in some ways from their other, more admirable roles as mothers, wives, or workers; some feel inhibited in bed by the sense that their sexual pleasure in some way demeans them. This set of beliefs is not a human constant—it is not even very old; it was essentially invented when cultural critics in Europe and America were alarmed by female enfranchisement, and female sexuality was assigned to a new profession, the male gynecologists. It was codified thoroughly for the first time about a hundred and sixty years ago. We are not stuck with this dualism.

The Victorian period saw a wholesale shift in how women's vaginas and clitorises were dealt with medically. This shift transferred a middle-class woman's sexual and reproductive health from the hands of midwives to those of male doctors. These doctors formed professional organizations in order to marginalize midwives. The midwives' approach to sexuality and birth had been to advise, and to support natural processes; the male doctors' model of dealing with the vagina and uterus was, rather, one of "heroic medicine," or impatient, sometimes violent, intervention.

In America, Ephraim McDowell, W. H. Byford, and J. Marion Sims also expanded the limits of the new male-dominated profession of gynecology. Sims perfected a technique for the repair of vesicovaginal fistulas; but his ambiguous legacy is that he did so by practicing on enslaved women—without the use of any kind of anesthesia. Meanwhile, in the United Kingdom, Robert Lawson Tait and William Tyler Smith pioneered British male-dominated gynecology. This male domination of a field of medical care that for millennia had been in the hands of female midwives was not challenged until the late 1890s when one of the first women gynecologists, Helen Putnam, began practicing in Providence, Rhode Island. In two generations, British and American male gynecologists transformed the ancient and characteristically gentle practice of midwifery. They introduced such innovations as reclining births, which were more comfortable for the doctor than the midwife's more active positioning of herself and her patient had been (reclining births require the baby to move against the force of gravity *up* the birth canal, a maternal posture in childbirth unknown outside the medicalized West), but that are far more damaging to women's perineums and birth canals. This positioning, which we damagingly inherit, ushered in an era of new kinds of gynecological injury among middle-class women who could afford doctors in childbirth. Victorian male gynecologists also established the convention of performing pelvic exams behind a veil or covering; it was forbidden to physicians to actually visually observe the vagina or cervix, and they had to manage their diagnoses by touch alone. Finally, a new discourse of medically authorized judgment and shame elaborated itself around this highly contested site, the vagina. William Acton's treatise promoting female passionlessness went through eight editions in twenty years; historian Carl Degler called it "undoubtedly one of the most widely quoted books" on female sexual issues "in the English-speaking world."[5]

As the nineteenth century progressed, more and more public discussion about women's role cast them as being mediated completely by their reproductive systems. Women's uteruses were increasingly viewed as negatively affecting their owners' moods, and their brainpower in general; women's monthly periods were presented, by gynecologists writing in popular journals, as being the reason that higher education would debilitate young women. By the 1890s, female education, in turn, was cast as affecting women's sexual nervous system, rendering "New Women" who insisted on a masculine education, infertile, in the views of some "experts," or sexually insatiable, in the words of others, and in either case, hairy and unmarriageable.

"Although the idea of separate spheres was not new to the nineteenth century," historians Ema Olafson Hellerstein, Leslie Parker Hume, and Karen M. Offen write, in *Victorian Women: A Documentary Account of Women's Lives in Nineteenth-Century England, France, and the United States,* "the obsessive manner in which [French, U.S., and British] cultures insisted on this separation seemed particularly novel. . . . [A]ny woman who, however tangentially, rejected the role that Victorian culture thrust on her, seemed as noxious and threatening to her contemporaries as the political revolutionary or the social anarchist."[6] Female sexuality, they argue, was seen as a threat as profound to a stable, ordered society as was terrorism or anarchism: "Just as Victorian society wanted to give a young woman educational experience but not the experience of being an educated person, so it wanted her to have (on the permitted marital basis and for reproductive purposes) sexual experience but not the experience of being a sexual person."[7]

From the 1860s to the 1890s, the brutality and punitive nature of masculine gynecological practices reached an apex. In this period, the use of cliterodectomy became, if not widespread, not unheard of, in "treating" girls who persisted in that dreaded vice, feminine masturbation. Dr. Isaac Baker Brown introduced cliterodectomy to England in 1858, and it was much practiced by him for ten years after that.[8] Dr. Brown became famous and sought after for his "cure," which took argumentative, fiery girls, and, after he had excised their clitorises, returned them to their families in a state of docility, meekness, and obedience—a result that we can now understand was doubtless the result of trauma, and also of interrupted neural activation.

And even for girls who were not threatened with actual excision of their clitorises as punishment for "the solitary vice," guidebooks, moral manuals, and even popular journals were filled with warnings about how a female masturbator, lured by "French novels" or "sensation novels," could be identified easily from her lassitude, listlessness, pallor, feverish eyes, and general air of furtiveness and dissatisfaction. It was understood that masturbation led girls on the downward path to other, even worse forms of "viciousness" and moral laxity; parents were advised to be vigilant and severe with those girls who persisted.

Jeffrey Moussaieff Masson examined three hundred European medical journals from 1865 to 1900: "These readings," he wrote, "all from standard, reputable professional journals—illustrate how men in positions of power over women's lives, especially their sexual lives, misused that power to warp, damage, inhibit, and even destroy women's sexual . . . selves."[9]

Women's ignorance of their own anatomy, coupled with the intense stigma surrounding female sexuality, often led to horrific outcomes. One French doctor, Démétrius Alexandre Zambaco, had a young female patient who, he believed, engaged in a "vice"—masturbation—which, he observed, "became more and more deeply rooted." He reported that he felt it "necessary to change tactics and treat her severely, even with the most cruel brutality. Corporal punishment was resorted to, in particular the whip."[10] Alfred Poulet, the surgeon-major of Val-de-Grâce Hospital in Paris, published, in 1880, the second volume of his *Treatise on Foreign Bodies in Surgical Practice*. In it, he listed the objects that he had removed from the vaginas of young women in his care, and he included in his report similar cases that had been written up in England and America. Poulet noted that he had had to remove from the uteruses, urethras, and vaginas of his patients, objects ranging from "spools of thread, needle-cases, boxes of pomade, hair-pins and hairbrushes and . . . objects like pessaries and sponges." He believed that "malice" and "insanity" addicted women to "the solitary vice," and led these women to masturbate with these objects.

Poulet tells an appalling story: a twenty-eight-year-old woman was masturbating with the handle of a cedarwood hairbrush. When someone came into the room suddenly, she quickly jumped up and seated herself in order to conceal what she had been doing, and the hairbrush—brace yourself—"was suddenly pushed through the posterior wall of the vagina into the peritoneal cavity." She was so ashamed, because a "modest woman" in the terms of Victorian medical discourse would never masturbate, that she kept her injury concealed for eight months, though the stick of wood had by then penetrated her intestines. Finally, when presumably the pain was too much to bear, she saw her doctor and confessed; the brush was removed, but she died of peritonitis four days later.

Poulet argues that nine out of ten of the perforations he dealt with, caused by sharp objects in the vagina, were introduced by the patient's masturbation. But contemporary scholars think that this is unlikely, and that in fact the many accounts from the period that seem bizarre to us, of women being injured by sharp objects in the vagina, resulted from their efforts to self-abort. In *Nymphomania: A History*, Carol Groneman claims that "the physical evidence . . .

might have led to multiple explanations, including sexual abuse or attempted abortion. Instead, many physicians saw these women as temptresses, not victims." Groneman points out that doctors see what they choose to see, and that Poulet saw "willfulness . . . vicious habits" and "lewd practices" leading to these injuries, not victimization or desperation, as "little distinction" in the medical profession at the time, Groneman notes, "was drawn between abuse, abortion, and masturbation."[11]

According to Yale University historian Dr. Cynthia Russett, uterine prolapse was extremely common throughout the nineteenth century because of the demands of fashion. From about 1840 to 1910, elegant women wore tightly laced whalebone corsets. Russett makes the case that corsets or girdles, in our experience, are made of elastic or rubber; but whalebone does not easily bend. These corsets—as you can visualize—constricted the waist, and in doing so they also forced the other abdominal and pelvic organs (small intestine, uterus, bladder) sharply downward, and exerted continual pressure upon them. Women were expected to lace tightly and keep their waists even when heavily pregnant, which of course forced the distended uterus downward as well, putting even more terrible pressure on the pelvic floor. Pessaries were round metal objects like diaphragms, which women suffering from prolapse introduced into their vaginas to take the place of the damaged pelvic floor and to mechanically prevent the uterus and other organs from collapsing into the vaginal canal. In their journalism, books, and poetry, many women writers made impassioned pleas for change in fashions, so that women's lives not be "deformed"—a frequently used term—into artificial models of propriety. They were talking about a physical as well as a psychological reality—a fashion that regularly led to the destruction of the integrity of the uterus and pelvic floor.

This epidemic of vaginal and uterine injury, and the invalidism it led to, was the background against which the great Victorian women novelists and poets—from the Brontës, to George Eliot, Elizabeth Gaskell, and Elizabeth Barrett Browning—fantasized about women's physical and emotional freedom.

## THE STATE VS. THE "BAD" VAGINA

In 1857, the first Contagious Diseases Act was passed in England, and it was expanded in 1864. This gave the state the power to round up any woman suspected of being a prostitute, and to forcibly incarcerate her in an institution in which she was compelled to submit to a vaginal and pelvic exam against her will—ostensibly to prevent the spread of syphilis, gonorrhea, and other venereal diseases.

The legacies of the Contagious Diseases Acts are much more influential in women's collective consciousness than histories usually suggest. All over England, especially in garrison towns, women who looked as if they might be prostitutes—a job category so loosely defined in the Victorian period that it described almost any woman who took care with her appearance, or looked or behaved as if she could be sexually active outside of marriage—could be seized by male agents acting undercover. Effectively kidnapped, they could then be held without due process in institutions much like prisons, called "lock hospitals." There, they were restrained and forcibly medically examined—by male strangers. They were then medically treated against their will. These women could be held—legally—for up to eight months and kept away from families and employment.[12]

The British government planned to expand this program of the arrest and detention of young women who looked as if they might have ever been sexually active. It was to expand city by city and reach London. As British historian A. N. Wilson points out in *The Victorians,* the immense scale of these kidnappings and the scope of the terror among women that they engendered is reflected in the fact that the medical officer tasked with expanding the program to London argued against it, because, to be proportionate with the number of arrests taking place in the rest of the country, there would have to have been twelve full-scale hospitals opened in the capital just to house the women who would have to be swept up and imprisoned.[13]

The terror of this situation, I believe, has deeply imprinted Anglo-American female consciousness, even though few of us actually know this history.

Why do we today in the Anglo-American West so often feel that if we report a rape or sex crime against us, our treatment will depend on whether or not we ever had any sexual agency in our pasts? That if we were to "admit" sexual agency at all in our pasts, in the context of a rape inquiry, some terrible, lasting public shaming will follow? Why do investigations of sex crimes themselves, and even prosecutions and convictions, so often mirror this situation, with conviction rates higher the more "pure" or "innocent" of sexual agency a woman can be proved to have been—in contexts quite separate from the rape itself? Why do we still feel somehow that to be open about our sexual wishes or agency is somehow to court catastrophe?

Josephine Butler, an early feminist, campaigned successfully against the Contagious Diseases Acts by casting the women imprisoned in a "seduction and betrayal" narrative—they were not sexual beings but abused innocents.

Given this imprinting cultural experience of a first major feminist political victory, it is not surprising that feminism, and women's campaigns in general, so often reflexively put their claims in a frame of women as "abused innocents," especially when it comes to sexual issues. Our history had no room for a more nuanced frame. This success became double-edged. Feminists learned that they gained social sympathy, status, and legal victories by constructing a narrative of helpless female sexual victimization by predatory, brutal men; I call this the "wrongs of" narrative. While there were many situations that certainly suited that narrative, the problem for us is that they almost entirely failed to develop a companion discourse that included female sexual desire and sexual agency.

We still live with the fallout from this intellectual history. When I sought in 2011 to tease out, in the rape accusations against Julian Assange, what happened after the woman's sexual consent on one level as well as her alleged lack of consent on another, I was attacked by feminists as "betraying the sisterhood." The trouble is that most date rapes today happen after a nuanced encounter—in which a woman wants *this*, but emphatically does not want *that*. If we are unable ever to talk about sexual agency without fearing that this makes us "fair game" for anything that follows, we will never be able to prosecute real rapes successfully.

## RESISTANCE

In spite of the brutal suppression of the vagina, uterus, and clitoris in this period, many female and male Victorians sought to create counternarratives to the toxic, medicalized vagina. Victorian women still sought out novels and art that represented the female self, female sexuality, and the vagina—however obliquely—in an appealing and positive light, and that sought to tell truths about female sexual desire and pleasure. Often these explorations and images were highly metaphorical.

In George Eliot's *The Mill on the Floss,* for instance, Maggie Tulliver is depressed and isolated; but she is drawn by her suitor, Philip Wakem—secretly and against her parents' wishes—to a part of the landscape that is called the Red Deeps. In this scenario, taking place in a vulval setting, female sexual desire is linked with female longing for learning, power, and a wider world:

> *In her childish days Maggie held this place, called the Red Deeps, in very great awe, . . . visions of robbers and fierce animals haunting every hollow. But now it had the charm for her which any broken ground, any rock and ravine, have for the eyes that rest habitually on the level. . . . In June time, too, the dog-roses were in their glory, and that was an additional reason why Maggie should direct her walk to the Red Deeps, rather than to any other spot, on the first day she was free to wander at her will—a pleasure she loved so well, that sometimes, in her ardors of renunciation, she thought she ought to deny herself the frequent indulgence in it.*

Eliot describes this "wandering" as intensely pleasurable, "the pleasure returning in a deeper flush." Maggie wonders if the secrecy with which she explores the Red Deeps is a "spiritual blight"—"something she would dread to be discovered in"—the same phrase that often describes female masturbation in this period; but "[y]et the music would swell out again, like chimes borne onward in a recurrent breeze. . . ." [14] Here female desire and self-knowledge are like music that "swells out"; as in so many such scenes, the female artistic or literary imagination, the sensual natural world, and an awakening vulval sensibility are all one.

Alluring holes, beautiful boxes, and valuable treasure chests appear with clearly suggestive implications throughout the classic women's novels of the mid-nineteenth century as well. Dr. Rees, in "Narrating the Victorian Vagina: Charlotte Brontë and the Masturbating Woman," explores the novel *Villette*—which tells the story of the quiet, humble governess Lucy Snowe, and how she triumphs over adversaries in a school in Belgium and finds passionate sexual and marital love at last—and looks at Charlotte Brontë's use of such vaginal metaphors. [15]

Dr. John, the "wrong" love interest who beguiles Lucy before she finds her better-suited mate, gives her illicit love letters, and Lucy furtively buries the letters under a pear tree: "I cleared away the ivy, and found the hole; it was large enough to receive the jar, and I thrust it deep in." "I was not," writes Lucy, "only going to hide a treasure—I meant also to bury a grief." "Lucy compulsively conceals objects in boxes, drawers and desks . . . like Poulet's patient, she must conceal her desires."

Lucy Snowe signals to Monsieur Paul—the "right" lover—that she is ready to begin a romantic relationship with him by handing him her precious "box," which "lay ready in my lap": "And taking from the open desk the little box, I put it into his hand. 'It lay ready in my lap this morning,' I continued; 'and if Monsieur had been rather more patient . . . —perhaps I should say, too, if *I* had been calmer and wiser—I should have given it then.'

"He looked at the box: I saw its clear warm tint and bright azure circlet, pleased his eye. I told him to open it."

A clearer sense of pleasure and ownership in the vagina could not be imagined, even if Victorian social convention ensures that these scenes unfold through metaphor and allegory.

As the nineteenth century progressed, the Pre-Raphaelite Brotherhood—which started publishing their magazine *The Germ* in 1850—developed explicit iconographies for the vagina. This theme was vivid in the wildly popular paintings of Dante Rossetti, Christina Rossetti's brother. Dante Rossetti often painted botanically incorrect, but anatomically correct, labial and vaginal pomegranates: his half-length portrait of Dante's Beatrice shows the beauty holding up such a pomegranate—with a cut in the skin of the fruit, and labial folds open on either side of the cut—and the same labial pomegranates appeared in his woodcuts for his sister Christina Rossetti's highly sexual epic of female temptation, "Goblin Market."[16] Just as the Pre-Raphaelites positioned themselves as social renegades and sexual dissidents, it is tempting to read their preoccupation with painting the vagina—indeed, graphically holding up and liberating the vagina from its usual repressed nineteenth-century context—as being part of their larger impulse toward social freedom and open creative expression.

In the 1860s, British women devoured genre novels called "sensation novels." In this kind of fiction, the heroine was not passive and dutiful—as she was in classic Victorian male fiction, like Dickens's novels—but was instead willful and determined. These novels gave readers many passages rich with sensuous description of these women's "voluptuous" feelings. Sensation novels were seen by the culture at large as being extremely threatening to women—especially to girls and young women—because they were understood to be arousing to them sexually. "Reading novels"—especially "reading French novels," which tended to be even more explicit about female sexuality and desire—surfaced as a metaphor for a gateway to moral perdition for women, described in terms very much like the terms used to warn young women away from masturbation. Indeed, women reading sensation novels and women's masturbation were often cast in terms that virtually linked them together.

## THE AESTHETIC VAGINA

As the 1880s and 1890s unfolded, aestheticism became an influential avant-garde movement, and aestheticist vaginas made their appearances. Illustrator Aubrey Beardsley used schematized vagina motifs as backgrounds for his lithographs for Oscar Wilde's plays, such as his censored play about overwhelming, even murderous female sexual desire, *Salome* (1892), as well as Wilde's folk tales. (There were even scary vagina motifs in this period as well: anonymous authors, including possibly Oscar Wilde, wrote the 1893 erotic novel *Teleny*, in which the vagina is portrayed at times as delightful, and at other times as being slimy, noxious, and monstrous.)

The 1890s, which saw massive shifts in terms of the education and social liberation of European and American women, also saw schematized vaginas, in the form of the iconic peacock feather motif and papyrus motif, which evolved into the art nouveau and art deco upside-down triangle motif. The peacock feather was represented vertically, as if an open vulva with the "heart" of the feather design the "heart" or what doctors would call "introitus" of the vulva.

The 1880s and the 1890s were a revolutionary period in Europe and America, as "aestheticism" and then "decadence," both of which were movements that subverted or questioned social and sexual conventions, became sweeping trends. "New Woman" writers such as Kate Chopin in *The Awakening,* Olive Schreiner, and George Egerton (a woman writing under a male pseudonym) began to write about female sexual desire. The New Woman figure, which became a focus of public discussion, was seen as sexually emancipated, and thus as very sexually threatening.

Toward the end of the nineteenth century, the curtain of repression of female sexuality was being lifted slightly by the sexologists, including Richard von Krafft-Ebing, whose *Psychopathia Sexualis* appeared in 1886—though Krafft-Ebing placed "excessive" female desire in the category of "nymphomania" and argued that most well-bred women's levels of desire should be "small"; "If this were not so," he wrote reassuringly, "the whole world would become a brothel"[17]—and the more liberal Havelock Ellis, who wrote *Studies in the Psychology of Sex* in 1889.

## THE FREUDIAN VAGINA

Sigmund Freud and his followers, of course, introduced a major shift in female sexuality and how the vagina was once again reunderstood. Though the Victorian conservative commentators saw the vagina as a mechanistic delivery system for reproduction, and had defined the clitoris as making women vicious and the uterus as making them crazy and unfit for higher education, Freud redefined the vagina in psychodynamic terms. In his *Three Essays on the Theory of Sexuality* (1905), he introduced the clitoris-vagina dualism that so engaged the 1970s and still so affects us: "If we are to understand how a little girl turns into a woman, we must follow the further vicissitudes of this excitability of the clitoris," he wrote.[18] Before Freud, the clitoris and the vagina were seen, even if not always admired, as different aspects of the same sexual/reproductive system. Freud popularized the idea that there was a kind of quarrel between them in terms of female development, and that there are morally "better" and morally "worse" kinds of female orgasm. In his terms, "mature" women had vaginal rather than "immature" clitoral orgasms, a position with which his disciples would concur and extend into the mid-twentieth century—thus making many women of our mothers' and grandmothers' generations self-doubting along the way.

But he also argued, in his essay on penis envy, that men see the vagina as a primordial castrator; elsewhere he depicted the vagina as the dark matrix of Oedipal psychodramas. After Freud, the notion of the devouring, castrating vagina as a source of male neuroticism became influential throughout the twentieth century.

Others—doctors and psychologists—picked up the argument that the vagina and the clitoris have political and psychodynamic relevance. In Wilhelm Stekels's 1926 book *Frigidity in Woman,* a chapter titled "The Struggle of the Sexes" assigns feminism the role of denying sexual pleasure to women; he believed that what he called female "sexual anaestheticism" was due to contemporary women's desires to be dominant over men. He also saw women's emotional and spiritual needs as being linked to their sexual responsiveness; a man must appeal to one kind of woman's spirituality, he wrote, before she could reach orgasm, whereas the "modern" woman can't reach orgasm unless she is treated like a "new woman," which is, he noted, "Ibsen's problem in Nora!" "With this requirement fulfilled," he concluded, "every inhibition that stands in the way of her sexuality is released."[19] It's remarkable that, well into the twentieth century, women's difficulties reaching orgasm were regularly assigned by authoritative commentators to women's emotional instability—rather than to men's seductiveness or technique.

But even as Freud and others were finding new terms—this time psychodynamic rather than medical—with which to control and sometimes condemn the vagina and clitoris, after the First World War, some women artists, dancers, and singers were looking for ways to liberate its meanings.

# Modernism: The "Liberated" Vagina

*Dear grey and white Janet . . . thank you for the bouquet. The pleasure is undescribable—like all enchantment and there is something sad about being unable to tell the secret of pleasure . . .*

—Dolly Wilde to Janet Flanner

Toward the end of the nineteenth century, women writers struggled to bring metaphors and narratives of female erotic desire, and even vaginal metaphors, into the light of day. Victorian women had referred to female sexuality in codes and allusions, but the female modernists, with their impulses toward breaking boundaries and establishing the new, began to articulate vaginal themes more directly.

In the first two or three decades of the twentieth century, a liberationist counterculture to reclaim female sexuality began in earnest. With modernism, women were making political, social, and artistic statements about their sexuality. From about 1890 to the 1920s, daringly many writers of marital advice literature began to decouple sex for women from reproduction. They decried male sexual selfishness and described techniques aimed at giving women more pleasure. Theodore van de Velde's huge bestseller, *Ideal Marriage* (1926), bemoaned the marital unhappiness that arose from not knowing "the

ABCs of sex" and repudiated the Victorian code of silence about these matters. The popularity of the book could also have been due to his championing in detail of cunnilingus, and the attention he gave to the details of how effectively to bestow on wives what he called "the genital kiss."[1]

Gertrude Stein, in her volume of poetry *Tender Buttons* (1912), made oblique references to the "tender button" of the clitoris.[2] Her famous line "a rose is a rose is a rose" is actually much more erotic and complex when read in its original setting. The line derives from a prose poem in which the context of the "rose" seems sexual—indeed multiorgasmic—and the rhythms of speech echo that escalating faltering of breath and cadence of waves of intensity that are so characteristic of female arousal, and which women poets have sought to capture since the time of Sappho's "thin fire":

> *Suppose, to suppose, suppose a rose is a rose is a rose is a rose.*
> *To suppose, we suppose that there arose here and there that here*
> *and there there arose an instance of knowing that there are*
> *here and there that there are there that they will prepare, that*
> *they do care to come again.*
> *Are they to come again.*

Here is another potential Steinian rose/vagina: "RED ROSES: A cool red rose and a pink cut pink, a collapse and a sold hole, a little less hot."[3]

Performer Josephine Baker, the African American dancer who was the darling of Parisian nightclubs in 1925, performed in a short skirt made of artificial bananas—a witty reference to her own sexual confidence, suggesting that one of "hers" was equal to any number of "theirs." Her glowing, self-possessed persona—which safely cast assertive female sexuality as exotic and "other"—was a new kind of iconography for female sexuality: a seductress who was not mincing or half ashamed, but who was open with her body, secure in its pleasures. Choreographer Loie Fuller's modern dance routines in the 1900s—in which she combined her innovative choreography with the movement of veil-like silks—caused a sensation in London and Paris. Contemporary critics interpreted her dance as a statement about female desire, as Fuller's waving, rippling, sensuous, almost labial cloth vortices swirled across the stage, with Fuller herself twisting at their centers. Contemporaries saw Fuller, writes literary historian Rhonda Garelick, as beginning and ending her performances with "a deeply female, birth-like violence," a "bleeding, floral wound": "As she whirls around in a spiral of blood-red light, Fuller seems to have set the air itself on fire, violently opening up a distinctly feminine, even vaginal rupture—a bleeding flower—in the planar space around her."[4]

Painter Georgia O'Keeffe left her family's farm in Wisconsin and built her own career and life as a young bohemian in Manhattan in the 1910s. She posed brazenly for her lover Alfred Stieglitz's geometrical, water-spangled nude photographs, leaving the viewing public and the art-criticism establishment shocked and titillated. Her flower paintings, often read as studies in a vaginal aesthetic, appeared in the early 1920s, when O'Keeffe was being personally identified as a free-spirited "muse" figure to male American modernists and Greenwich Village rebels, and she was identified with that subculture's interest in female sexual freedom. Both male and female art critics responded to her flower paintings breathlessly, claiming that the paintings were telling truths about female sexuality that no woman had dared to reveal before, even though her biographer Hunter Drohojowska-Philp makes it clear that O'Keeffe at least overtly denied these images' sexual content. O'Keeffe distanced herself from the vaginal nature of the images, according to Drohojowska-Philp, because she herself felt that the highly sexualized image of her persona, promoted by critics, obscured the seriousness of her intention as an artist.[5]

The poet Edna St. Vincent Millay, also a bohemian participant in the 1920s demimonde of Greenwich Village, "branded" herself consciously as an artistic advocate of female sexual freedom. She was among the first women to pick up the banner of transcendentalist, liberationist sexual advocacy that had been raised first by Walt Whitman sixty years before, in his 1855 publication of the scandalous prose poem, *Leaves of Grass*—though other male writers, from Walter Pater to Oscar Wilde, had developed this liberationist, mystical view of sexuality following Whitman. Millay famously wrote the female-liberationist quatrain, suggestively titled "First Fig" (1922), in her collection *A Few Figs from Thistles:*

*My candle burns at both ends;*
*It will not last the night;*
*But ah, my foes, and oh, my friends—*
*It gives a lovely light!*[6]

This caution-to-the-winds image of a rapturous and careless female sexual renegade, who makes her own choices and regrets none of her mistakes—because she welcomes the value of the experience—stood at the opposite end of the spectrum from the staid, victim-focused tradition of "seduction and betrayal" sexual narratives in Victorian women's fictions. The female narrator who would willingly, even gladly, throw it all over—social role, identity, life itself—for the sake of, or in allegiance to, overt sexual passion was a long way from the demure sonnets of Elizabeth Barrett Browning seventy years before, when female sexual passion had smoldered far below the surface of the language.

These artistic trends coincided with the latest iteration of vaginal motifs in art and architecture: the art deco papyrus was schematized into a repeated upside-down triangle, the icon for the exterior of the feminine pubis dating from humanity's earliest visual art. These images were incorporated into buildings, wallpaper, household objects, and advertising posters. In the 1910s and 1920s, when "New Women" and then flappers began to rebel against the social and sexual mores of their mothers' generations, the craze for Egyptiana in architecture, film, and furniture design also saw schematized triangle-pubis motifs everywhere.

A sudden explosion of accurate and sympathetic information about female sexuality now replaced the Van de Velde moralistic and inaccurate medical discourses of the Victorian period. Women were starting to be able to make love on their own terms for a very simple reason: technology. In the 1920s, reliable contraception became readily available: Marie Stopes opened her first birth control clinic in London in 1921, during the same era that Margaret Sanger opened her own clinic on Manhattan's Lower East Side.[7] Casual sex became far less dangerous for women, simply because of advances in rubber processing, which led to the greatly increased availability and effectiveness of both condoms and diaphragms. Dr. Marie Stopes's bestsellers *Married Love, What Every Girl Should Know* and *What Every Mother Should Know* also appeared in the 1920s. Women were learning from public, noncensorious sources accurate information about their own sexual responses, for the first time in Western history.

But not all male modernists moved as fast. They certainly saw sexuality as connected to creativity—but it was *male* sexuality and *male* creativity that interested them. Dr. Michael H. Whitworth, in an Oxford University lecture in 2011 on "Modernism and Gender," quotes from Ezra Pound's "Translator's Postscript" to the 1922 edition of Remy de Gourmont's *The Natural Philosophy of Love.* Pound identified creativity as sexual and male: "the brain itself, is, in origin and development, only a sort of great clot of genital fluid held in suspense. . . . There are traces of it in the symbolism of the phallic religions, man really the phallus or spermatozoid charging, head-on, the female chaos. . . . Even oneself has felt it, driving any new idea into the great passive vulva of London, a sensation analogous to the male feeling in copulation."[8]

For Henry Miller, similarly, the whole matrix of reality was a "womb" upon which he inscribes himself: "When into the womb of time everything is again withdrawn chaos will be restored and chaos is the score upon which reality is written . . . I am still alive, kicking in your womb, a reality to write upon."[9] When modernist men own and inseminate the cosmos's vulva with their ideas, the vulva and the womb are seen as positive; but when women, with their own ideas, seek to possess their own vulvas and wombs, those same organs degrade them. In Miller's *Tropic of Cancer* (1961), when women are creative, he tends to reduce them to "cunts" and to sexual appetites;

Elsa, a visitor to his quarters, plays Schumann, and Miller writes, "A cunt who can play as she does ought to have better sense than to be tripped up by every guy with a big putz that happens to come along." Or he describes women expatriate artists as "rich American cunts with paint boxes slung over their shoulders. A little talent and a fat purse." [10]

Dr. Whitworth points out that the male modernists identified "the feminine as submarine, and the masculine as dry land." [11] In contrast to Pound's and Miller's dynamic images of erect masculine ideas, Pound, as well as T. S. Eliot, tended to characterize the work of female colleagues in wet, flaccid, or quivering *negative* vaginal metaphors: Eliot accused Imagist poet Amy Lowell, for instance, of a "general floppiness," a floppiness that had, he argued, in terms of the literary movement of Imagism, "gone too far." Dr. Whitworth notes that critic Conrad Aiken encouraged readers to "pass lightly over the . . . tentacular quivering of Mina Loy" in favor of the "manly metres" of Eliot and Stevens. [12]

When the male modernists actually did write about female sexuality or about the clitoris and vagina, they did so in responses that showed an emerging Freudian dualism: their responses ranging from a chilly awe—as in Samuel Beckett's reference to "The great grey cunt of the universe"—to D. H. Lawrence's seeming amazement at the transcendental potential of female sexual ecstasy, as in the love scenes in which Mellors awakens Lady Chatterley's vaginal responses, to irritable resistance, as in Lawrence's description of New Woman clitoral "beak pecking" in another lovemaking scene in *Lady Chatterley's Lover* (1928). But in addition to the anxious male response to the clitoris and the sometimes admiring male description of vaginal sensuality in this era, a new place on the spectrum appeared, established first by Henry Miller: the dismissable, contemptible, pornographic "hole." In its not-important-ness, it differed from Tertullian's hellish snakepits of sin; it is the modern pornographic vagina: something tawdry, that simply doesn't matter.

In Lawrence's work, scenes of clitoral excitement often have a threatening quality, and are often linked to what Lawrence describes as the overly intellectualized nature of New Woman social renegades and feminists: "You want a life of pure sensation and 'passion,' " the character Rupert says to the New Woman Hermione in *Women in Love* (1920), "but your passion is a lie. . . . It isn't passion at all, it is your will. . . . You haven't got any real body, any dark sensual body of life. . . . If one cracked your skull perhaps one might get a spontaneous, passionate woman out of you, with real sensuality. As it is, what you want is pornography—looking at yourself in mirrors . . . so that you can . . . make it all mental." [13] The "New Woman," with her liberated, even demanding sexuality, was not an easy image for male modernists to welcome.

## THE MODERNIST DIVIDE:
## TRANSCENDENTALISM OR "JUST PUSSY"?

This dualism—is the vagina a locus of transcendentalism or "just pussy"?—is the dualism we inherit today. Since the 1940s, the "just pussy" interpretation has—temporarily, one can hope—gained the ascendancy.

In the 1940s, Anaïs Nin, Henry Miller's lover and contemporary, worked in the sexual-transcendentalist tradition of the female modernists, who revered the imaginative potential of the vagina. For Nin, the vagina enhances the woman; it expresses, rather than being separate from, her will and her sensibility, and is itself an object that is framed in a cherishing and tender context. Nin contributed the first extended female sexual voice to the canon of English literature when she began writing erotica for money, at so many francs per page. In her short story collection *Delta of Venus,* written at various times in the 1940s, but published posthumously in 1978, she frequently linked female Eros to female consciousness, and she sought to explore all the dimensions of sexuality hidden in women. Her stories reveal in attentive detail all the delights of the sexual feast that constitute the Goddess Array (which I explore in the last section of this book)—gazing, stroking, admiring, lubricating, melting, opening, and so on—and stand very much in contrast to Miller's work, and to that of Nin's male contemporaries.

In her story "Mathilde," Nin narrates the sexual adventures of a woman who falls in love with a drug addict, Martinez. Mathilde "remembered Martinez, his way of opening the sex like a bud, the flicks of his quick tongue covering the distance from the pubic hair to the buttocks, ending on the dimple at the end of her spine. How he loved this dimple, which led his fingers and his tongue to follow the downward curve and vanish between the two full mounds of flesh." Mathilde asks herself how she appears to Martinez, sits in front of a mirror, and opens her legs: "The sight was enchanting. The skin was flawless, the vulva, roseate and full. She thought it was like the gum plant leaf with its secret milk that the pressure of the finger could bring out, the odorous moisture that came like the moisture of sea shells. So was Venus born of the sea with this little kernel of salty honey in her, which only caresses could bring out of the hidden recesses of her body."[14]

Mathilde changes position before the mirror. "She could see her sex now from another side. . . . Her other hand went between her legs. . . . This hand stroked her sex back and forth. . . . The approach of orgasm excited her, she went into convulsive gestures, as if to pull away the ultimate fruit from the branch, pulling, pulling at the branch to bring down everything into a wild orgasm, which came as she watched herself in the mirror, seeing the hands move, the honey shining, the whole sex . . . shining wet between the legs."

Nin's treatment of the vagina—delicate and reverent—stands in stark contrast to Miller's. Miller helped to introduce the "pornographic frame" around the vagina that has prevailed to the present day—in which the vagina is debased and debasing to the woman, and decontextualized from the rest of the woman. This frame is so familiar to us we take it for granted, but it is really quite historically recent. Miller created the template for this frame in a famous passage from *Tropic of Cancer*—read breathlessly by generations of schoolboys—in his description of the prostitute Germaine's vagina. Germaine "advanc[ed] toward me leisurely," Miller writes;

*"she commenced rubbing her pussy affectionately, stroking it with her two hands, caressing it, patting it, patting it. There was something about her eloquence at that moment and the way she thrust that rosebush under my nose which remains unforgettable, she spoke of it as if it were some extraneous object which she had acquired at great cost, an object whose value had increased with time and which she now prized above everything in the world. Her words imbued it with a peculiar fragrance; it was no longer just her private organ, but a treasure, a magic, potent treasure, a God-given thing—and none the less so because she traded it day in and day out for a few pieces of silver. As she flung herself on the bed, with legs spread wide apart, she cupped it with her hands and stroked it some more, murmuring all the while in that hoarse, cracked voice of hers that it was good, beautiful, a treasure, a little treasure. And it was good, that little pussy of hers. . . . And again that big, bushy thing of hers worked its bloom and magic. It began to have an independent existence—for me too. There was Germaine and there was that rosebush of hers. I liked them separately and I liked them together. . . . A man! That was what she craved. A man with something between his legs that could tickle her, that could make her writhe in ecstasy, make her grab that bushy twat of hers with both hands and rub it joyfully, boastfully, proudly, with a sense of connection, a sense of life. That was the only place she experienced any life—down there where she clutched herself with both hands . . . It glowed down there between her legs where women ought to glow, and there established that circuit which makes one feel the earth under his legs again. When she lay there with her legs apart and moaning . . . it was good, it was a proper show of feeling."*[15]

I am not making an argument about which kind of text is "hotter." Some women will respond to Nin, some to Miller—some, no doubt, to both or to neither. My intention is to point out, rather, that they represent very different cultural ways of seeing what the vagina represents. The male-modernist view of women is all here in how the narrator sees the vagina of Germaine. The woman is sexually desiring, but makes no distinction between purchased and freely given sexual favors. She is portrayed as dead everywhere but in her sexual center. She is identified with life and vigor and there are some appealing metaphors—"rosebush," "treasure"—but she has no existence separate from her vagina and its relationship to the male narrator, and the vagina itself is separate from the woman rather than integrating another dimension of the woman, as it does so delicately in the "transcendentalist gateway" Nin passages.

## THE BLUES VAGINA

The early years of the twentieth century prepared the way for another thread: the flowering of ragtime at the turn of the century and then African American jazz and blues in the 1920s and 1930s. This musical development transfixed the United States and also swept over Britain and Western Europe. Ragtime, jazz, and blues were seen as harbingers of the new and the free. The spontaneous styles of dancing that accompanied these new rhythms were identified with other kinds of avant-gardism, including new kinds of classlessness, rejection of traditions, and of course sexual freedoms. White sophisticates listened in new ways to African American voices and lyrics, as well as new musical forms.

Ragtime, and then jazz and blues, also introduced a new frankness about discussing the vagina, and female sexuality in general. Blues lyrics in particular were filled with African American slang for *vagina*. Through this slang, a great deal of direct discourse about the vagina and about female sexual response in general made its way into the drawing rooms and salons of American and European society. These slang terms were usually encoded in metaphors: the clitoris was a bell that needed to ring; the vagina was a hot frying pan, or a butter churn that needed to be beaten, or a hot dog bun in need of a hot dog. So middle-class and upper-middle-class white audiences outside of Bohemia—men and women whose social norms still forbade them to discuss the vagina or female sexuality in public—could sing the lyrics, and enjoy and repeat their double meanings, without social penalties.

The crossover of blues lyrics from African American into white and mixed society was so important partly because the blues "frame" around the vagina is so very different from the frame created by the dominant Western traditions. Unlike the gynecologists of the era, blues slang does not medicalize the vagina. Unlike Freud, it does not psychologize a "better" or "worse" sexual response for women. In contrast to Freud's theory of male castration anxiety, and also in contrast to modernists such as Lawrence, blues slang is not fearful of the vagina. Rather, the metaphors that both male and female blues singers used about the vagina consistently cast female desire as strong, steady, positive, sometimes very funny—just as male sexual desire is often portrayed as very funny—and obviously in need of gratification, as well as deserving satisfaction. The blues vagina is not a shameful vagina. The words surrounding it are not associated with neurosis. The blues vagina is virtually never described as a "gash," a "nothing," or a source of shame and disease. Rather, blues vagina metaphors describe something that is delicious, appealing, or just amusing. Metaphors for the vagina in the blues tradition include jelly, jellyrolls, sugar and candy, seafood, frying pans, butter churns, bells, buns, and bowls. In blues lyrics, women are not victimized by having vaginas, but they are generally portrayed as being in full possession of their own sexuality and *liking* their vaginas. African American women's sexuality had been brutally owned and traded by others for four hundred years, but in spite of—or perhaps because of—this, the sexuality of women in blues lyrics is emphasized as belonging to the women themselves. So very unlike the white, Victorian women's novel and its "seduction and betrayal" theme, in which a "good" woman is a passive sexual victim and there is almost no narrative of positive female sexual agency, in the blues tradition, female sexual agency is the story line that predominates. Women are almost never portrayed as victimized via their sexuality, though love can certainly break their hearts.

In the blues, male lyricists tend to cast the women as being fully in control of "that thing"; a woman is often depicted as having a kind of artistry in handling her "thing," and the male observer/narrator in the song is often cast as an appreciative audience of her sexual skill and power. One can't say that these roles—the female demonstrator of her skill and mastery of her "thing"; the male troubadour touting the woman's skill with "her thing"—are inherently misogynist. I think that they are actually philogynist, if you will—the male narrators of these songs often seem to love women. Blues lyrics are often philogynist lyrics.

In the lyrics of the famous women blues singers of the 1920s through the 1940s are dozens of code terms for *vagina*. Lil Johnson sang about female frustration in "Press My Button (Ring My Bell)," a song in which she laments an overconfident lover's inability to locate her clitoris:

> *My man thought he was raising Sam*
> *I said, "Give it to me baby, you don't understand*
> *Where to put that thing,*
> *Where to put that thing,*
> *Just press my button, give my bell a ring!"*
> *Come on, baby, let's have some fun,*
> *Just put your hot dog in my bun,*
> *And I'll have that thing, that thing-a-ling.*
> *Just press my button, give my bell a ring!*
> *My man's out there in the rain and cold*
> *He's got the right key, but just can't find the hole.*
> *He says, "Where's that thing? That thing-a-ling?*
> *I been pressin' your button, and your bell won't ring!"*
> *[Spoken] "Beat it out, boy! Come on and oil my button! Kinda*
> *    rusty!"*

*Now, tell me daddy, what it's all about*
*Tryin' to pinch your spark plug and it's all worn out.*
*I can't use that thing,*
*That thing-a-ling,*
*I been pressin' your button, and your bell won't ring!*
*Hear my baby, all out of breath,*
*Been working all night and ain't done nothing yet,*
*What's wrong with that thing? That thing-a-ling?*
*I been pressin' your button, and your bell won't ring.*
*Hear me, baby, on my bended knee*
*I want some kind daddy just to hear my plea,*
*And bring me that thing*
*That thing-a-ling,*
*Just press my button, give my bell a ring.*[16]

In her 1936/1937 song "Hottest Gal in Town," Lil Johnson describes strong female desire in a richly domestic, even "foodie," set of metaphors, in which the eager vagina is described variously as milk, cream of wheat, and biscuits, and in which female desire is compared to a furnace being stoked. In the song, Johnson describes her ideal male lover, who will take the time to wake up early every morning to stoke said furnace, amping up the intensity of its heat, and who should be good-looking and well built; in her series of metaphors, he will churn her milk, cream her wheat, and toast her biscuits. She dwells on his physical characteristics—his height and his strength—and insists that he be similar to a cannonball. She explains that all of these qualities are the reasons that she wants him in her life—after all, she boasts, she is the hottest woman around. The repetition of different metaphors that characterize mutual desire and mutual sexual pleasure underscores the centrality of reciprocity in a satisfying sexual experience and the multiple ways in which female desire seeks and manifests pleasure.

The great female blues singers' lyrics sometimes mourned lost sexual pleasure. In 1936's "If You See My Rooster," the legendary Memphis Minnie sang:

*If you see my rooster, please run him on back home.*
*If you see my rooster, please run him on back home.*
*I haven't found no eggs in my basket, eeh hee, since my rooster*
    *been gone.*[17]

Memphis Minnie's hit mourned her "empty basket." A year later, Bessie Smith, a crossover sensation, sang "I Need a Little Sugar in My Bowl." She needs sugar, but she also needs a hot dog between her buns, she needs her lover to move his finger a little, she needs something that "looks like a snake," and she needs something to be dropped in her bowl:

*Tired of bein' lonely, tired of bein' blue,*
*I wished I had some good man, to tell my troubles to*
*Seem like the whole world's wrong, since my man's been gone*
*I need a little sugar in my bowl,*
*I need a little hot dog, on my roll*
*I can stand a bit of lovin', oh so bad,*
*I feel so funny, I feel so sad*
*I need a little steam-heat, on my floor,*
*Maybe I can fix things up, so they'll go*
*What's the matter, hard papa, come on and save your mama's*
    *soul*
*'Cause I need a little sugar, in my bowl,*
*Doggone it,*
*I need a little sugar in my bowl*
*I need a little sugar, in my bowl,*
*I need a little hot dog, between my rolls*
*You gettin' different, I've been told,*
*Move your finger, drop something in my bowl*
*I need a little steam-heat on my floor,*
*Maybe I can fix things up, so they'll go.*
*[Spoken] Get off your knees, I can't see what you're drivin' at!*
*It's dark down there!*
*Looks like a snake!*

*C'mon here and drop somethin' here in my bowl!*
*Stop your foolin', and drop somethin', in my bowl!*[18]

Bo Carter sang back to these assertive female voices with his own counterpoint of sexual metaphors. In contrast to the "wrongs of" or "seduction and betrayal" of white Victorian women's ways of seeing sexuality—male dominance, female reticence—the penis-and-vagina pairings in blues lyrics play together equitably: they are interdependent and work together; each needs the other. The sexual world of the blues is one of affection and intense mutual physical need, in which neither man nor woman is necessarily "on top." In "Banana in Your Fruit Basket," Carter pleads with his audience, begging for a woman who will, in burning his bread, make use of his "brand-new skillet." He swears that if the woman in question would just let him put his "banana" in her "fruit basket," than that would be enough for him. A series of other metaphors that describe paired objects follow, objects that operate not only reciprocally, but fit together. Carter notes that he is the owner of a washboard, and that his beloved has a tub—and that when the two are put together, the couple can "rub, rub, rub"—and of course, a washboard without a tub (into which it is placed) is not useful. Carter makes a similar comparison when he continues on to sing about his "dasher"—a dasher is the staff used to churn butter. His baby, no surprise, is the owner of the churn. The song goes further in its bawdy but loving descriptions: Carter has a needle and his lover has some cloth, together they can stitch "till we both will feel it." These series of couplets describe reciprocal relationships in which neither object is useful absent its partner; the metaphors underscore a mutual need in sex. Carter closes the song singing that whereas his baby has the "meat," he has the "knife"—and if she will let him do "her cutting," it will "solve" his life.

The blues singer Blu Lu wrote and performed the sensuous "Don't You Feel My Leg" in 1938—a song so steamy, and the lyrics so obviously about sexual desire from a female point of view, that it was banned for a time.

*Don't you feel my leg, don't you feel my leg.*
*Cause if you feel my leg you're gonna feel my thigh.*
*And if you feel my thigh, you're goin' to go up high*
*So don't you feel my thigh.*
*Don't you buy no rye, don't you buy no rye.*
*Cause if you buy some rye you're goin' to make me high.*
*And if you make me high you're goin' to tell a lie.*
*So don't you make me high.*
*You said you'd take me out and treat me fine*
*But I know there's something you've got on your mind.*
*If you keep drinking you're gonna get frayed*
*And you will wind up asking for fine brown turkey . . .*
*Don't you feel my leg, don't you feel my leg . . . [refrain].*
*Don't you feel my leg now, you know why,*
*Cause I ain't goin' to let you feel my thigh.*
*Yes, you might go up high . . . [refrain]* [19]

Some female artists made the same version of a sexually explicit song even more graphic in subsequent renditions. Georgia White recorded "I'll Keep Sittin' on It (If I Can't Sell It)" in 1936. The song employs a "chair" motif to express pride and sexual self-respect as well as humor—a motif that also allowed it to pass the censors. The song describes a woman contemplating selling a chair, but only for the right price. If she can't sell her chair, White sings, she'll make the decision to just keep sitting on it. The listener *must* purchase the chair if he wants it so badly—White isn't giving it away, regardless of her prospective buyer's desire; in fact, she adamantly refuses to even entertain the possibility. The song exhorts the buyer to step up and show that he values it. White sings with bravado about the chair's lovely bottom, built to last. She notes that if a buyer desires something of high quality in general, he is expected to part with money for it, and she promises that he won't ever regret his decision. She stresses that she is not speaking lightly: she means to draw this line. In context, the idea of exchanging "money" for her "chair" does not read as a metaphor for sex work, for a literal exchange of sex for money, but a statement, rather, of the value White places on her own sexuality—she is not going to treat it as if it were worthless.

Ruth Brown's rendition of four years later is much more explicit.

> *I own a second-hand furniture store*
> *And I think my prices are fair.*
> *But this real cheap guy came in one day*
> *Saw this chair he wanted to buy*
> *But he wouldn't—claimed the price was too high.*
> *So I looked him straight in the eye,*
> *And this was my reply . . .*
> *If I can't sell it, I'm gonna sit down on it.*
> *I ain't gonna give it away.*
> *Now darlin', if you want it, you gonna have to buy it.*
> *And I mean just what I say.*
> *Now how would you like to find this*
> *Waitin' at home for you every night?*
> *Only been used once or twice, but it's still nice and tight . . .*
> *Now you can't buy a better pair of legs in town*
> *And a back like this? Not for miles around. . . .*
> *Because it's made for comfort,*
> *Built for wear and tear.*
> *Where else would you find such an easy chair?*
> *It's lush, plush, slick and sleek.*
> *Darlin', a high-class piece like this at any price is cheap . . .*
> *Now look at this nice bottom.*
> *Ain't it easy on the eye?*
> *Guaranteed to support*
> *Any weight or size.*
> *If I can't sell it . . .*[20]

The African American blues tradition continued to change American popular music: its descendants include rock and roll and hip-hop. But the humorous and explicit lyrics of the blues that took for granted the essential goodness of female sexual desire did not survive into the musical traditions that descended from the blues. White producers who packaged African American music for white audiences in the 1950s cleaned up the references in the lyrics they were mainstreaming, and by the time rock and hip-hop seized their own initiatives in singing about sex, this woman-friendly lyrical tradition was long gone.

## THE SELF-DEFINING VAGINA OF THE SECOND WAVE

The postwar years, as Betty Friedan documented in her 1963 classic, *The Feminine Mystique,* were years of regression.[21] Freudian analysis loomed large in the United States and middle-class white women, at least, and much to their frustration, struggled to fit into domesticity and sexual "fulfillment" centered around a Freudian (that is, non-clitoral) model of "maturity" and "adjustment." Nonetheless, the ground shifted again with the 1965 discovery of the birth control pill, and the beginning of what came to be called the "sexual revolution."

In 1976, Shere Hite published *The Hite Report: A Nationwide Study of Female Sexuality.*[22] This book created a radically different perspective from all that had preceded it, particularly the Freudian model, since it looked directly at what women experience during intercourse and presented their experiences in their own words, rather than prescribing to them what they *should* experience. What Hite found, as noted above, was that two-thirds of women could not have orgasms with penile thrusting alone. This conclusion was a revelation to millions of women who had felt themselves, having read Freud and the neo-Freudian Karen Horney, to be insufficiently mature if they were unable to reach orgasm through intercourse.

Hite's quotes from women who do have orgasms from intercourse—versus women who need clitoral stimulation to reach orgasm—set up a political duality that is still with us. We should now understand, as I noted in the first section, that the clitoris, the vagina, and indeed all the many sexual centers in the female sexual area (for lack of a better term; it is more than an "organ" and more than just one organ) are all part of the same complex neural nexus. And the latest data show that the G-spot is probably *part* of the structure of the clitoris.

But in the 1970s, in a newly fierce argument with Freud, many feminist commentators addressed the clitoris as if it needed to be championed in opposition to the vagina. Feminists such as Anne Koedt, in the *The Myth of the Vaginal Orgasm* (1970), sought to dismiss Freud's elevation of the vagina over the clitoris. These feminists, in their reasonable championing of clitoral attention, made the case that the idea of vaginal pleasure was a sinister patriarchal plot. This plot, they argued, sought to persuade women that the vagina is the locus of true femininity, and the clitoris insignificant. If women could be persuaded of this, they maintained, then they would be brainwashed into dependency on men—and men would have carte blanche to be lazy, and to ignore women's needs for attention to the clitoris.

Shere Hite's 1976 success in reglamorizing the clitoris reinforced the many ways of teasing and stimulating the clitoris in Alex Comfort's *The Joy of Sex* (1972), which also imprinted a generation. With all this rebranding, the vagina ended up, for the thirty years that followed, suffering a bit of a cultural downgrade. From the 1970s on, the vagina was recast as rather retro, housewifey, and passé—until the rediscovery of the G-spot in 1981 by Beverly Whipple. (In the twenty-first century, porn-driven interest in female ejaculation drew attention back to the vagina.) This polarization assigned to two parts of women's sexual systems—which turn out to be part of a single network—are two very different cultural identities. For thirty years, the clitoris was seen as sort of *cooler* than the vagina, and once again women were faced with a false choice that minimized their own sexual complexity. The clitoris, if it had a persona, was a glamorous, miniskirt-wearing Gloria Steinem; the vagina was the slightly ridiculous, out-of-date-hairstyle-wearing Marabel Morgan, who wrote the regressive bestseller *The Total Woman* (1970).

Soon, Second Wave feminists were on a mission to teach repressed middle-class women to locate their clitorises, to demand orgasmic parity, and by all means to masturbate. In 1973, Betty

Dodson, a feminist activist and sex educator, began to run work-shops for women to help them "appreciate the beauty of their geni-tals as well as to explore the varied experience of orgasm through practicing masturbation skills."[23] Her mission was to teach "pre-orgasmic" women how to masturbate to orgasm, and she has been successful. Dodson's is a down-to-earth, unthreatening presence; her workshops were widely covered in the mainstream press and in *Ms.* magazine, leading women to become familiar with the idea that it is empowering to sit with open legs before a mirror and become familiar with one's own vulva and vagina.

The 1970s also saw a great deal of feminist reclamation of the vaginal complex—that is, the vagina, labia, and clitoris. Germaine Greer, who had garnered international attention with her feisty man-ifesto *The Female Eunuch* (1970), understood the vagina-freedom connection implicitly. She devoted a chapter in her book *The Mad-woman's Underclothes* (originally published in 1986) to "The Politics of Female Sexuality," published in 1970, to the vagina and the poli-tics of its derogation, and exhorted, in a much-mimeographed essay in *Suck* magazine, "Lady, love your cunt."[24]

Assertive and self-defining feminist vaginas debuted in literature as well in this key feminist decade. Erica Jong, of course, published *Fear of Flying* in 1973, coining the famous term that she jokes will be inscribed on her tombstone: the "zipless fuck," which, she argues in the novel, is the fantasy goal of every liberated woman: hot sex with no emotional entanglements and no baggage. Jong's heroine, Isadora Wing, also links her vagina's awakening to her own creative awaken-ing, and to her individuation as an agent of her own life rather than as the passive hanger-on to various men. Jong's novel was published in fourteen countries. It was so popular precisely because it was the first female *bildungsroman* to identify in parallel terms a journey of female sexual awakening with a journey of psychological and cre-ative awakening. The dry, physically repressed Dr. Wing, Isadora's husband, whom she flees at length for more sensuous male lovers, can never, we understand, awaken the latent adventuress/writer in Isadora. The final scene of the book, in which Isadora—now deeply engaged with her own sexual and creative journey—contemplates her own blond pubic hair as she lies in the bathtub, is a trope for the vagina's connection to the imagination: "I floated lightly in the deep tub, feeling that something was different, something was strange. . . . I looked down at my body. The same. The pink V of my thighs, the triangle of curly hair, the Tampax string fishing the water like a Hemingway hero, the white belly, the breasts half floating. . . . A nice body. Mine. I decided to keep it. I hugged myself. It was my fear that was missing . . . whatever happened, I knew I would survive it. I knew, above all, that I'd go on working. . . ."[25] The newly liberated and creative heroine contemplates her own body, her own vagina— and thinks about a rededication to her creative work: this scene is a metaphor for a sexual awakening that is creative as well as physical, and a creative awakening that is as sensuous as it is cerebral.

In the visual arts, Judy Chicago took her exhibit *The Dinner Party* to museums around the country in 1974. Chicago portrayed thirty-nine mythic and real women from throughout history by depicting different vaginas painted on dinner plates and placing them on a triangular dinner table—the triangle being an archetypal feminine or vulval shape. She spoke of the "butterfly-vulva" motif as a trope of women's creativity. The various vaginas were meant to convey these women's individual characters and to represent their work. She published the collection of plates as a book of photographs in 1979. This exhibit and the book were shocking at the time, drawing a range of virulent critical responses. These portraits of the hypothetical vaginas of Mary Wollstonecraft and Emily Dickinson could not have portrayed the vagina-creativity connection more literally— even if the nature of that connection still remained intuitive.

So it was a pretty good decade for the vagina, if one that superficialized its importance as a locus of pleasure strictly defined. The results were positive for women: in the late 1970s, *Redbook* magazine reported that 70 percent of female respondents self-reported "satisfaction with the sexual aspect of their marriage"; 90 percent reported taking an active role in sex at least half the time, and often "always"; 64 percent said they regularly reached orgasm during lovemaking;

most of the subjects said they often initiated sex, and that they felt they could communicate their sexual needs clearly to their partners. (The numbers of women who reach orgasm during lovemaking have not gone up in the subsequent decades of "sexual revolution" and the proliferation of pornography; and the data for women who self-report that they are honest in expressing sexual needs to their male partners has actually gone down.) [26]

The feminist movement to reclaim the vulva and vagina was not restricted to literature, painting, and nonfiction prose. The marketplace also stepped in enthusiastically: the culture saw "sex-positive" consumer attention to the vagina in woman-centric erotica such as Vive productions, which made (slower-paced, more emotionally involving, more romantic) pornographic videos for women—a genre soon to become almost obsolete, as women acclimated to masturbating to conventional porn—and woman-friendly sex toy emporia opened, such as New York City's Babeland boutiques and San Francisco's pleasant, brightly lit store Good Vibrations. (A manager at the Brooklyn branch of Babeland—formerly Babes in Toyland—reports that new sex-play products designed to stimulate the G-spot and to encourage female ejaculation are being designed continually, and that the stock is flying off the shelves. Why the trend, I asked? She replied that pornography had begun to focus intensely on female ejaculation, leading women to wish to explore stimulation of their G-spots.)

But there was a real difference in tone between this mode of reclaiming female sexuality and that of the early twentieth century, which had, as we saw, also witnessed a stirring of women's voices and imagery around female sexual pleasure. Loie Fuller, Edna St. Vincent Millay, Georgia O' Keeffe, and Edith Wharton were writing or painting or dancing as ways to express truths about female desire; but sexual desire, in their work, is not separate from female transcendence, inspiration, and joy in other areas of women's lives. It is a means to a larger, fuller, all-encompassing transcendence and creativity. The post-1970s "reclamation" of female sexuality, in contrast, is quite mechanical. It is not about the spirit. It is much debased. It is about what vibrates how. It is diminished, I believe, by the influence of medical discourses such as Masters and Johnson's, which reframes female and male sexuality as "just flesh," and it is also distorted by the pressures of the porn industry that boomed alongside the sexual revolution.

Historian of sexuality Steven Seidman notes that the 1960s and 1970s introduced the notion of "fun"—not just pleasure—as an important part of sexual life, especially in best-selling sex manuals.[27] He cites David Reuben, M.D.'s *Everything You Always Wanted to Know About Sex (But Were Afraid to Ask)* (1969), Alex Comfort's *The Joy of Sex,* and "M" 's *The Sensuous Man* (1971) as recasting consensual sex as "an adult form of play"; all sexual practices, including flagellation, aggression, and fetishism, he writes, were now seen as equally valid, and any kind of fantasy—no matter how "wild or bloodthirsty"—was to be valued and explored. This of course is a radically different model than the gateway to heaven or hell of the Renaissance, or the sober duty of the Victorians, or the connection with the Divine of the Aesthetic sexual transcendentalists. "This sex ethic may be termed libertarian," he writes persuasively.

This is our sex ethic. There is nothing wrong with "fun," of course; but this model of what sex is for—what the vagina is for—has left many with deeper questions about the role of sexuality as a medium of profound intimacy or profound alterations of consciousness. And the "sex as play" model also raises all the questions that any "anything goes" ethic raises—why not, even if one is in a relationship, get hooked on porn? Why not go to a strip club, or frequent sex chat lines? Why not have a threesome, or share details with one's mate of a fantasy involving someone else? What, in a libertarian model of what sex is, is the rationale for drawing any kind of line keeping sexual energy "sacred," in a sense, between two people?

This "libertarian," "sex as play" view of sexuality and the vagina's role in it is our complicated inheritance. Sexual libertarianism may not be the same thing, as it turns out, as true sexual liberation. "These manuals [such as *The Joy of Sex*]," Seidman continues, "encourage the reader not to resist [any kind of fantasy] since the sexual sphere represents an ideal setting for probing tabooed wishes and fears. . . . [D]on't block [your own fantasy] and don't be afraid of your partner's fantasy; this is a dream you are in."

In these manuals, Seidman notes, "to put the reader at ease," he or she is assured that sexual behavior is not a marker of a person's true nature. This ideology—descending from Walt Whitman and Oscar Wilde, via, in debased form, Friedrich Nietzsche—argues that sensation, even extreme sensation, is good for its own sake alone. This sexual "will to power," adorned with a dollop of Freud's argument that the individual gets a "pass" for whatever the subconscious comes up with—since one can have no responsibility for, and hence no guilt about, subconscious desires—fit perfectly with the heady, consumerist postwar economy in the West. It prepared a fertile ground for the entrenchment of the pornographic experience of sex and of the vagina in particular. It came to be how we thought "sex was"—rather than letting us understand that this way of thinking about sex is just one of many possible sexual ideologies. And it cleared the way in the minds of both women and men for the rise in the next few decades of wider and wider acceptance and then internalization of the moral flatness, distractedness and fixatedness of pornography.

But is what one does in bed with someone else—with all the hopes, intimacies, and possibilities for grief involved—really just "a dream you are in"? The next three decades would call this worldview's vision of consequence-free sex and fantasy into question.

————

So 1970s feminist activists were trying to express a new relationship to the vagina that quickly became decontextualized by mass-produced pornography, by libertarian sex manuals, and by sexual scientists. (*Playboy* centerfolds were "pink"—meaning open legs and inner labia visible—by the early 1970s.) As the so-called sexual revolution of the '70s got under way, even feminist discourses about the vagina were framed in ways that were rather sterile or "porn-y," since the modernist and blues associations around female sexuality—echoes of mystery that went deeper than mere carnality, and ecstasy that was more than physical—had been lost.

The upbeat discourse about female sexuality that characterized the work of Germaine Greer and Erica Jong did not last long. Things turned dark in the 1980s. In 1985, Andrea Dworkin's *Intercourse* cast the vagina as being—intrinsically—a site for male sexual violence. In an argument dense with sexual pessimism, she argued that heterosexual intercourse is always about male dominance and female submission: "The small, intimate society created for intercourse, one time or many, the social unit that is the fuck in action, must be one that protects male dominance. . . . The penis needs protection of the law, of awe, of power. Rebellion here, in intercourse, is the death of a system of gender hierarchy premised on a sexual victory over the vagina."[28]

By this point the ebullient 1930s and 1940s bananas and fruit baskets, the needles and cloth, the hot dogs and buns, and the churns and butter of blues lyrics—metaphors that are about mutual dependency or mutual energy rather than about dominance and submission—had been lost to time. To Dworkin, male penetration of the vagina was always inherently an act of aggression. In her view, it was impossible for a woman freely to want to be penetrated. If she did indeed desire penetration, it was a result of her having internalized a "false consciousness" about the nature of her desire because she had internalized the norms of her oppressor. Paradoxically, just as women had been charged by misogynists in the Elizabethan era with being "wounded," Dworkin made—from a pro-woman position—the very same claim. In Dworkin's work, the vagina is demoted back to its Elizabethan status as an allegorical injury, a "gash," a ready-made wound awaiting the ready-made male wounder.[29]

Other kinds of advocacy did surface in the 1980s and 1990s. In 1993, Joani Blank edited *Femalia,* a collection of close-up color photographs of many vaginas, including those owned by some well-known women. (The book was published by Down There Press.) This was an update of activist Tee Corinne's 1973 vagina coloring book. Both women wished to send images of the immense variation among vaginas out into the culture, as they felt that women were too often ashamed of their own unique labial and vulval shapes. *The Vagina Monologues,* originally a 1996 play by Eve Ensler, made a great impact: Ensler used real women's monologues about their vaginas to call attention to still-taboo issues of female sexuality and rape. In 1998, Inga Muscio wrote *Cunt: A Declaration of Independence*—and sought to reclaim the word and concept, turning it from a negative to an emblem of power.

And today? Depending on where one looks, there is a widespread movement of female musicians, artists, and writers painting, taking pictures of, narrating, championing, and "problematizing"—as they say in the academy—the vagina. E-mails have alerted me to a knitting circle in Toronto in which young women, seeking a sense of empowerment, knit woolen vulvas. A female Danish artist bikes around Copenhagen with a six-foot plaster-of-paris vagina sculpture attached to her bicycle. The young-feminist website Feministing.com runs a feature titled "I Love My Vagina." A website called Vulvavelvet .com, rather charmingly, encourages women to post images of their own vaginas so that no woman will feel "weird." The range of labial diversity that women send in to the site is truly astonishing, and the wide range of what is "normal" for women certainly challenges the surgical uniformity, as well as the creepy childlikeness, of the pornographic vagina. Like Tee Corinne and Joani Blank, the site's founders, too, want women to accept in themselves the very broad range of normal variations and complex symmetries and asymmetries in labial arrangements. (Vulvavelvet.com also has a fascinating page in which women write in with tricks and tips for satisfying masturbation. Suggestions range from the use of varieties of vegetables—not the usual suspects—to creative ways to sit on washing machines and complex arrangements involving showerheads. With its chatty, informative tone—try this at home!—it feels much more like "Hints from Heloise," the housekeeping tips column, than like "Penthouse Forum.")

It is as if the zeitgeist is at work, and women in the public eye and all over the cultural map want to join an inchoate and unspecified movement toward a new kind—a funnier, or tenderer, or gentler kind—of reclamation of the vagina.

This is all positively motivated, no doubt. But is it a reclamation that is profound enough?

# three

## *Who Names the Vagina?*

## 10

## *"The Worst Word There Is"*

---

*"What is cunt?" she said. . . .*
*"It's thee, dost see: and tha'rt a lot besides an animal, aren't ter?*
*Even ter fuck? Cunt! Eh, that's the beauty o' thee, lass!"*

—D. H. Lawrence, *Lady Chatterley's Lover*

*Our self-contempt originates in this: in knowing we are cunt.*

—Kate Millet, *Sexual Politics*

If we understand the vagina-brain connection, and how liberated vaginas relate to potentially liberated female minds and
spirits, we can also start to see why words, when deployed in relation
to the vagina, are always more than "just words." Because of the sub-
tlety of the mind-body connection, words about the vagina are also
what philosopher John Austin, in his 1960 book *How to Do Things
with Words,* calls "performative utterances," often used as a means
of social control. A "performative utterance" is a word or phrase that
actually accomplishes something in the real world. When a judge
says, "Guilty," to a defendant, or a groom says, "I do," the words
alter material reality.[1]

Words about the vagina create environments that directly affect women's bodies. The words women hear being used about their vaginas change, for better or worse, what they purport to describe. Because of their effect on the female autonomic nervous system (ANS), words about the vagina can either help or hurt actual vaginal response. New studies, as we saw, show that the autonomic nervous system in women is directly connected to optimal sexual arousal functionality in vaginal tissue, circulation, and lubrication itself—so verbal threats or verbal admiration or reassurances can directly affect the sexual functioning of the vagina. Another new study, which we explore below, suggests that a stressful environment can actually negatively affect vaginal tissue itself. This "bad stress" affecting the vagina can also, as it inhibits orgasm, lower the levels of women's confidence, creativity, and hopefulness overall.

Women react strongly to male verbal abuse of their vaginas or to implied threats of rape, even when these are "just jokes," for these very reasons—though most of us are unaware of the science behind our "gut reactions" that this kind of abuse is somehow really bad for us.

This tactic is common: The film *North Country* (based on the 2002 book *Class Action: The Story of Lois Jenson and the Landmark Case That Changed Sexual Harassment Law,* by Clara Bingham and Laura Leedy Gansler, which chronicled the case of *Jenson v. Eveleth Taconite Company*) centers on male coal miners in a Pennsylvania mine who resisted female miners' incursions into their world. At one point, the women miners entered their locker room to find that the word *cunts* had been spray-painted in massive letters on the wall of lockers. In Oxford University in February of 2012, a college club established a "game" in which young men hunted down young women scantily dressed as foxes (in British foxhunts, riders on horseback chase the fox with packs of hounds; when the fox is captured, the dogs destroy it). On a UK college humor website, in 2012, the editors posted a joke pointing out that few rapes get prosecuted and so "your odds are good." "Who has put pubic hair on my Coke?" Clarence Thomas was alleged in 1991 to have asked Anita Hill, something which he denied. But if true, then it surely would have made her uneasy. Comedienne Roseanne Barr described male TV writers' behavior when women made inroads into their profession: she noted that she hated going up to the writers' house because there would be a "'stinky-pussy' joke" within three minutes. When a woman faces a workplace in which her male peers want to show her she is unwelcome, similar words or images targeting or insulting the vagina will often surface: centerfolds with legs spread, for instance, and the face of the woman in question superimposed on the naked body, will appear somewhere in public.

Of course, cultural and psychological motivations play a part in this form of harassment. But the role of manipulating female stress in targeting the vagina should not be ignored. This behavior—ridiculing the vagina—makes perfect instinctive sense. These acts are often impersonal and tactical—strategies for directing a kind of pressure at women that is not consciously understood but may be widely intuited, and even survive in folk memory, as eliciting a wider neuropsychological "bad stress" response that actually debilitates women.

In 2010, male Yale students gathered at a "Take Back the Night" event, where their female classmates were marching in a group, protesting against sexual assault. The young men chanted at the protesters, "No means yes and yes means anal."[2] Some of the young women brought a lawsuit against the university, arguing that tolerating such behavior created an unequal educational environment. Ethically they are in the right, and neurobiologically they are right as well. Almost all young women who face a group of their male peers chanting such slogans are likely to feel instinctively slightly panicked. On some level they are getting the message that they may be in the presence of would-be rapists—making it impossible to shrug off immature comments, as women are often asked to do. They sense there is a wider risk to them that is being threatened, and indeed there is, but it is not just the risk of sexual assault. If they are stressed regularly in this way, they will indeed depress the whole subtle and delicate network of neurobiological triggers and reactions that make them feel good, happy, competent, and as if they know themselves.

In many cases of sexual harassment in school settings or in the workplace, the vagina is targeted, threatened, or ridiculed. Why should this be so uniform a tactic, appearing in elite universities and blue-collar labor settings, crossing class and other boundaries?

It is common because it is a form of verbal aggression against women with effects—actual physical effects—that go deeper than other kinds of name-calling. Dr. Burke Richmond, as we saw, pointed out the mind-body connection in terms of lasting damage to some women's sensory perceptions as a result of sexual trauma. Even more research is identifying new kinds of lasting damage or dysfunction to many other female body systems as a result of sexual "bad stress"—what one recent study called, using a new nomenclature for what is emerging as a newly recognizable medical pattern in some women—"multisystem dysregulation."

The female body reacts in the same way to "bad stress" whether the context is the birthing room or the university or the workplace. If the female brain senses that an environment is not safe, its stress response inhibits all the same organs and systems, regardless of setting. Many of the signals that either stoke or diminish female desire have to do with the female brain's question: Is it safe here?

So if a woman goes to work or to study in a sexually dangerous or threatening atmosphere day after day, she risks—because of the cumulative, long-term effect of that "bad stress"—having the letting-go, creative "relaxation response" inhibited even outside her work or school environment. A woman's reproductive and mothering life can be affected by chronic sexually threatening stress; stress inhibits not just a woman's ability to become aroused and to lubricate and reach orgasm, but also her ability to give birth effectively and to nurse her child, and so on. Over time, if her vagina is targeted verbally, her heart rate, blood pressure, circulation, and many other systems will suffer chronically. Sexually threatening stress releases cortisol into the bloodstream, which has been connected to abdominal fat in women, with its attendant risks of diabetes and cardiac problems; being on the receiving end of sexually threatening "bad stress" also raises the likelihood of heart disease and stroke.

If you sexually stress a woman enough, over time, other parts of her life are likely to go awry; she will have difficulty relaxing in bed eventually, as well as in the classroom or in the office. This in turn will inhibit the dopamine boost she might otherwise receive, which would in turn prevent the release of the chemicals in her brain that otherwise would make her confident, creative, hopeful, focused—and effective, especially relevant if she is competing academically or professionally with you. With this dynamic in mind, the phrase "fuck her up" takes on new meaning.

H. Yoon and colleagues, Korean researchers who published "Effects of Stress on Female Rat Sexual Function" in the *International Journal of Impotence Research* in 2005, concluded that "chronic physical stress modifies the sexual behavior of female rats through a mechanism believed to involve complex changes in sex hormones, endocrine factors, and neurotransmitters."[3] They point out that "Many women with stress experience some forms of sexual difficulty, such as a decreased libido, arousal difficulty, or orgasmic difficulty. However, no research has been conducted related to changes in the clitoris and vagina when female subjects are subjected to prolonged stress. Is it that only a psychological phenomenon occurs at the cerebral cortical area controlling sexual activities? Or are there any significant changes in the vagina, clitoris, or other sexual response organs that lead to arousal or orgasmic difficulties?"

This first study to look at the effect of "bad stress" on female rat arousal—though many studies had looked at how stress inhibits the sex lives of male rats—found the chemical "smoking gun" that explains why women need to relax to become aroused. Evidently nitric oxide (NO) and nitric oxide synthase (NOS) play important roles in vaginal and clitoral engorgement—helping the smooth muscle of the vagina relax and the vaginal tissues swell in preparation for arousal and orgasm—and these chemicals and their actions are inhibited when females are negatively stressed.

"In this study, we undertook to investigate the effects of physical stress on sexual function by measuring changes in sexual behaviors, serum hormonal levels, and in neuronal NOS (nNOS) and endothelial NOS (eNOS) concentrations in vaginal tissues, both important mediators of smooth muscle relaxation and vascular engorgement, and therefore sexual arousal," the authors explain.[4]

They divided sixty-three female rats into three equal groups, all of them in estrous (that is, under ordinary circumstances, eager to mate). A mucosal smear was taken from every rat's vaginal tissue. "A male rat was then gently introduced into the cage and sexual behavior was observed. All sexual behavior tests were recorded on video camera and the results were scored and analyzed by one observer who was blind to the study details." The researchers checked the female rats' "receptivity" by recording their responses of "lordosis"—the arched-back, paws-up signal that a female is interested in mating. "Any defensive kick, push, run or roll onto the back was considered as a rejection response." Fair enough.

All the way down the mammalian ladder, scientists such as the Yoon team are confirming that getting females "in the mood" is scientifically a more complex and more "mind-body" process than is the analogue in males: "In general, sexual response in the female requires mental–physical reciprocal reactions, which are more complicated than in the male. Therefore, the effects of psychological and physical stress on sexual activity could be much larger in female than male subjects. . . . We hypothesized that chronic physical stress may affect female sexual function and aimed to identify pathophysiologic changes induced by chronic stress. Furthermore, we investigated how these changes could bring about arousal and orgasmic difficulty."[5]

Well, the scientists found exactly what they were looking for: the stressed-out female rats were not nice to their mates, and did not want to make love: "female rats under stress showed significantly decreased receptivities to their male partners," wrote the scientists; the female rats also displayed measurable "aggression" and "irritability." Stress diminished the female rats' physical ability to get aroused; it decreased their genital blood flow:

*In animal model studies, mental or physical stress increases the level of serum catecholamines, thereby causing vascular con-*

*traction, which in turn reduces blood flow and leads to sexual dysfunction. . . . Since stress is concomitant with an increased output of catecholamines in blood . . . it is reasonable to assume that blood flow to the genital organs reduces during periods of stress. . . . [W]e measured norepinephrine as an indirect index of catecholamine level and found that it increased in the stress group and decreased in the recovery group. This result indirectly supports the suggestion that stress affects female genital blood flow.*[6]

Stress messes with the sex hormones of female rats, and, the authors hypothesize, causes interference in the baseline vaginal actions—neurotransmission, smooth muscle relaxation, and blood vessel engorgement—necessary for female sexual arousal: "[E]stradiol level was significantly reduced in the stress group. It is widely known that sex hormones play important roles in sexual response in males and females. . . . Our data show that vaginal nNOS and eNOS expression in the stress group reduced compared to the control group. . . . Therefore, it is postulated that reduced nNOS and eNOS levels cause reduced neurotransmission, less smooth muscle relaxation, and a lowered vascular blood flow in response to sexual stimuli in the vaginal tissue. Furthermore, this is clinically expressed as a difficulty in arousal response and orgasmic response."[7]

Not only did they find that "bad stress" lowered female rats' sex hormones and interfered with their arousal processes, they also projected that such changes on that physiological level could, if sustained over time, affect vaginal tissue itself. The cranky, stressed, and sexually rejecting female rats, and the more receptive, unstressed control female rats, were all killed, and all the rats' vaginal tissue prepared for sampling: "Tissues were snap-frozen in liquid nitrogen and stored . . . until required." The results of the vaginal tissue analysis showed *biologically measurable* changes in the female rats' vaginal sexual functioning; the Yoon team scientists even projected that changes in the rats' vaginal tissue, caused by stress, would escalate over time: "If such abnormal hormonal profile changes persist for a long time, secondary tissue changes could occur in the vagina."

This is a version of the insight reported anecdotally by Mike Lousada, Katrine Cakuls, and other vaginal-work therapists: *"bad stress" can apparently affect the very tissue of the vagina.*

Lousada did not speculate on the science of this change in vaginal tissue. But these scientists do have a hypothesis: "In the present study, physical stress in female rats induced hormonal and vaginal NOS expression changes and caused observable sexual behavioral changes. We believe that these changes result from multifactorial reactions." In other words, stress in female rats affects the neuroendocrine system and this induces the various secondary changes in the vagina that affect sexual function. "In female rats under chronic stress, sexual behaviors were changed. We suggest that changes of serum sex hormones, catecholamines, and NOS subtype expressions in the vaginal tissues participate in a multifactorial response in chronically stressed female rats."[8]

In other words: stress out female rats, and sooner or later the sexual functioning of their vaginas—with its potential to release pleasure hormones to the female mammalian brain—will suffer as well.

———

Women experience a sense of something like panic when they realize they are trapped inside an environment in which sexually degrading remarks will be directed at them at random. They intuit that they will suffer from this situation when they are present in it, or away from it, when they are trying to relate to their children and friends, when they are trying to turn to their husbands or lovers in bed, or when they are facing their easels or their journals. They are right.

As we have seen with the difference in the protection of the male and female pelvic nerves, a woman is quite vulnerable physically when she has opened her legs—more vulnerable than a man is. Because of this, and because males are generally larger and often stronger, the sense of safety may not be as important to male sexual response as it is to female sexual response. The vagina responds to the sense of female safety, in that circulation expands, including to the vagina, when a woman feels she is safe; but the blood vessels to the vagina constrict when she feels threatened. This may happen before the woman consciously interprets her setting as threatening. So if you continually verbally threaten or demean the vagina in the university or in the workplace, you continually signal to the woman's brain and body that she is not safe. "Bad" stress is daily raising her heart rate, pumping adrenaline through her system, circulating catecholamines, and so on. This verbal abuse *actually* makes it more difficult for her to attend to the professional or academic tasks before her.

Title IX in America is gender-equality legislation that forbids the creation of a "hostile working environment." When women face jokes, images, insults, or implied threats related to their vaginas in the workplace or at school, it *actually* becomes more difficult for them to focus on their work or on their books as well as their male peers can who are not being distracted in this way. It *actually* does create a material disadvantage to them that is bound to be discriminatory, simply because of the way the female brain and body are wired. It *actually* does create a "performative utterance"—words that have real effects in the real world.

Repeated trauma or verbal threats, contemporary neuroscience points out, rewire the brain: a brain that hears verbal abuse often becomes more reactive. Hearing the vagina debased feels, on an amygdala level, like a threat of sexual assault or other kinds of danger. Verbal abuse and threats of violence hurt the brain. This rewiring effect is another reason why language aimed at the vagina and at female sexuality is so abusive. Verbally abusing the vagina is a way—a socially acceptable way—to abuse and affect the wiring of the female brain. If women never hear sexually abusive language, their brains will be less reactive to threats. One could read this politically as: if you don't bully a woman by insulting her vagina, her brain is less intimidated than is the brain of the woman whose vagina is insulted regularly.

And the word widely considered to be the most derogatory, the most violent, the most abusive? *Cunt.* "Somehow every indignity the female suffers ultimately comes to be symbolized in a sexuality that is held to be her responsibility, her shame. . . . It can be summarized in one four-letter word. And the word is not *fuck,* it's *cunt.* Our self-contempt originates in this: in knowing we are cunt," writes Kate Millet in *The Prostitution Papers.*[9] Philologist Matthew Hunt's doctoral dissertation traces the etymology of how *cunt* became equated with "the worst possible thing you can ever call anyone." "Censorship of both the word 'cunt' and the organ to which it refers is symptomatic of a general fear of—and disgust for—the vagina itself," Hunt concludes.[10] Or is it, as I would argue, also a symptom of fear of and disgust for the potential of female power? If you name something in a way that deters pride, exploration, and discovery, you deter the likelihood of women unlocking the chemicals of confidence, creativity, and so on that such discovery might entail.

The citations from Hunt's thesis bear out the fact that the vagina is considered, philologically, "the worst possible thing," in the Western tradition at least: "The vagina, according to many feminist writers, is so taboo as to be virtually invisible in Western culture," writes comparative mythology scholar Lynn Holden. " 'Cunt' is probably the most offensive and censored swearword in the English language."[11] Ruth Wajnryb commented in 2004, "Of all the four-letter words, cunt is easily the most offensive." Journalist Zoe Williams wrote, "It's the rudest word we've got, in the entire language," and commentator Nick Ferrari echoed this as well: "[It's] the worst word in the world . . . I think it's an utterly grotesque word . . . it's just a gutteral, ghastly, nasty word."[12] In her study of Australian prison graffiti, Jacqueline Z. Wilson writes that cunt is "the most confronting word in mainstream Australian English, and perhaps in every major variety of English spoken anywhere." Sarah Westland calls it "the worst insult in the English language," "the nastiest, dirtiest word," "the greatest slur," and "the most horrible word that someone can think of."[13] In her 2011 article "The C-Word: How One Four-Letter Word Holds So Much Power," Christina Caldwell calls *cunt* the "nastiest of nasty words."[14]

Got it? It's the worst of the worst. But the word *cunt* did not be-

gin in all this infamy; indeed, its etymological origins are, like the
vagina itself, quite context specific, and it has ranged from neutral to
very positive to very negative. Linguist Eric Partridge wrote that the
prefix *cu* is an expression of "quintessential femininity": "in the un-
written prehistoric Indo-European . . . languages 'cu' or 'koo' was a
word base expressing 'feminine,' 'fecund' and associated notions."[15]
Linguist Thomas Thorne points out that "the Proto-Indo-European
'cu' is also cognate with other feminine/vaginal terms, such as the
Hebrew 'cus'; the Arabic 'cush,' 'kush,' and 'khunt'; the Nostratic
'kuni' ('woman'); and the Irish 'cuint' ('cunt'). 'Coo' and 'cou' are
modern slang terms for vagina, based on these ancient sounds."[16]

The same root relates to *gud,* which is Indo-European for "enclosure"; it also refers to a *cucuteni* or "womb-shaped Roman vase."
*Cu* has associations with "knowledge" as well: *can* and *ken*—both of
which mean "to know" and possibly even "cognition"—are, Thorne
points out, related to this *coo. Sex* and *knowledge* share a strong linguistic connection: *ken* is "know" and "give birth." *Ken*—which relates to the Old English *cyn* and the Gothic *kuni*—also connotes the
vagina: "['Kin'] meant not only matrilineal blood relations but also a
cleft or crevice, the Goddess's genital opening."[17] Historian Gordon
Rattray Taylor explores the links between femininity and knowledge: "The root cu appears in countless words from cowrie, Cypris,
down to cow; the root cun has two lines of descent, the one empha-
sising the mother and the other knowledge: Cynthia and . . . cunt,
on the one hand, and cunning, on the other."[18] In India, the name of
the goddess Cunti-Devi suggests that "cunt" variants originated not
as insults but as terms of great respect. *Quefen-t,* a "cunt" variant,
was used by the Egyptian pharaoh Ptah-Hotep when he spoke to a
goddess. The earliest *cunt* citation in the *Oxford English Dictionary*
features the word as part of a London street name: around 1230, in
the neighborhood called Southwark, a street called "Gropecunte-
lane" was where prostitutes worked.[19]

Charmingly, many *cunt*-connected words were originally water
related: *cundy* is an "underground water channel"; less charmingly,
*cuniculus* means "passageway" and was used by the ancient Romans

to describe their drainage systems. (*Cunnilingus,* or "vagina tongu-
ing," is one of the *cuni*-related words, of course.) Sanskrit *cushi/
kunthi* meant both "ditch" and "vagina." But the neutral and positive
echoes of *cunt* do not survive widely in our slang. Even Greek and
Latin language around the vagina began as fairly neutral, if male-
centric: *vulva* simply means, in Greek, "matrix"; *vagina* is Latin
for "sheath"; *labia* is Latin for "lips." (Though, granted, *pudendum*
is Latin for "shame.") Outright contempt and disgust do not pre-
dominate in Western vagina names until Victorian slang made words
about the vagina cognate with "the worst." There have always been
negative names for the vagina, as well as positive; but disgust is not
necessarily embedded in the language of the vagina.

Many of us feel a kind of existential shudder when we see the re-
iterated modern connection between *cunt* and *disgusting, stupid,* or
*hateful*—or when women are reduced to just *cunts.* We are continually told to "just relax" about such demeaning language, but there
are good reasons, related to the power of such words to represent
sexually threatening acts that can wreak "multisystem dysregulation" upon us, why we physiologically *can't.*

I experienced firsthand the powerful impact that the words used
to communicate about the vagina can have on the female brain. This
book had just been signed by a publisher, and I was euphoric, in
creative terms, about the research and writing ahead. At the same
time, I was anxious about grappling with such a strong social taboo.
At that point, a friend—a man whom I will call Alan, and describe
as a businessman, who has a complicated sense of humor and enjoys
creating social spectacles that heighten tension—said he wanted to
throw a party celebrating my book deal. The party became a topic of
conversation among his friends, often with a ripple of amusement—
with something oblique in it—as an undercurrent.

"Alan" told me that he was going to do a pasta party, at which
guests could make vagina-shaped pasta. I thought that was a funny
and sort of charming idea, possibly a tribute to the subject matter, or,
at the very least, not awful, though it was not a thematic twist I would
have chosen myself.

When I arrived at the party, though, there was a slightly ominous, mischievous stir at the far end of the loft where the kitchen was located. Alan was in the kitchen, surrounded by a crowd of guests. I made my way there, with some trepidation.

As I walked toward Alan, I passed the table where the pasta maker had been assembled. A group of people stood around the pasta maker—fashioning, indeed, little handmade vulvas. The objects were rather sweet-looking: like the real thing, the little pasta sculptures varied—each person's experience (or body, perhaps) informing his or her interpretation. There was an energy of respect and even would-be celebration from that table, from both the men and the women. So the platter of pasta resting on the table seemed to me to be assembled with a kind of love: flowery or feathery, fluted or fanned, each small sculpture was detailed and distinct: lovely little white objects against a handpainted blue Italian ceramic tray.

Alan appeared at my side. "I call those 'cuntini,'" he said, laughing, and my heart contracted. A flash of tension crossed the faces of many of the women present. The men's faces, which had been so open, and some so tender, became impassive. Something sweet and new, that had barely begun, was already closing down.

I heard a sizzling sound. I looked to the kitchen: the sound was coming from several dozen enormous sausages, ranged in iron skillets on the big industrial stove. I got it: ha, sausages, to go with the "cuntini." I noticed that the energy of the mixed-gender crowd was now not simple. The room had become more tense—the tension that I was familiar with by now, as I was recognizing those moments when women feel demeaned but are expected to "go with it" and have a "sense of humor." My heart contracted further.

Finally, someone called my attention to the final featured item on the evening's menu. On the back burners of the stove, several immense salmon fillets were arranged on another platter. Again: I got it. I got the joke. Women are smelly. Fish-smelling. I flushed, with a kind of despair that was certainly psychological—depression that a friend would think this was funny—but which also felt physical.

But that was not what was really interesting to me about that night. I can deal with a misfired joke, if that was all that the event entailed. What is really interesting to me is that after the "cuntini" party, I could not type a word of the book—not even research notes—for six months, and I had never before suffered from writer's block. I felt—on both a creative and a physical level—that I had been punished for "going somewhere" that women are not supposed to go.

Because of the evidence of physical consequences to women of sexualized stressors, I understand better now what constituted the connection between the visual "comedy," the olfactory public insult, and my fingers being unable to type. But at the time, the six months of writer's block was a mystery.

The theme of the "uppity woman" having her vagina targeted in lieu of her brain is a universal theme still—both in emerging democracies and in the "advanced" West. In Egypt, once part of the British Empire, this practice had an echo: women protesters have played prominent roles in the "Arab Spring" and the uprising in Tahrir Square in 2011–12—and these "unruly" women are being targeted by the state for forced vaginal exams.

Samira Ibrahim, twenty-five, a young Egyptian protester, brought suit against that country's military in 2011, asserting that after the army had arrested her in Tahrir Square during a protest, she was forced to undergo a vaginal examination against her will. And human rights groups report that this is systemic: many women protesters, they confirm, have been forcibly vaginally "examined"—that is, assaulted—by the Egyptian military upon being taken into custody. Ibrahim posted a moving account of her ordeal on YouTube, describing how she and other female protesters had been first beaten, electrocuted, and accused of being prostitutes (echoes again of the Contagious Diseases Acts of 1864–66 in Britain); then forced to undergo a vaginal exam, a "virginity test," performed by a soldier in army fatigues in front of dozens of strangers. An army spokesman defended the forced vaginal "exams": "We didn't want them to say we had sexually assaulted or raped them, so we wanted to prove they weren't virgins in the first place," a military source explained to the news site Al Jazeera.

"When I came out, I was destroyed, physically, mentally and emotionally," Ibrahim said.[20]

Could that, given the delicate workings of the ANS in women, and the connection of vagina to brain, of emotional sexual trauma to the biology of chronic suffering—have been the point? Is this not a sign of random brutality—but a technique to suppress revolution, and tamper with the very chemical makeup of potential revolution?

In the West, where actual vaginal assault or traumatic sexual "exams" are not legal, female verbal insurrection is also routinely met with threats against the vagina and verbal rape. (Though the United States may be moving toward physical aggression by the state against women's decision making, via violation of the vagina, in the form of recent American states' proposals to legislate a mandatory invasive transvaginal ultrasound if a woman is considering choosing an abortion.)

Women in the West who "speak out" experience this sex-directed aggression: Vanessa Thorpe and Richard Rogers, in the UK newspaper *The Observer,* reported that female commentators regularly receive threats of sexual assault. Caroline Farrow, a blogger for *Catholic Voices,* reports that she receives "at least five sexually threatening emails a day," which she sees as the result of her taking responsibility for her own views by posting under her own name, with a photo that, she says, seems to make her harassers see her as "a legitimate sexual target." She notes, "One of the 'least obscene' emails read: 'You're going to scream when you get what you've asked for. Bitch.' " *Guardian* commentator and novelist Linda Grant and feminist nonfiction writer Natasha Walter both report that, as a result of sexually violent comments directed at their writing, they now write less often online. The *New Statesman* journalist Helen Lewis-Hasteley confirms that rape threats are the most prevalent form of online harassment of women writers in Britain: "I know many people will say that every commentator on the Internet gets abuse, but what really came through to me when I was looking at this [in the experience of other female journalists] was the modus operandi of the attackers, which was to use the rape threat." "The threat of sexual violence is an attack in itself," concludes the *Observer* article.[21] The science is now in as to why that is correct.

Sexualized fear drives out creativity in women because fear elicits a tension response, and our creativity in particular, because of the role of the ANS, demands a relaxation response. Whenever a woman's sexuality is insulted, her creativity suffers—because the same relaxed and focused state needs to be protected in order for the irrational wellsprings to be tapped: the same relaxation and focus supports arousal and orgasms, babies, books, artwork, criticism, and music. When you honor a woman's sexuality and her very sex, you support the optimal functioning of the physical systems that support her intellectual creativity; when you threaten and insult her sexuality and her very sex, you do exactly the opposite.

# How Funny Was That?

---

*Q: What's the difference between a pussy and a cunt?*
*A: A pussy is a sweet, juicy, succulent, warm, fun and useful*
*thing. The cunt is the thing that owns it.*

—jokes4us.com, "Vagina Jokes"

The more I understood about the vagina, and how sensitive it is to the emotional environment—and also how frankly creatively and intellectually precious its well-being is—the less able I was to screen out, dismiss, or numb myself to the casual insults and abuse that even the nicest people in our culture take for granted as normal in commonplace discussion. After I had traveled to England in the spring of 2011, had finished my interviews with Dr. Richmond, Nancy Fish, and Mike Lousada, and seen the stress research by H. Yoon and colleagues about the effect of stress on the vagina, and the research by Alessandra Rellini and Cindy Meston on how sexual trauma elevates women's baseline nervous system responses, and the new data on sexual trauma and multisystem dysregulation and its relationship to chronic pain in many women, I felt that I had a deeper understanding of the vagina's emotional sensitivity and its connection to emotional and intellectual sensitivity in women in general. And I was continually reassessing the meaning of rape and reperceiving its effects in an increasingly complicated and far more enduring light.

I had been very deeply affected by my Skype interview with Lousada under the trees at the beautiful medieval college, and I felt that it had changed me, in a way. I returned to New York in June of that year feeling unusually open and free myself. I was not at all romantically interested in Lousada—I was very much in love with someone else. But there was something about his being a man who was so committed to actually witnessing the sexual suffering of women, and so dedicated to their sexual liberation, that made me feel existentially more hopeful that men and women could understand one another at last around these issues. Something about his discussion of how trauma "locks" the female body and mind had unlocked something in me. Though I have never been sexually assaulted, I have experienced the typical share of harassment and a couple of scary situations. I am surrounded, as any woman is, by a sexually (and vaginally) contemptuous culture. I had returned feeling hopeful, but also strangely vulnerable and undefended.

One night I went down to the docks near Battery Park to join friends on the same sailboat on which I had first interviewed Dr. Richmond the year before. It was a fresh, late-spring night. Two young women were guests for that evening's sail, and three male friends of mine, who were older than the young women, were on board as well. The young women were not dating any of the men, but that possibility was in the air. We motored out of the mooring ground by the park and sped onto the dark Hudson under a nearly full moon. I remember how I felt—renewed, in an odd way; light, rich, fertile with ideas, but unguarded.

We sailed alongside the glittering lights of the city, past the sparkling canyons of lower Manhattan. Clouds sped across the neon-bright face of the moon. I chatted with a friend I will call Trevor, one of the three men on board. He is a kind and caring man, a solid citizen, with three kids and a lovely wife. My friend Alex was handling the ropes. I asked Trevor what he was reading these days.

"War stories," he confessed. "I had to stop reading modern fiction. I found that most modern fiction is written for women, and I couldn't really get into it. I had to face the fact that that wasn't for me, that I like war stories. I like stories about combat, and tactics, and sex."

"There isn't usually sex in a war story," remarked our friend Stephen, who was steering the boat.

"There's rape," joked Trevor and Alex, simultaneously.

Both of these men are nice men. And part of my brain immediately, routinely declared: "That was just a joke. Dismiss it." But something had happened to me in England: I had had a glimpse of a world in which men respected what, for lack of a better language, I was starting to think of as the Sacred Feminine—or even as "the Goddess"—and I glimpsed the harm such language did, to me and to the women around me. For once, I was not numbed to those eternal jokes, those rape jokes, those pussy jokes. I felt the slashing harm of it. A great lump rose in my throat; I excused myself to go down into the hold.

I lay down on one of the bunks. The hold swayed beneath me, as I was held over the dark, open river. I closed my eyes. I felt the pain of the words cutting again, like a scimitar, ripping into what I can only describe as my energy field; pain that I never would have even noticed before in brushing those words off, or "arguing" with the jokers, intellectually. I was in touch with my own "pelvic emotions," I suppose, in an unmediated way, and so felt the violence of those words—words that were not even intended as malicious—a carelessness that only made it worse, in a way; words that were "merely" as insensitive to harm to the feminine as I had been myself.

I took deep breaths—but something very odd happened. Tears started to slide from under my closed lids and down my cheeks. I wasn't sobbing. I was just almost too full of feelings. I lay perfectly still, but the tears slid and slid from under my lids, and splashed down my neck and throat, in a way that I had never experienced before. I lay like that—relaxed, without sobbing, just tearing up again and again, welling over with tears—for fifteen or twenty minutes. I thought of the young women above deck, who had also heard those words and who now, I knew, would be ever so slightly changed by them; who would be ever so slightly more closed down physically, or ever so slightly more spiritually or creatively dampened by them. I felt the grief of it.

The sexual threats encoded in hostile language centered on the vagina do more than trigger stress reactions in our bodies. Cultural concepts become embedded in a woman's body and her brain perceptually. As University of Michigan psychologist Richard E. Nisbett demonstrated, in his book *The Geography of Thought,* the brains of people from different cultures *neurally encode cultural differences in perception* through daily practice over time. For example, his research showed that Westerners tend to perceive through a narrow focus on singular objects, while Easterners used a wide-angle lens and see objects as contextually embedded.

So a woman's cultural "take" on her vagina also shapes her brain.[1]

If a woman hears about her vagina as a "gash" or a "slit" all her life, then that perception of her vagina will become neurally encoded in her brain; whereas if she hears about it, for example, as "the jade gate," her brain shapes itself and her perceptions around that sensibility.

In Han dynasty China (206 BCE–220 CE) or India fifteen hundred years ago or in thirteenth-century Japan, when the vagina was portrayed as the most sacred spot in the most sacred temple in a sacred universe, that was how woman's brains experienced their vaginas. When, as in medieval Europe during the witch hunts, the culture cast the vagina as the devil's playground and the gateway to hell, a woman in that culture felt herself to be built up around a core of existential shame. If, as in Elizabethan England, a culture portrays the vagina as a hole, a woman in that culture will feel that she is centered around emptiness or worthlessness; when, as in Germany and England and America after Freud, a woman's culture portrays the vagina's response as a test of womanliness, she is likely to feel herself insufficiently womanly. When a woman's culture—as in today's women's magazine-type sexual athleticism in the West—casts the ideal vagina as a producer of multiple orgasms on call, she will feel herself put to a continual, impossible test. When mass culture represents any given vagina as just one in ten million available orifices, as in today's porn industry, a woman will feel her sexual self to be replaceable, not important and not sacred.

And all this is not superficial: these perceptions are constructed at the level of neural synapses. In other words, the female brain changes physically over time in response to these kinds of repeated triggers in the environment.

These triggers also affect her confidence and sense of hope. In a lecture I give on female sexuality, there's a moment when I ask the women in the room to recall the names they first heard used in relation to their vaginas, when they were fourteen or fifteen—passing by construction sites, or while walking in the street. I can feel the deep discomfort of, say, eight hundred women all at once remembering where they were at the moment when, just coming into womanhood, they first heard—directed toward them—such phrases as "sit on my face" or "give me some of that thing" (or, as at least one young Asian American woman has recalled, "Give me some of that slanty pussy"). "How did that make you feel?" I ask. "Did it make you feel: 'Is this what I am, this shameful—or this vulgar—thing?' " Then—those emotions still raw in the room—I have the pleasure of reading them a list of other terms for *vagina* from other cultures. "Golden lotus," I read, from the Chinese Han and Ming dynasties' love poetry. "Scented bower." "Gates of Paradise." "Precious pearl." Chinese Taoist terms are always just as poetic: the vagina is referred to in Taoist sacred texts such as *Art of the Bedchamber* as "Heavenly Gate," "Red Ball," "Hidden Place," "Jade Door," "Jade Gate," "Mysterious Valley," "Mysterious Gate," and "Treasure."[2]

One could go much further: in sacred Tantric texts, vaginas are classified into categories, but all the categories are fairly affectionate: the Chitrini-Yoni (the yoni of a "fancy woman") is "rounded and soft, and easily and quickly lubricated, with little pubic hair. Her love-juice is said to be exceptionally hot, to smell sweet and to taste as honey." The Hastini-Yoni "is large and deep, and enjoys much stimulation of the clitoris." The yoni of the Padmini ("lotus-woman") is "like a flower and loves to absorb the sun's rays—that is, to be seen in daylight—and the caress of strong hands. Her juices have the fragrance of a freshly blossoming lotus flower." The yoni of the Shankhini (the "fairy" or "conch-woman") is "always moist . . . covered with much hair and . . . love[s] being kissed and licked."[3] Hindu vagina iconography sometimes referred to a vagina-mind connection that the West seemed determined to obscure: one Hindu synonym for vagina is "Lotus of her Wisdom."

"What if it were always like that?" I ask my audience. "What if the words you heard as a girl and young woman made you think of yourself—in the most intimate, sexual sense—as a source of wisdom, as precious, fragrant, a treasure?" To be surrounded by comparably reverent or appreciative language about one's sexuality would make women not only more open sexually, but it would also make them more able to function in the world in ways that increased their creativity, strength, and sense of connection.

I often read the women in the room a passage from the Ming dynasty–era Chinese masterpiece *The Golden Lotus,* and it is really erotic.[4] But it's a different kind of Eros than they are used to: the philosophers and courtiers of the Han dynasty saw gratified female sexuality as the force that kept the universe in harmonious order. They believed that men's greatest health, wisdom, and potential could be developed only by becoming masters at pleasing women, and thus enjoying the potent yin essence that emanated only from the intimate parts of a truly aroused and ultimately fulfilled woman. When I am done with the passage—when my audience has heard the language of admiration with which the Han poets describe the art of love, and in the midst of it, their adoration of the vagina—everyone's face is flushed, and the women tend to burst into a spontaneous cheer.

There is certainly something steamy in thinking about our own sexuality—our own vaginas—in such a tender, admiring context; but there is also something empowering in the act. Having gone on an imaginative journey to other times, places, and contexts in which the vagina is spoken of reverentially, these contemporary women leave the room feeling different. They walk out energized and slightly giddy, as if newly in possession of a wonderful secret. You can feel that they will make different decisions, enjoy themselves in new ways.

Language is powerful. As Virginia Woolf said, talking about another kind of arousal—intellectual arousal—"One cannot think well, love well, sleep well, if one has not dined well. The lamp in the spine does not light on beef and prunes."[5] She meant—and she was right—that the body and the imagination are interdependent.

In our culture, the female body's sexual imagination must ignite itself with meager linguistic kindling: the very word *vagina* is hard to say. It is an antierotic word, in a way (that annoyingly buzzy *v*, that unpleasantly soft *g*). When you think *vagina* in our culture (or search for it on Google, or look on Amazon), you get associations that are either coldly, repellently clinical ("vaginal herpes," "vaginal discharge") or at least tediously health related ("vaginal tone"). At the other end of the spectrum of associations, it's just porn. It is almost impossible to daily feel one's essence as a woman to be exciting, mysterious, profound, and complex if the language swirling around the center of our being is tacky or medicalized, hostile or reductively hard-core.

Do your own experiment, if you are a woman. Reread the excerpts of Anaïs Nin and Henry Miller earlier in the book. Observe what happens inside of you as you read the text—even if it might cause you some stress. As you compare the Nin to the Miller, note what happens to the sense of relaxation or tension in your muscles, to your heart rate—is it lowered or elevated, or is there no change? Pay attention to your vaginal pulse, if you are aware of it; pay attention to your breathing, and to whether you feel a generalized sense of calm or anxiety.

Over the course of researching this book, I noticed that as I read texts that described the vagina in different ways, the descriptions directly affected my sense of energy and general well-being. After a morning reading Nin, for example, the world glowed. After an afternoon—in the same chair in the sun, with the same bougainvillea waving over my head—of reading Miller, I felt ill and weak, and very much like taking a shower.

How far we have come from the honey and seashells of the female modernists. Onlineslangdictionary.com, a website that aggregates slang terms, lists the following contemporary violent slang for *vagina:* "axe wound," "hatchet wound," "open wound," and "wounded soldier."[6] In response to the query "What are slang terms for vagina?" the answers at Yahoo.com included the violent-sounding "hole," "gash," "slash," "slit," and so on.

The following conversation occurred on a mixed-gender discussion site when it asked for slang terms for *vagina.* It did not ask for "hostile slang terms for *vagina.*" While the respondents are self-selected, the site is a mainstream one. I repeat the discussion intact, punctuated for clarity. Listen for the language of violence and derision.

ANDY: I saw a few nominations for best slang word for "vagina" dotted about so I thought it'd be best to put them down in one place. My two favourites are "gash" and "clunge." The best thing about gash is you can add other words to it to describe a lady's level of arousal . . . "frothing at the gash"; "she must have turned the temperature of her clunge up to gash mark 6."

. . .

DAVID: "Meat curtain."

ZOE: "Half eaten steak sandwich," "gutted rabbit," "vertical seafood taco," "corned beef curtains in white sauce," . . . "motor," "minge," "pouch."

LEWIS: "Butcher's dustbin."

STEVE: "V-hole."

STEVEN: "Cock-holster," . . . "Poonany," . . . "Quim," . . . "Snatch. . . ."

ANNA [one of the few women on the site, interjecting wailingly]: "clunge": bahahah.

JOSH [undeterred by this self-deprecating gentle protest]: "Beef eating spunk bubble."

KIN: "Hairy mussel," "the Snack That Smiles Back."

STEVE: "Cockpocket."

DANIEL: Of course the normal "minge," "tuna bap [sandwich]," "the fish plate," "doner kebab," "trout pouch"; but personally I think there should be more words for "fanny batter [vaginal lubrication]."

ANDY: A "sleeping fruit bat" could be used for a lady with rather large, dangling flaps. "Pink velvet sausage wallet," "quim."

STEVE: "Quim" is definitely awesome, as is "quinny" which I saw in that movie *Elizabeth*.

ANDREW: I like "badly packed kebab," for an untidy one. The old ones are the best though: "pussy," "fanny," and "twat." "Hairy fish pie" is nice.

ANDY: I haven't seen "mott" or "motty" (or is it "motti"?) anywhere on here yet. . . . "Get motty out for us, Petal."

DANIEL: Oh, forgot: "flange."

I think most women would agree that the terms above range from kind of awful to really awful—to hear or even to think about. (Another site adds the equally repellent "ass mate" and "bearded oyster.")

It is striking how many of the young male slang terms for vagina on these discussion boards have to do with meat: violent images of meat prepared for consumption, as in "butcher's dustbin" (in British usage, a *dustbin* is a garbage can; a "butcher's dustbin" is where unwanted, discarded meat scraps would end up) or else low-grade, junk-food, industrialized meat, also prepared for consumption:

"badly packed kebab," "sausage wallet," "pink taco," "beef eating spunk bubble." One is not invoking champagne and caviar here, but neither do these terms have the heavily socially insulting echoes ("cunt") of the recent past. Rather, most of these half-gross, grossly half-funny terms just connote something fleshy with which it would be unappetizing to be sexual. Other sites list contemporary slang terms that are not violent or meatlike, but that are a bit silly: "bikini bizkit," "cherry pop," "chuff," "furburger," "beaver," and "grumble." The only even slightly positive or endearing terms that I saw on contemporary slang websites were "honeysuckle," the Elizabethan "quim"—mentioned above—the affectionate "hush puppy" and "lick-me-please," and the rather dear "passion fruit" and "Southern Belle." "Map of Tassie/Mapatazi [Map of Tasmania]" is popular in Australia, apparently—the island of Tasmania is an upside-down triangle. Other sites note the wretched "panty hamster," "vertical bacon sandwich," and "Velcro triangle."

A very few other slang sites have a very few less appalling terms. From Blackchampagne.com, we learn about slang terms for *clitoris* that include "the sugared almond" and, from African American slang, the rather lovely "pearltongue." [7]

This slang suggests that Western young men today do not identify vaginas with the dark magic of the past nor with its more viciously insulting associations; instead, most of the terms connote low-grade, mass-produced junk food and don't carry much of an emotional wallop. Does this shift have something to do with the way pornography portrays the vagina: that is, exactly like "sausage wallets"? Does it have to do with the way pornography is produced—in mass units, like junk food—or with the way sex is represented in pornography—as fast and interchangeable, like junk food? And with the way in which pornography is consumed, especially by this generation that was sexually initiated on it—casually and repetitively, like junk food?

Does this slang reveal that pornography has achieved the opposite of what Andrea Dworkin feared? Rather than frantically driving men to rape the vagina, does pornography lead many young men raised on it today to view the vagina with relaxed or even desensitized emotional distance, as something only slightly more compelling, and perhaps slightly less efficiently packaged, than a microwavable burrito?

Women are trying to "talk back" or "name back." A girl-power website, Tressugar.com, lists woman-friendly terms for the vagina—doubtless to counter all the negative slang terms that exist in abundance. The site was assembled by Western women in their twenties. You can clearly see from it that these young women in our post-sexual-revolution, postfeminist context see their vaginas not as dark and foreboding, nor as potently alluring and overwhelmingly compelling. Rather, they see them as cute and nonthreatening: the vagina is a little fluffy Hello Kitty buddy, or a sweet treat; metaphors merge, like a box of Jujubes wrapped in glitter and fur.

The site also encourages women to send in their own terms for *vagina* to counter hostile or unpleasant male-derived slang. Some of these young women's favorite terms evoke deliciousness: "yum yum," "honey pot," and "goodies"; others refer to furry accessories or fluffy pets: "muff," "beaver," "kitty." Other young lexicographers seem to name their vaginas as if they were funny little siblings, the way some men have affectionate nicknames for their penises: "cooter," "poon."

A current women's magazine ad for vaginal deodorant, repackaged as vaginal "wash"—yes, that product from the benighted 1960s has resurfaced—shows a grinning redheaded model in a very short bright-yellow frock with her arms in the air, in a kind of "lady bits power" salute, cheering, "WooHoo for my FrooFroo!" The ad continues: "mini, twinkle, hoo haa, flower, fancy, yoni, lady garden . . ." and goes on to warn (always the warning)—"Did you know that some regular shower gels and soaps, if used on your privates, could strip it of its natural defenses, causing dryness and irritation? With its ph-balanced formula, especially developed for intimate skin, Femfresh washes are one of the kindest ways to care for your vajay-jay, kitty, nooni, lala, froo froo! Whatever you call it, make sure you love it." The sloganeers sign off by adding that Femfresh offers "Extra Care for Down There."

The your-vagina-smells-bad shame of the douche ads of the 1960s has been replaced with cheery faux empowerment language for yet another invented product, but is "hoo haa" and "froo froo" (I couldn't help thinking of the characters from the children's television show *Teletubbies*, brightly colored infantile creatures named Tinky Winky, Ditsy, Laa Laa, and Po)—or even "muff," "kitty," or "yum yum"—as far as we want to get on our "lady garden" journey?

Elsewhere in the recent tabloid or popular press, other girl-power approaches to the naming of the vagina have surfaced: Marian Keyes, the popular Irish novelist, called her vagina, hilariously, the "growler." An American tabloid reports that Jennifer Love Hewitt, the star of the hit television show *The Ghost Whisperer*, "vajazzles" her "vajayjay"—that is, puts crystals around it—before a big date.

Why speak out in a media context and offer more positive names for the vagina? Naming in public is different from private action—it has an element of the political; naming constructs reality. And just as women have suffered quietly for centuries, so now they understandably wish to assert the right to name in ways that are affectionate, or charming, or at least not quite so awful.

There is gain and loss in how these apparently empowered women name the vagina: for the better, the vagina is no longer the abyss, or the gateway to hell; for worse, neither is it any longer very powerful, let alone the center of the universe.

Alarming or dismissable or "cute," vaginas are now everywhere in the culture, like wallpaper, but the magic and power of the vagina are almost nowhere in Western culture or Western naming—or are very hard to perceive.

According to anthropologists, some people in Sri Lanka believe that with the arrival of electric light, ghosts, with their omens, fled. In Ireland, some people say that the fairies, with their blessings, have retreated in the face of modern life. In our contemporary lexicon, the vagina has been similarly denuded of its mystery, no longer haunted by ghosts and demons, nor any longer charmed with magic.

# The Pornographic Vagina

*There have probably been days when I saw 300 vaginas before I got out of bed.*

—Rock musician John Mayer, *Playboy*

Not only has the vagina lost some of its magic: the men who are engaged with the vagina are losing some magic of their own. It is becoming clear that a plethora of vaginas on call makes some men slightly crazy, and not in a good way; porn, now ubiquitous, is, it appears, rewiring the male brain.

An increasing problem for the vagina, and the whole life of the woman who owns that vagina, is that porn affects men neurologically, to their detriment. There is evidence that it is also habituating many men to become bored with "the Goddess Array"—the many gestures and caresses women's autonomic nervous systems (ANSs) need—and to fast-forward past it.

"Ordinary" sex is no longer stimulating enough to many men who are heavy porn users. So there is a trend toward anal (often violent anal) penetration and anal climax as the "goal" of the sexual action.

I began to realize what a systemic problem this might be turning into when I spoke on two very different college campuses within a space of a couple of months. At a liberal, anything-goes Massachusetts state college—after a discussion focused on the campus culture of drunken anonymous sex, colloquially called "hooking up"—an anguished student health counselor stood up and asked me what I could do to help her with a terrible problem she was seeing: the number one medical issue young women presented in her clinic was, I was amazed to learn, anal fissures.

"Anal fissure" is the euphemism for anal tearing, an injury that young women can sustain in the unskilled, often drunken, impersonal, sometimes unsafe sex that is common in a "hookup" culture. These young women had repeatedly told the counselor that young men on campus expected that kind of sex because of porn, and that they felt obliged to make themselves available for it accordingly, especially if they wanted a "hookup" to turn into a potential date or relationship down the road.

The following month, I spoke at a buttoned-down, highly religious Mormon university in the Midwest. Another anguished student body health counselor stood up and asked me what I could do to help her with the number one health issue young women presented in her clinic—anal fissures. On that campus, there was strong social pressure for girls to maintain their virginity until marriage. Young men were urging anal sex to the young women as a way to have sex, while still preserving the young women's "virginity."

I am not stigmatizing anal sex for consenting adults who know what they are doing (though pelvic tearing of any kind is not good for the female or male neural network). But there is increasingly substantial evidence that the ubiquity of and ease of access to contemporary pornography—which has turned away from the kinds of caressing and stimulation that turn women on, demoted the vagina, and emphasizes often violent penetration—promotes the kind of lovemaking that increases the sexual and emotional dissatisfaction of women—dissatisfaction that we saw in the 1997 and 2004 national sexual satisfaction surveys. Male exposure to pornography (and, increasingly, female exposure to it) has increased in amounts so meteoric as to be scarcely meaningfully measurable since the *Hite Report on Female Sexuality.* Female sexual satisfaction, and sexual honesty about female needs, have decreased. Could there be a connection?

If, as the study reported above in the *Daily Mail* suggests, in any group of one hundred couples, 85 percent of the men think their female partner has reached climax—but only 61 percent of the women have actually done so—could it be that porn's often bizarre or theatrical representation of female sexual response could be leading many men to misread their own intimate situations?

The danger here is not just about how men's consumption of pornography may affect their perceptiveness about the signs of female desire, arousal, and satisfaction in the immediate sex act. Pornography also appears to be presenting another less obvious, though major, problem to heterosexual women as well: the evidence is in that chronic masturbation to porn sexually desensitizes men overall. When many women react instinctively against their male mate's porn use, they may feel irrational—especially as our culture has a "relax and enjoy it," or "it's harmless," or even "it's positive; it spices up your sex life" attitude to porn consumption. But, in fact, recent data show that the exact opposite turns out to be the case: pornography leaches men's virility, and watching it is now confirmed to be potentially addictive for many men who have a vulnerability to this kind of addictive response in general.

A happy heterosexual vagina requires, to state the obvious, a virile man. Currently, the general assumption is that what happens in the male brain as a man masturbates to porn is no one's business but his own. But in fact, neurologically, what happens to a man's brain at that moment is eventually likely to have a negative effect on his body and thus on his partner's body—and then on her brain as well. Women are not wrong if they react instinctively—often jealously— against their partner's interest in porn, since pornography is actually, neurologically, a woman's destructive rival for her man's sexual capabilities. The more attuned a man is to masturbating to porn, the less sexual vigor he may have, eventually, for himself or for his human lover.

In 2003, I wrote an essay in *New York* magazine called "The Porn Myth," which pointed out that therapists and sex counselors were seeing a correlation between the rise in porn use among healthy young men and a rise in impotence issues and problems with delayed ejaculation in the same group.[1] These young men, who had no organic or psychological reason to have problems with virility, were, their physicians and therapists reported, having trouble sustaining erections; and ejaculations were often difficult for them to achieve, or were delayed. The hypothesis among these experts was that heavy porn use was progressively desensitizing these men sexually. The science behind this anecdotal evidence was not yet fully established.

After the article's publication, I was flooded by distressed—and distressing—e-mails from men who reported that what I described had happened to them. They were distraught. They wrote to me that, over time, they felt a need to watch more and more porn to achieve arousal at all; they felt less and less choice about whether or not to use it; and they were experiencing escalating sexual difficulty in bed with their girlfriends or wives, to whom they had previously been very attracted. These men were a perfectly "normal" cross section of people with no apparent axe to grind; they had no ideological objections to porn use in general, and were not "crusaders"—they were just suffering, and frightened. What really struck me about their e-mails was that haunting sense many had of a loss of choice; these were often men who were perfectly in control in most or all other areas of their lives, and they were writing to me about feeling themselves to be at the mercy of something in their lives over which they felt powerless.

Since that piece was published, a great deal of new data on the effect of pornography on the reward system of the male brain have accumulated, which explains these men's self-reported sexual unhappiness and loss of virility more concretely. Masturbating to porn delivers a strong short-term dopamine boost to the male brain, which, for an hour or two afterward, lifts men's mood and makes them feel good in general. This effect works along the same neural circuitry as, say, gambling or cocaine use. But, just as gambling and cocaine use can trigger addictive behavior, so can porn use when it becomes part of what Dr. Jim Pfaus calls "an OCD-type response" of chronic masturbation to porn that researchers are finding to be not uncommon.[2] This may sound like Victorian language, but researchers on male porn addiction describe "OCD-type chronic masturbation" to porn in which men feel compelled to masturbate many times in succession, or finally lose interest in other aspects of their lives and feel no ability to constrain their need to view porn in the context of compulsive masturbation.

Dr. Pfaus explains the neuroscience of porn addiction:

> [W]*ith each ejaculation, as with orgasm, you are turning on refractoriness. You've got the hit of opioid, serotonin, and endo-cannabinoid. This produces ecstasy, satiety, and sedation. With each successive ejaculation, for chronic masturbators, the inhibition gets stronger—because of the increased serotonin—making it less likely for these men to achieve another erection, much less another ejaculation. To counteract this, these individuals require access to stimuli that will activate increasingly their SNS [sympathetic nervous system]. That is why people who chronically masturbate to porn habituate to erotic material and need more and more intense imagery that more arrestingly activates the SNS. The reason this happens to some people and not others is the frequency of use. It's like smoking or drinking—occasional use is fine, but frequent or neurologically chronic use can get you addicted. And addiction is always a risk of use at all. The danger here is "chronic" and the OCD nature of the masturbation. It's not the porn per se but its use in chronic or obsessive masturbation. The addiction is not actually to the porn but to the orgasm and the predictability of the reward.*[3]

Add to that picture the fact that some men (and women) are born with what is called by those who treat porn addiction "a dopamine hole": their brains don't produce reward with the same efficiency as other brains, so they are much more likely to become addicted to more extreme porn (and other stimulants) more easily. This situation can make some men who have this vulnerability impotent, or suffer delayed ejaculation, after consistent masturbation to porn. But in other men, this vulnerability, combined with high levels of masturbation to porn, can affect sexual impulse control. Some unfortunate men can suffer from *both* problems as a result of their dopamine dysregulation.

As with any addiction, it is very difficult, for neurochemical reasons, for an addict to stop doing even very self-destructive things that allow him to get that next reward. A man with dysregulated dopamine processing, chronically masturbating to porn, might become more addicted to sex chat lines than other men, or engage in other kinds of sexual acting-out that he is ashamed of and wishes to control. But far more seriously, in terms of our focus here, masturbation to porn can lead men in general to develop sexual "habituation" problems—desensitization that leads to problems getting hard and staying hard, or problems with ejaculation. The more vaginas a man masturbates to in an unmediated, online, click-through format, the more habituated to this stimulus he will become, and the less able he is to engage in the sustained, patient, slowly arousing attention to "the Goddess Array" that "deep orgasm" for women requires.

As biologist Robert Sapolsky explained in his book about the biology of desire and satiation, *Why Zebras Don't Get Ulcers:*

> *Unnaturally strong explosions of synthetic experience and sensation and pleasure evoke unnaturally strong degrees of habituation. This has two consequences. As the first, soon we hardly notice anymore the fleeting whispers of pleasure caused by leaves in autumn, or by the lingering glance of the right person, or by the promise of reward that will come after a long, difficult, and worthy task. The other consequence is that, after awhile, we even habituate to those artificial deluges of intensity. . . . Our tragedy is that we just become hungrier.*
>
> *Thanks to the way our brains work, chronic over-stimulation fails to satisfy; it can leave a person nearly insatiable [for more*

*levels of stimulation]. Someone may find himself wondering automatically about every woman, "Would she engage in . . . ?" Also, any resentment that arises from the mismatch between his virtual reality and his physical reality may raise doubts about his partner/union, making him uncharacteristically irritable and self-absorbed. He'll focus on what his relationship doesn't offer, not on what it does. Nor does dissatisfaction necessarily stop there. Humans tend to project such feelings automatically onto other aspects of life as well . . . sadly, distorted perception born of neurochemical dysregulation can make a person extremely resistant to understanding what's really driving him or what would ease his misery. His limbic brain has him firmly convinced that only his drug of choice will restore his good feelings.*

 *It can take an uncomfortable month or two to restore normal perception after habitual overstimulation. But as ravenous feelings ease, it's easier to find satisfaction in every aspect of life.*[4]

This escalation of the need for stimulation to achieve the same level of arousal is why trends in porn are for images that are more and more extreme. The relatively soft lighting and nonviolent pacing of the Emanuelle-branded adult films of the 1980s have given way to porn sites that render mainstream desires for quite violent sex, or sex with apparently very young girls, or incestuous situations, which used to be considered quite marginal or fetishistic. Some of this change in content may be because our culture is more sexually open overall, and less invested in moral judgments about individuals' sex lives than it once was; but some of this escalation of extreme images is also, according to the science, the result of porn users' overall desensitization. The OCD nature of chronic masturbation to porn means that the next time a porn user sees that image that last turned him on, it is not going to turn him on as much. This is why pornography trends tend to become more and more extreme over time—to migrate, say, from missionary position consensual sex to violent anal rape, or to images that arouse the SNS through breaking such taboos as incest taboos or taboos against sexualizing minors.

Even strip club ads have evolved rapidly in the direction of more extreme imagery. In Manhattan, the Private Eyes Gentlemen's Club advertises with signs on top of taxicabs. A few years ago, the women's faces in such ads simply looked fetching and seductive. About a year ago, the women began to gaze into the camera with an expression that was slightly frightened or angry, as if they were confronting some kind of violation. Recently, I noticed, faintly but unmistakably, on a sign for the Private Eyes strip club on a yellow taxicab on a city street—that is, not on a fetish website or buried in a grimy publication—that on the upper cheekbone of a lovely model advertising the club, there was now a single drop. Was it a tear?

It is common to condemn heterosexual men for their interest in looking at women who are not their partners. But, according to Christopher Ryan and Cacilda Jethá's *Sex at Dawn,* men have to contend with the "Coolidge effect," a biological phenomenon in which men may respond sexually to a new partner with greater arousal. (Females have a similar spike in arousal with a new partner.) The Coolidge effect has been demonstrated in male rats; nothing perks a male rat up more readily than the introduction into his cage of an unfamiliar female. In humans, as Dr. Helen Fisher has demonstrated also in *The Anatomy of Love,* erotic excitement shoots up when a man or woman has sex with a new partner, but that excitement subsides over time.[5] (Fewer people know that while, all things being equal, male rats choose novelty, if they are primed to associate scent with postorgasmic good feeling, they will choose their familiar scented partner—who is associated with that good feeling—over a more novel or younger "wife."[6])

The problem for contemporary men is that the novelty effect of new partners did not evolve in an environment in which hundreds or thousands of naked or copulating women emerged at a signal to make themselves visually available to men until men were done masturbating to orgasm at the sight of them. Rather, the male brain evolved in a context in which the sight of a naked or copulating woman was extremely rare, and typically arrived at arduously—thus making it very, very exciting. This arousal and dopamine response was keyed to having actual sex with an actual woman after a specific courtship hunt, raising dopamine levels.

YourBrainOnPorn.com, which tracks the science of porn use and addiction, presents findings that make the case that porn has a similar effect on the brain that junk food has on the body, as does the book *Cupid's Poisoned Arrow* by Marnia Robinson, who manages the site with Gary Wilson.[7] Gary Wilson also presented a summary of the research on porn and male sex problems in a TED talk: "The Great Porn Experiment." The science shows that with dopamine activation and opioid release, men who use porn are bonding with the porn.

Robinson writes, "As psychiatrist Norman Doidge recounts in *The Brain That Changes Itself,* adults have no sense of the extent to which pornography reshapes their brains. His patients report increasing difficulty in being turned on by their actual sexual partners, girlfriends and spouses, though they still consider them objectively attractive. They try to persuade their lovers to act like porn stars, and they are increasingly interested in 'fucking' as opposed to 'making love.' Humanity is running a massive, uncontrolled experiment, and we don't yet know the results. However, there's increasing evidence that there's no free lunch."[8]

Porn sites, by offering abundant "free samples," intentionally seek to engage this addictive response, to use it to boost profits. The tactic is successful: the porn industry is now larger than conventional film, records, books, and video combined (and Viagra sales constitute a multimillion-dollar-per-year industry in the United States alone). The mass-produced, fast-forward, pornographic vagina is to the real vagina what highly processed or GMO food is to slow-grown or to organic food, and it has parallel negative effects on the consumer.

We should deal with the dilemma of modern men—urged by massive industries into an addictive relationship to porn—with empathy rather than hostility. Almost no one has warned men adequately about the problems they may have with their virility—let alone their free will—once they introduce this free, compelling image stream into their neurological environment. The men who wrote to me about their porn addiction and potency problems were not monsters; they were suffering men who were loving husbands and boyfriends, who hated the pain they were causing their partners, and who were ashamed of what they now felt to be their sexual inadequacy.

After I wrote a new article on the subject of porn's addictive effect on the male brain in 2011, I received a number of e-mails from concerned high school counselors and counselors at boarding schools, asking me for more information about dehabituation programs, as they were seeing younger and younger male teens who were suffering from porn addictions so severe that, by sixteen or seventeen, these addictions were interfering with other aspects of the teenagers' lives, such as school, sports, and friendships.[9] At one college in Virginia where I spoke in 2012, an undergraduate woman asserted that most of the young men she knew were, in her view, addicted to pornography by the time they had graduated from high school and that there was strong pressure on young women to accept this situation as "the new normal."

On Reuniting.info, a website that offers concerned porn users science and information for dehabituation, Marnia Robinson and Gary Wilson report, confirming Robert Sapolsky's analysis, that their community members describe "gradual" and "subtle" shifts in their perception after weaning themselves from pornography addiction. They note that similar shifts in perception can arise with recovering from erectile dysfunction, which they call "a very tangible symptom that more and more heavy porn users report since free Internet videos became widely available some five years ago."[10] The authors sought to compare users' self-reporting after several months of scaling down or ending their porn use completely, with self-reports of men who were using pornography intensively, to see what if any differences arose.

After several months of following steps to dehabituate themselves to pornography use, many of the men found looking at the same porn videos, which had so aroused them in the past, curiously dissatisfying or even unpleasant.

One man turned off his browser and noted his own emotional

reaction: "I now realize that much of the pornography I've been watching is either not really exciting or is basically exploitation. My attitude is changing. In the past, I have typically fast-forwarded past any vaginal sex or emotionally positive interactions to the anal bits. Also, in the past, I have often felt strong resentment toward my wife for her unwillingness to emulate porn. But today I feel remorse at how I have treated her, and gratitude that she still seems to unconditionally love me. Well, not unconditionally, but rather unselfishly."

Another porn addict who is dehabituating from masturbation to pornography reports on the site:

*Until recently, I believed that I could never get enough sex, and that I was unlucky because I married a woman who prefers sex not more than once every other day and does not accommodate indiscriminate penetration of every orifice. But then I successfully got through 31 days without watching pornography, masturbating only minimally, genuinely trying to appreciate my wife for her sexuality on its own terms, and actively suppressing the fantasy/obsessive urges that have progressively insinuated themselves on my personality over the last decade.*

*Following this experimental reduction of my "sexual expression," it has become evident that the emphasis our culture places on . . . sexual activity that I was "free" to develop as a member of our culture, has been detrimental to my emotional development, to my marriage, to my fundamental attitude toward women as a category, and has restricted my breadth of experience.*

*I have not yet calculated the amount of time I devoted to masturbating, pornography, fantasy, projecting sexual dissatisfaction as dissatisfaction with life, etc., but I have probably lost years. I'm not yet free from sexual compulsion, but I truly feel, for the first time in probably 16 years, that my life still has the potential to offer deep, meaningful experience without also including a hyperactive sexual component. This vision of freedom from compulsion is completely novel.*

*The fantasies and the basic dissatisfaction with my sex life have not returned with any of their usual force. My perception of my wife is changing, too. She looks increasingly attractive. That can only be a positive development!*[11]

Add to all this yet another complication: the centers for aggression and sexual desire are close to each other in the brain. Many of the women who have written to me or confided in me about their boyfriends' or husbands' porn use were upset less by the nakedness of the women involved than by their degradation; they could not believe that their kind, caring male partners got off on watching men urinating on women, or degrading them in other ways. When men see, over time, images that connect sex to violence or degradation, they may become more and more aroused by the connection of sex to violence or degradation. This may be true for women as well. The vulnerability to this kind of limbic deregulation is not an existential moral flaw in men, as feminist writers Catharine MacKinnon and Andrea Dworkin posited. It is not because most men like, as a rule, to be violent to or to degrade women in real life. Many men who are on "dehabituation community" websites, trying to deescalate their porn addiction with the support of other sympathetic men, do not even like that aspect of their masturbatory lives. The potential link between sexual desire and aggression is an aspect of the male brain that a new technology is cynically manipulating, for profit, at men's expense.

Heterosexual women are adapting—at some sacrifice to their own sexual richness—to the onslaught of male-paced pornography in the environment. We saw how masturbation to porn can desensitize men to the vagina. But does it also desensitize women to their own vaginas? Recent studies indicate that it does. Female masturbation to porn *can desensitize women themselves to their own vaginas.* Women who contacted me also reported their own desensitization after masturbation to porn. As a result, they no longer respond sexually to the more simple versions of erotic imagery. They, too, need to "fast-forward" to get to hard-core fucking, or to more violence, to become as aroused as women used to become, in studies of a generation earlier, by scenes showing female nakedness, kissing, stroking, genital caressing, and so on. Female sexual response is adapting to male-porn's pacing—with consequent problems for women in libido and arousal under less intense sexual triggers, and to the detriment of both genders' sexuality and sense of connection.

Marnia Robinson sent me a comment that a female reader posted under her last *Psychology Today* post on erectile dysfunction:

*I have this exact problem except I don't have a penis.*

*When I read this it made me realize this is what I have been suffering. I did not know porn was my problem. I have been looking at porn, and addicted to it since I was very, very young. I am only 24 and my love life is a struggle at best. My husband understands somewhat but I have never really been able to tell him what it was from. I didn't tell him about my addiction. Mine started normal, where my sensitivity to touch decreased exponentially, since I started looking at porn. Also as the paper said, the porn I viewed also increased in "harshness." I used to get turned on over nakedness and now [am] at a stage where I am concerned about my mental sanity.*

*I have a hard time achieving any type of orgasm without clitoral stimulation and some hard thought processing on my part. I miss being able to have sex and have it feel good without much effort.*

*I have not looked at porn for a long time, and have just started again, and the time away did not increase my libido but might explain why I had no libido. I used to have a very extreme libido and could barely control it, now I don't even like being touched.*

*I think in my case, giving up porn and visual aids would be difficult and a long journey. I have a feeling it might be years before my sensitivity would come back, if that. Here is for hoping! Thank you for writing this and bringing it not only to my attention but many others'!*

*I hope the authors understand that women, along with men,*

*use porn to masturbate too. In secret I bet women are pretty close to the amount and severity that men use and maybe that's why many women need some type of stimulation to achieve anything. Vibrators are the devil and I will be getting rid of mine, that's for sure.*"[12]

This may not be a rare situation: according to a study published in the *Journal of Adolescent Research,* while nine out of ten young men say they use pornography, so do a third of young women.[13]

I checked with Pfaus about the reports I was getting from women that porn use and vibrators seemed to correlate to desensitization in them as well; he noted that vibrators desensitize women over time because of a natural habituation phenomenon—the spinal circuit itself habituates to the same repeated stimuli. So truly, for women, porn and vibrator technologies offer no long-term neurobiological substitutes for an attentive, inventive lover or inventive, attentive, imaginative self-care. Technology is creating its own problems.

There are more negative ways in which porn intervenes in and distorts women's sense of their own vaginas. Labiaplasty—the surgical reconstruction of a woman's labia—is a major new industry in cosmetic surgery. Natural variation in the folds and arrangement, and even the symmetry, of the outer and inner lips of the vagina is quite extensive among women. It is very common for a woman's labia to not look remotely like the standardized versions of labia that appear in porn magazines and on websites; consequently, many women who are completely normal think that there is something very unusual, or even deformed, about their "too" long, "too" complicated, or "too" asymmetrical labia.[14]

Dr. Basil Kocur, of Lenox Hill Hospital, a highly principled and accomplished specialist in pelvic floor problems who does "real" licensed, credentialed, medically justified vaginoplasties and pelvic floor repair to help women recover from pelvic floor collapse (the loosening of vaginal walls after childbirth and with middle age, which can involve the collapse of other organs), explained in an interview that pelvic floor surgery is the wave of the future in surgery: the population of women is aging, and more and more women want to reclaim the positive sexual feelings of their youth, and have better pelvic floor function, which can be returned to them with a corrective tightening of the vaginal walls and support of the pelvic floor. (He also warned that there were uncredentialed "butchers" out there, exploiting women's desires for this kind of reconstruction.) But he also noted that in the last few years, sometimes a patient who is scheduled for a pelvic floor surgery or a vaginoplasty will hand him a page from *Penthouse* or *Playboy* and ask for a labiaplasty as well, so she can "look like that"—when there is absolutely nothing wrong with her labia. He believes that pornography has given many women an unrealistic idea of what their vulvas should look like, because the neat, symmetrical labia of porn models have often been reconstructed surgically themselves.[15]

## PORN AND VAGINAL ILLITERACY

In lectures I give that elucidate the distinction between addictive male-centered pornography as opposed to erotica and Eastern discourse that tease out "the Goddess Array," young women and young men talk very frankly about how the wave of porn around them has short-circuited their sexual and emotional lives. It seems clear from what I now understand about the importance of the female ANS that porn can short-circuit female orgasmic response as well.

Young women are also direct, in these talks, about how the portrayal of female sexuality in porn—and the portrayal of the vagina itself in pornography—has had, in their opinion, a sharply negative effect on their young men's understanding of vaginas, and on what young men should ideally be doing to women sexually. Porn is leading men to become poorer lovers to women, and, more specifically, training young men to mishandle or ignore the vagina.

A group of young women who spoke to me at what I will call, to protect identities, a community center on the West Coast, were even more concrete: "I get so angry," said Lisa, a lovely, slight young woman in biker boots and skinny jeans. We were sitting with cups of coffee around a folding table, and as she spoke she whacked increasingly savagely at a coffee spill on the table.

"I had a lover," she said, "whom I really liked in every other way. But he always wanted to make love with a video on, and he always fast-forwarded the video right to the climax of the intercourse. And I just wanted to take the remote from him and make him watch it all the way through—that is, including the foreplay—or even just *slow it down*." I was surprised that she did not apparently mind that the video had to be on in the first place. The other young women at the table did not react with any surprise at all to what Lisa was saying. I, of course, being two generations older, was astonished that Lisa seemed to feel the video and its timing mediated what was going to or what could happen to her sexually, rather than her sexuality being inflamed or distracted by the video. But from comments I have heard from many young women (and young men) now, it is indeed the porn video—its timing, its options for activities, its positions—that is the dominant "script" for what is expected between contemporary young Western lovers. Now, for young people, a struggle over porn and even over the remote control often actually *is* a struggle over sexual behavior and pacing.

While we are told we live in a time of sexual liberation, this may only mean more sex, or even just more images of sex—and not better or "freer" sex. For there is a good case to be made that in fact the sophistication of skill sets, and the skill level overall, taught to men, generation by generation, by their culture and by their peers, about how to please women in bed, has gone precipitously downward since the middle of the last century, when public porn became widespread, and when male sexual education went from peer stories and their own experiences with real women to the model presented in the new mass-market medium.

John Cleland's *Memoirs of a Woman of Pleasure*, written and published as pornography in 1748, is full of "the Goddess Array": it was clearly considered a guide to eighteenth-century men on how to turn women on, and the vagina could not be described with more appreciation in both male and female voices: "[t]hat now burning spot of mine," Fanny Hill says, describing her own vagina; sexual love "inflamed the center of all my senses . . . the curling hair that overspread its delightful front . . . the powerfully-divided lips of that pleasure-thirsty channel . . . so vital a part of me . . . so strict a fold! A suction so fierce! . . . that delicate glutton, my nether-mouth . . ."

On beholding a lover's vagina, the male narrator describes

*That delicious cleft of flesh . . . a moist inviting entrance . . . delicately soft and pouting . . . Now with the tenderest attention not to shock, or alarm her too suddenly, he, by degrees, rather stole . . . up her petticoats. . . . Then lay expos'd, so to speak more properly, display'd the greatest parade in nature of female charms. The whole company . . . seem'd as much dazzled, surpriz'd, and delighted as any one could be. . . . Beauties so excessive could not but enjoy the privileges of eternal novelty . . . no! Nothing in nature could be of a beautifuller cut than the dark umbrage of the downy spring-moss that over-arched it . . . a touching warmth, a tender finishing, beyond the expression of words . . . with one hand he gently disclos'd the lips of that luscious mouth of nature . . . the soft laboratory of love . . . he awaken'd, rouz'd and touch'd her so to the heart . . . till the raging stings of the pleasure, rising toward the point, made her wild with the intolerable sensations of it . . . as she lay lost in the sweet transport. . . .*[16]

Eighteenth-century and early Victorian erotica—which was the equivalent of porn in its day, designed for men, without literary or moral pretensions, for the purpose of arousing them to orgasm—is striking in terms of how much of "the Goddess Array" you naturally find within it. Even though the vagina had been downgraded in public discourse, in private male-consumed erotica, it was still receiving plenty of positive attention. The women in these anonymously published illicit novels are continually deeply kissed, sensuously stroked, passionately caressed and fondled; their breasts and nipples are admired; their vulvas are touched and manually penetrated, kissed, and licked; they are gazed at and described in admiring tones; their own arousal is carefully noted, and their own climaxes are described, with great delicacy and attention. About a third of the description of the sexual activity in general consists of attention to "the Goddess Array" and the pacing does not cast that attention as being part of the dreaded concept of "foreplay," but as a sensuous, lingered-over and delicious part of the sexual feast itself. Men, writes Cleland, should ply the beloved with a "thousand tender little attentions, presents, caresses, confidences, and exhaust them with invention . . . what modes, what refinements of pleasure have they not recourse to. . . . When by a course of teasing, worrying (stroking), handling, wanton pastimes, lascivious motions . . . they have . . . lighted up a flame in the object of their passion. . . ." Only then may the men seek their own satisfaction. And the female voice in *Memoirs of a Woman of Pleasure* confirms this attention to female arousal: "Kissing me in every part, the most secret and critical one so far from being excepted . . . his touches were so exquisitely . . . wanton, and luxuriantly diffus'd, and penetrating at times, that he made me perfectly rage with titillating fires." [17] But on PornHub or Porn.com, there is little of this kind of touching that, two hundred sixty years before the "sexual revolution," drove Fanny Hill to "perfectly rage with titillating fires."

The sexual revolutionaries of the 1960s, including advocates for "adult" material such as Hugh Hefner and Al Goldstein, represented porn to us as a great social radicalizer. But a nation of masturbating people who are looking at screens rather than at one another—who are consuming sex like any other product and who are rewiring their brains to find less and less abandon and joy in one another's arms, and to bond more and more with pixels—is a subjugated, not a liberated, population.

It is no wonder that advanced corporate capitalism, which truly liberates neither men nor women, likes porn so much, and allows porn to colonize public space. Virtually nude images that would have been considered fit for *Playboy* in the 1980s are now five stories high in Calvin Klein ads in Times Square, fairly graphic sex scenes are not elided in R-rated movies on planes where children are seated, and porn is visible to children passing newsstands. Internet filters are difficult for parents to understand and install. Porn thus intrudes on the imaginations of children and seeps systematically into mainstream entertainment. Parents are not really free to instill a model of sex into their children's education that is not *this* model, which got there first and more graphically. There is a great deal of money at stake, but part of the reason that almost no backlash has taken place against the colonization of public space by porn—even though until the 1960s active community debates set limits on obscene material— is that porn addiction abundantly serves the status quo. Porn puts people to sleep, conceptually and politically as well as erotically.

Social conservatives have always feared real sexual awakening because erotic aliveness has the power to lead people into other kinds of resistance to deadening norms and rigid political, class, and social oppressions. Eros has always had the potential to truly rouse people, spiritually and politically as well as physically. Porn really is a drug, but it is the kind of drug that diminishes individuality, imagination, and pleasure rather than releasing it. Porn, it turns out, eventually takes the sexiness—that is, the wildness—out of sex.

The sexual "revolutionaries" of the 1960s branded porn as being a great liberator of libido—a lifter of repression, a great demystifier of the "shame" of sexuality. But—in the greatest of great ironies—we are discovering that porn diminishes rather than heightens libido over time; that its effect on the phallus is ultimately unmanning and depressive; and that its effect on the vagina is a short-circuiting of the intense erotic potential—which means, also, the intense creative potential—inherent in every woman.

four

# The Goddess Array

## "The Beloved Is Me"

---

*Seated upon a lotus, with lotus in hand, is Lakshmi, the goddess . . . riding in chariots the goddesses appear . . .*

—Devyāḥ Kavaçam, Hindu sacred scripture

*How answer you,* la plus belle Katherine du Monde, mon très cher et divin déesse?

—William Shakespeare, *Henry V*

*L*et's look back again at the 1970s, where the feminism of a Betty Dodson and a Shere Hite, and the market opportunity grabbed by Hugh Hefner and his fellow pornographers in the following decades, "set" our model in the West of female sexuality.

This model of the feminist vulva and vagina—joined eventually by pornography's elaboration of this model—was the one that was formative for women of my generation. The vagina and vulva were primarily understood as mediating sexual pleasure. What was important was technique—one's own masturbatory technique, and the skills one taught to a partner. Feminists and pornographers alike defined the vagina and vulva in terms of the mechanics of orgasm.

But while technique is important, this model leaves a great deal out of the "meaning" of the vagina and vulva. It leaves out the connections to the vagina of spirituality and poetry, art and mysticism, and the context of a relationship in which orgasm may or may not be taking place. It certainly leaves behind the larger question of the quality of a masturbating woman's *relationship to herself.*

The Dodson model of the empowered female did a great deal of good, but also caused some harm. The good is that feminism of that era had to break the association of heterosexual female sexual awakening with dependency on a man. The harm is that the feminism of this era successfully broke the association of heterosexual female sexual awakening with dependency on a man. "A woman needs a man like a fish needs a bicycle," as one seventies-era feminist bumper sticker insisted. The feminist model of heterosexuality—that straight women can fuck like men, or get by with a great vibrator and no other attention to self-love, and be simply instrumentalist about their pleasure—turned out to have created a new set of impossible ideals, foisted, if through the best of intentions, upon "liberated" women. Feminism has evaded the far more difficult question of how to be a liberated heterosexual woman and how to acknowledge deep physical needs for connection with men. As nature organized things, we ideally have a partner in the dance. If we don't have a partner, there is attention we should give to self-love as self-care. It does not solve straight women's existential dilemma, the tension between our dependency needs and our needs for independence, simply to declare that the dance has changed.

The harm of this model of female sexuality is that it reaffirms a fractured, commercialized culture's tendency to see people, including "sexually liberated women," as isolated, self-absorbed units, and to see pleasure as something one needs to acquire the way one acquires designer shoes, rather than as a medium of profound intimacy with another, or with one's self, or as a gateway to a higher, more imaginative, fully realized dimension that includes and affects all aspects of one's life.

Recent data collected in 2009 by sociologist Marcus Buckingham, drawn from multicountry surveys, show that Western women report lower and lower levels of happiness and satisfaction, even as their freedoms and options have grown, relative to men.[1] Both feminists and antifeminist commentators sought to find answers for this broadly confirmed trend: feminists sought to argue that it was inequality or wage differences in the workplace and the "second shift" at home—but the surveys were adjusted to account for sex discrimination. Antifeminist commentators argued, of course, that this was all the fault of feminism, making women seek fulfillment in professional spheres unnatural to them.

I think it is very possible, judging from the tremendous amount of data we have seen about what women need psychologically, which they are generally not getting, that they are saying they are dissatisfied because the "available models of sexuality"—the post-Dodson, post-Hefner, post-porn, married, two-career, hurried, or young and single drunk-with-a-stranger-in-a-bar-or-dorm-room models—are, long term, just plain physically untenable. These models of female sexuality—left to us by a combination of pressures ranging from an incomplete development of feminism in the 1970s, to a marketplace that likes us overemployed and undersexed, to the speeding up of sexual pacing set by pornography—doom women eventually to emotional strain caused by physiological strain. These models of female sexuality are simply extremely physically, emotionally, and existentially unsatisfying. (This model of sex may well doom Western heterosexual men in other ways, deserving of their own book.)

Now that we know that the vagina is a gateway to a woman's happiness and to her creative life, we can create and engage with an entirely different model of female sexuality, one that cherishes and values women's sexuality. This is where the "Goddess" model comes in, a model that focuses on "the Goddess Array"—that set of behaviors and practices that should precede or accompany lovemaking. But where is a "Goddess" model to be found in contemporary life?

My search to locate a working "Goddess" model led me first into the past, into the historical differences between Eastern and Western attitudes toward female sexuality. Of course, women were subjugated in the East as well as in the West, but in two cultures in particular—the India of the Tantrists, about fifteen hundred years ago, and the Han dynasty of China about a thousand years ago—women were, for a time, elevated and enjoyed relative freedom. These two cultures viewed the vagina as life-giving and sacred, and, as I noted, they believed that balance and health for men depended upon treating the vagina—and women—extremely well sexually. Both cultures appear to have understood aspects of female sexual response that modern Western science is only now catching up with.

Tantra, from the Sanskrit, best translated as "doctrine," emerged in medieval India. Tantra sees the universe as a manifestation of Divine Consciousness in a state of joyful play, as expressed through the balancing of feminine and masculine energies: *Shakti* and *Shiva*. A subset of Tantra developed, which used sexuality as a path to the realization of the Divine. In Tantra, the vagina is the seat of the Divine, and the fluid (*kuladravya*) or nectar (*kulamrita*) that helps initiates reach transcendence is perceived as flowing naturally from a woman's womb. Tantra even sees the source of female vaginal fluid (especially female ejaculatory fluid, or *amrita*) as originating in heaven.

From the second century CE until as late as the 1700s, a Taoist tradition of related sexual practices, and a related sexual philosophy, developed in China. In Tao, the vagina was also seen as life-giving and divine. Men were encouraged to bring women to orgasm with great skill and care, in order to benefit from their energizing "yin" essences. The penis was seen to draw life-enhancing qualities from women's vaginal juices. Men were trained in the classic sexual Yoga texts ("the education of the penis") to ensure that they sexually satisfied their wives and concubines with long foreplay and carefully timed thrusting, since personal and cosmic harmony, as well as healthy offspring, were all seen as being dependent on female sexual ecstasy.

As historian Douglas Wile describes it in his book *Art of the Bedchamber: The Chinese Sexual Yoga Classics,* "At the very least, a man must delay his climax to adjust for the difference in arousal time between 'fire and water' and to ensure the woman's full satisfaction." Wile elucidates the Taoist philosophy further: "The woman was said

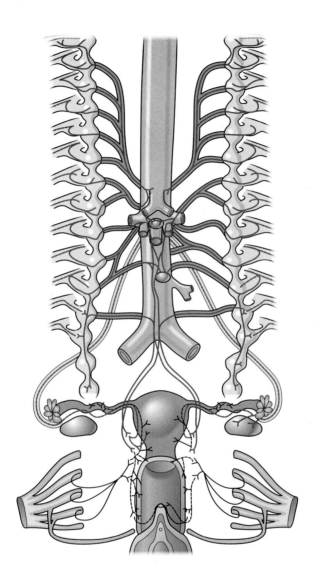

$\mathcal{T}$he innervation of the female pelvis: This
illustration shows how the complex
pelvic nerves in women branch from the spinal
cord. [Oxford Designers & Illustrators]

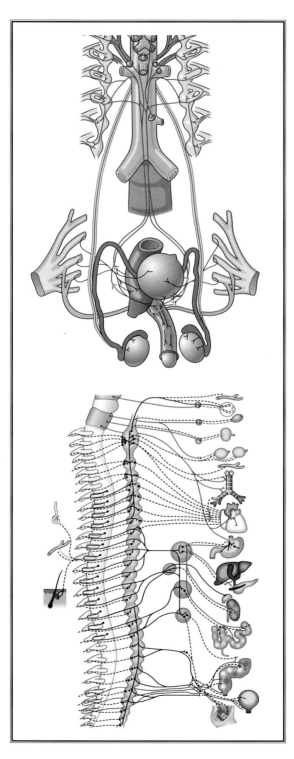

*T*he innervation of the male pelvis: This illustration shows a comparatively simpler neural "grid." [Oxford Designers & Illustrators]

*T*he Autonomic Nervous System: The lower right schematizes its relationship to the female pelvis. [Oxford Designers & Illustrators]

# Dopamine Levels
## *(or altered sensitivity to dopamine)*

| DEFICIENT | "NORMAL" |
|---|---|
| Addictions | Healthy bonding |
| Depression | Feelings of well-being, satisfaction |
| Anhedonia—no pleasure, world looks colorless | Pleasure, reward in accomplishing tasks |
| Lack of ambition and drive | Healthy libido |
| Inability to bond | Good feelings toward others |
| Low libido | Motivated |
| Erectile dysfunction | Healthy risk taking |
| Social anxiety disorder | Sound choices |
| ADHD or ADD | Realistic expectations |
| Sleep disturbances, "restless legs" | Parent/child bonding |
| | Contentment with "little" things |

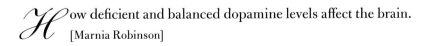

How deficient and balanced dopamine levels affect the brain.
[Marnia Robinson]

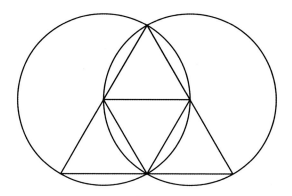

*S*acred geometry: The *vesica piscis* is derived from the intersection of two circles signifying the overlap between the divine and the worldly.

*T*he "mandorla" or divine feminine symbol is a *vesica piscis* that represents liminality—the meeting point between heaven and earth. A medieval mandorla showcasing the Virgin Mary enthroned in an almond-shaped frame.

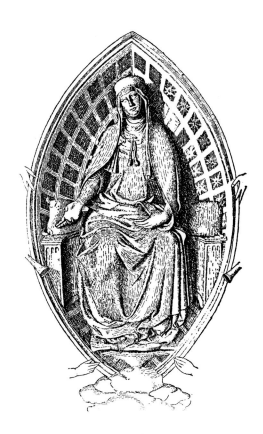

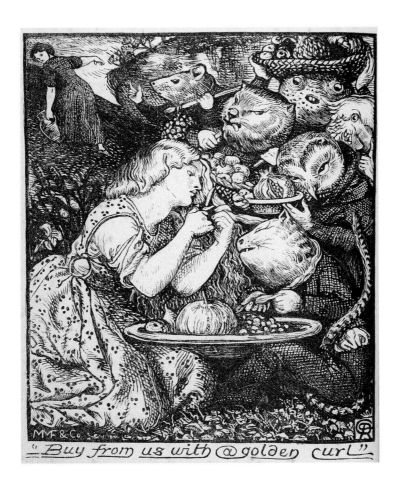

"Buy from us with @ golden curl"

$O$ne of Dante Gabriel Rossetti's illustrations for the first edition of his sister Christina Rossetti's 1862 poem "Goblin Market." The pomegranate, always a feminine symbol in pre-Raphaelite iconography, is inaccurate as a literal rendition of a fruit, but is anatomically accurate.

*D*ancer Loie Fuller creating the vortex shapes with her costume that scandalized audiences, c. 1902.

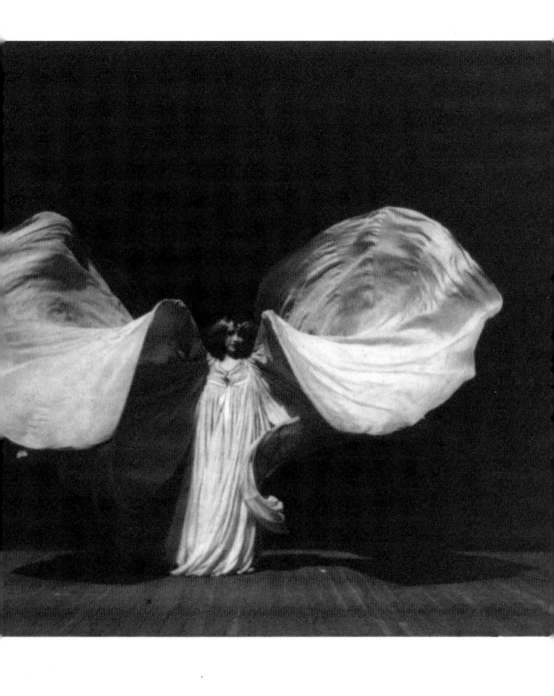

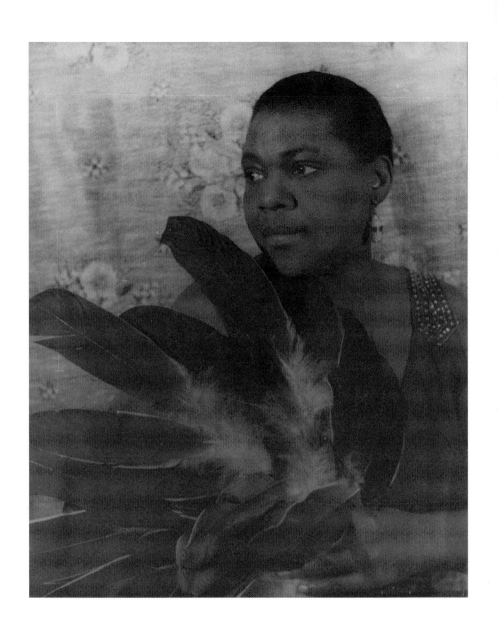

*Portrait of Bessie Smith Holding Feathers* by the photographer Carl Van Vechten, circa 1936.

to love slowness (hsu) and duration (chiu), and abhor haste (chi) and violence (pao). . . . The woman expresses her desire through sounds (yin), movements (tung), and signs (cheng or tao). In her sexual responses she is compared to the element water, 'slow to heat and slow to cool'. . . . Prolonged foreplay is always presented as the precondition for orgasm."[2] The Taoist sexual texts take it for granted that female sexual intensity is stronger than its male counterpart, and so the sexual training of men was necessary to harmonize those innate disharmonies. Learned techniques cultivated male sexual control and the eliciting of a woman's health-giving "jade fluid."

In Taoist sexual texts, women were understood to emit medicinal fluids from various parts of their bodies, including from under their tongues, from their breasts, and from their vaginas. The man's goal for the sake of his own health was to stir the release of these precious fluids: the Taoist sacred text *The Great Medicine of the Three Peaks* explains that a woman's breasts issue "jade juice," which, if a man sucks on them, nourishes the man's spleen and spinal cord. By sucking her nipples, he also opens "all of the woman's meridians" and "relaxes the woman's body and mind." This action penetrates to the "flowery pool" and stimulates the "mysterious gate" below, causing the body's fluids and chi (energy) to overflow. "Of the three objects of absorption," writes the author, "this is your first duty." When intercourse takes place, the woman's emotions are voluptuous, her face red, and voice trembling. At this time her "gate" opens up, her chi is released, and her secretions overflow. If the man withdraws his "jade stalk" an inch or so, and assumes the posture of "giving and receiving," he then accepts her chi and absorbs her secretions, thereby strengthening his "primal yang" and nourishing his spirit.[3]

These terms, so alien to our culture, bear thinking about. A woman who experiences her vagina and her sexuality in this framework—one in which the very essences that flow from her during oral sex are considered health-giving to her partner; one in which it is that partner's first duty, he has been taught, to relax her body and mind in his lovemaking with her—would be liberated from the pressures many Western women experience when they receive sexual attention, from anxiety about how long it takes to reach orgasm to anxiety about sexual selfishness. And the ensuing relaxation, as we've seen again and again, is the key to sexual opening for women.

Islam, which the West stereotypes as being repressive to women, has a rich tradition of erotic literature and of careful attention to the vagina: the sixteenth-century erotic classic *The Perfumed Garden* recounts at least twenty different kinds of vaginas: *El addad* is "the biter"; *El aride,* "the large one"; *El cheukk* means "the chink," or "the hard yoni of a very lean or bony woman" with "not a vestige of flesh." *El hacene* is "the beautiful," or a vagina "that is white, firm and plump without any deformity" and "vaulted like a dome." *El hezzaz,* or "the restless," is "the eagerly moving" vagina "of a woman starved for sexual play." *El merour,* or "the deep one," "always has the mouth open." *El neuffakh* is "the swelling one." *El relmoune* is the vagina of a virgin who is experiencing her first act of lovemaking. *El taleb* or "the yearning one," means the vagina of "a woman who has been abstinent for too long, or, who is naturally more sexually demanding than her partner." *El keuss,* or "the vulva," is "usually used for the "soft, seductive, perfect" and pleasantly smelling organ of a young woman; plump and round "in every direction, with long lips, grand slit." In this culture, when one dreamed of a woman's vulva, it was a positive omen: *The Perfumed Garden* asserts that the person who dreams of having seen the vulva, *feurdj,* of a woman, will know that

> *if he is in trouble God will free him of it; if he is in a perplexity he will soon get out of it; and lastly if he is in poverty he will soon become wealthy.*
>
> *It is considered more lucky to dream of the vulva as open. . . . If the vulva is open so that he can look well into it, or even if it is hidden but he is free to enter it, he will bring the most difficult tasks to a successful end after having first failed in them, and this after a short delay, by the help of a person whom he never thought of.*
>
> *Generally speaking, to see the vulva in dreams is a good sign; so it is of good augury to dream of coition, and he who sees him-*

*self in the act, and finishing with the ejaculation, will meet suc-*
*cess in all his affairs. . . .*[4]

While not all of these terms are poetic or positive, this vista into a different cultural frame around the vagina shows a non-Western directing of elaborate levels of male cultural attention to the subtleties and aesthetics of different women's vaginas, their moods, varying appetites, and their relationships to the life of the woman in question; and a very non-Western awareness that vaginas are pluralistic, individualistic, and have wills and intentions of their own.

Having seen how much sexual suffering Western women still experience, according to the data, even after the "sexual revolution," and having learned from my research more about how Tantra and its related Taoist traditions regard the vagina so differently than does the West, I became convinced that Tantra had some answers to the question of how female sexuality was best understood, especially in terms of the brain-vagina connection. Increasingly, many signposts—both historical and now neurobiological—point to the centrality of the "G-spot"—or "sacred spot," in Tantric terms—in mediating the relationship between a woman's sexuality and her consciousness. In Tantra, understanding the "sacred spot" is fundamental to understanding the nature of "the Goddess," which is seen as being an innate part of every woman.

So, looking for where a Tantric trove of wisdom might be found, I went to one of the best-known and most highly regarded regularly recurring Tantric workshops that centers specifically on "sacred spot massage." The workshop, which takes places over two days, is taught by Charles Muir—whose booming recorded voice had swiveled the heads of all those undergraduates in the college library—along with his ex-wife, Caroline Muir (the couple is amicably divorced). The couple has been teaching "sacred spot massage" workshops for twenty-five years.

I confess that before I attended the Muirs' workshop, I thought of Tantra primarily as intimidating; whatever treasures it might yield seemed, before I looked into it more deeply, to be obscured by esoteric mumbo jumbo, and people with startling amounts of facial hair. I didn't doubt that there must be interesting or useful things to know, but Tantra just seemed to me—an overscheduled Western woman—like an alienating, labor-intensive *hassle,* involving not just my own mastery of a whole new set of approaches, but the roping in of my equally overscheduled mate. Could I glean the basics of what Tantra knew about female sexuality—and communicate them in an accessible way to women who did not want to take on a major new time-consuming life path?

On the weekend I attended, the workshop was being held at a big hotel in Midtown that, while still genteel, had seen better days. All weekend long, the forty male and female participants would learn Tantric skills centered on women's well-being. On Saturday night, after a day of conversation and instruction, the women would walk among the gathered attendees and select a man (or men) who would give them "sacred spot massage" that night in a private hotel room. The massage would proceed according to careful earlier direction in an all-male seminar taught by Charles Muir. The theme of the seminar? Sacred spot massage is all about the woman.

It seemed clear from the discussion leading up to the deed itself that this model—of a male Tantrist completely focused on releasing female sexual and emotional energies, in all their variability and wildness, and the woman supported in simply receiving this care and not worrying about reciprocity—was what was so apparently transformative for all the participants involved. People who had gone through the training did indeed, in a noncultish way, describe this experience as changing their lives in ways far beyond the "merely" sexual. It seemed to confirm what I had learned about women's neurophysiologic needs.

Early Saturday afternoon, I joined a group of workshop participants for lunch at a nearby vegetarian Indian restaurant. I saw a gathering of men and women, mostly in their late twenties to early fifties, speaking intently to one another, a sheen of eroticism lifting up over the table like the shimmer from a heat mirage. I took in the scene, with its highly excited atmosphere, and tried to figure out just what was so different about it. Then it hit me: all of the men were gazing deeply into the eyes of the women, and gave the impression, at least, of giving the women their undivided attention.

There was something else I noticed: while all of the women were quite conventionally attractive, many of the men were not at all conventionally attractive. But they were mesmerizing the women nonetheless. Did men who were at some kind of physical disadvantage in the mating game find themselves drawn to weekends and practices such as this, which would give them additional skills to bring to the table? The not-conventionally-attractive men, I could not help noticing, all appeared to approach the women, no matter how conventionally attractive they were in turn, with a rare kind of confidence—not arrogance, but a kind of certainty of their own value to women. Tall geeky men with pens clipped to their shirt pockets gazed confidently into the eyes of sleek sophisticates; grizzled older men gazed into the eyes of women of all ages; men of all shapes, sizes, and physical conditions were deeply attentive to women and quietly self-assured, and so, in spite of whatever they were or were not endowed with by nature, did come across as unusually charming. Amazing what an understanding of sacred spot massage must do for a guy's confidence level, I thought.

I started chatting with a modest, dark-haired entrepreneur from Australia, who was married to a Belgian woman. He had flown halfway around the world to be at this event: he explained that his wife, after twenty-four years of marriage, had confessed that she no longer felt desire for him; she was belatedly getting in touch with her own sexuality and had awakened to this catastrophe for them both—she was parched in some way. I was amazed at the man's forthrightness in facing the couple's problem.

"Because I love my partner," he said, "I lived in hope of things improving. It was very painful. This journey has taken many steps."

Not wishing to lose the marriage, the man was here at the sacred spot massage weekend to see what he could learn about stoking the fire between them.

Tantra, he said, was already helping the couple. "We started with healing touch—nonsexual massage," he confided, surprisingly ready to share his insights and not flinching as I took out my yellow legal pad and a pen. "It's a way to connect without the expectations and demands of having to perform, of sex. The giving and receiving of nonsexual touch is so powerful," he explained. The Tantric approach of nonsexual massage had helped him "become better friends with his wife." Their marriage, he said, had, over time, become "an illusion— not real on the intimate love part. We were so busy with a family, rais- ing children—living the expectations of the world around us. I was always the warm, giving one; she was colder. It's great that [Tantric practice] is finally allowing her to receive; sexually and in general.

"I'm here," he continued, "because I want to know more about the art of loving: I want to learn this skill. As boys, as men, we are actually taught a lot more about having the ejaculation than about en- joying the moment. We are taught that frequency is everything. The idea of wanting to create intimate moments becomes the last priority, when it is the very thing to which we should look forward."

Another man I interviewed echoed this desire for nonsexual in- timacy, a desire that formed the basis of his Tantric approach. We started talking after I noticed him smiling mischievously at me—he was completely bald and rather stocky, and altogether charmingly inoffensive in his approach. I folded my arms, identified myself as a journalist—that universal antiaphrodisiac—and asked him what had drawn him to the weekend.

He smiled even more broadly.

He had taken the workshop four times already, and he was back, he declared, because, "My lovers tell me I'm getting better and better."

"What's the secret?" I asked him. I couldn't help smiling, too, at his boyish bravado.

"I transmit energy, love, and affection in my touch without doing something necessarily sexual," he said. "It's about the art of enjoying the moment rather than wanting to just 'get it.' To hold and experience a connection, not to go in a programmed way to please this one or that one, or to please yourself. Every man should learn a Tantric approach at twenty."

Why had he begun to investigate these skills in the first place, I asked him?

"I found that sexual intimacy without love makes me feel empty. I don't want to go back into situations like that. I found that it's not about ejaculating [primarily]."

With a Tantric approach to a woman's desire, he said, "You're paying attention. . . . You're not in your own world. How can you not be more successful?" He said that men often complain about women being emotionally volatile. But sacred spot massage, he said, helps to ground women emotionally: "If you [as a man] are present and can hold space for their emotions, how can you not be successful in relationships with women? Women [who receive sacred spot massage from men] are better able to ground themselves sooner, not hold on to their stuff, not create new stories, like: 'You never pay attention to me.'

"You're paying attention, asking permission to enter. Tantric teachers talk about how many nerve endings there are in the vaginal lips—most nerve endings are in the first inch. You're paying more attention. It's a whole different experience. You're appreciating that area, not just trying to just get in as fast as you can, as deep as you can. . . . What is porn? Deep; fast; ejaculate. In contrast, Tantra is: slow; connect; explore every inch of what you're doing."

"Do you think most men in our culture understand the vagina?" I asked.

"Men in our culture don't understand the penis *or* the vagina," he said. "Because how often have men in our culture explored either? Get in, release, get out. Most of our sensitivity, too, is that first inch—the crown. Charles Muir talks about seven sections to the penis—each one relates to a chakra. But men don't learn control in our culture in relation to their own pleasure either. Orgasm can be longer—for some men it stays for days. Do you think most men in our culture learn that the female sacred spot can be reached in different ways—you may have to curl around, or come from a different angle? Why would you learn that?" He laughed. "Angle, depth, rhythm: each creates a different response. Even when [one's penis] is soft you can part her lips with it. Even if you don't have a hard-on at that moment, you are exploring; it's a game; that can be one of the most intense parts of an evening.

"These days especially," he said, "young men learn from porn. You're watching people put themselves in rather weird positions. Being subjected to all these images, you compare the person you're with to a pair of breasts, or legs; you get into this whole comparison thing; and you also compare yourself to the hundred guys in the world with ten- or twelve-inch penises.

"Men don't talk that much about sex—that is, about technique, detail, or emotions. You might say, 'Hey, we were on the rooftop, it got crazy,' but you don't communicate much that is that useful about women. Most men don't know about this stuff. It's nowhere in the culture."

I asked my new Tantra friend: What comes to mind when he thinks about the vagina? Like many people to whom I had put this question, he laughed. Then he said: "It's great. It's wonderful fun—a mystery to explore. A place of fun, enjoyment, magic—confusion at times: if they [women] are not quite reaching an orgasm—us guys are very process oriented, and it can be like: 'This worked *last* time!' It's a wonderful space; on the other hand, at the same time, it's be-deviling."

He mused, "If more women knew themselves better, the more they could explain what is going on: communicate to themselves, or to a partner, how to connect more. It would feel really good if more women communicated what they wanted—offer, invite positive rein-forcement."

————

On Saturday night, I entered the hotel ballroom where the sacred spot massage selection was to take place, my curiosity intensely piqued by that afternoon's conversations.

A *tangka,* a sacred fabric tapestry, hung on the wall by the stage. The *tangka* featured the goddess Shakti standing in an inverted triangle, the universal feminine symbol. The Shakti had long black wavy hair; she held open pink lotuses in each of her four hands; and a corona of light surrounded her. She looked like the darker, earthier sister of the radiant Mary of New College.

The expansive, shabby ballroom in the hotel's basement had been set up with a podium ranged with banks of yellow roses, and comfortable cushions were scattered over the floor. Women and men of all ages lounged on them or sat up attentively throughout the proceedings. Charles Muir stood at the podium, delivering a lecture—in a dry, Borscht Belt accent, ready with a grin for every punch line—about how men should approach "the yoni." He made the same general points that Mike Lousada had made in our conversations and that I had heard in Muir's own audiotapes: cherishing, patience, respect, care, attention.

"There is a point called the yoni-nadi," he said, "in the woman, which is found inside of her: behind her pubic hair is the pubic bone. On the backside of the pubic bone—if you go inside her vagina, curl your finger back against her pubic bone—there is erectile tissue there that swells up. About two square inches of it. When the area is activated, the point comes to the surface and manifests in vaginal orgasms. It is the point that connects 'down there' to your brain—so many neural circuits are there. This is the South Pole of the clitoris, which in turn is the north side of her sexual energy." (I would note that this phrasing confirms the latest Western anatomical discoveries about the actual relationship of the clitoris to the G-spot—they are North and South Poles of the same anatomical structure.) "We stop at the clitoris because there is so much pleasure there. But on the other side of the clitoris is the G-spot."

Throughout the workshop, I noticed that whenever sacred spot massage was discussed, it was presented as a practice more about releasing emotion than primarily about accessing pleasure. Caroline Muir explained that Charles would teach the men "how to be present for a woman as she releases whatever she needs to release—to stand in his love even if she is raging at him. . . . The men will be trained in this art of sexual healing. . . . The encouragement, permission, and invitation from a man to express authentically whatever she's feeling is a step to amazing foreplay, because she can actually trust you. If some damage happened to us at the hands of a man, as it has for almost every woman, we need to trust that a man can be with our bodies and our yonis without having to fuck us. It's your hands, heart, lips, spirit that bring healing."

Charles Muir added, speaking to the men: "Your message is: 'Tonight I will serve you. No matter what you look like or how big your breasts are, I will serve the Goddess in you. And the women will be asking: 'Does Goddess move me to choose one of these men to have sacred spot massage from?' " The men perked up.

"Science says it takes fourteen days to experience new neural pathways. I say bullshit. This spot is a fulcrum with so many nerve endings to the brain. Will this develop into something serious? It is a healer, not a beloved. This is a one-night hand." Laughter.

Charles Muir led the men out—they were all going to room 1750. "When they come back they will know things," he smiled to the remaining women. "You can look at them with new respect."

The men trooped off behind Muir. As I watched them pass—a group of men about to gather together to watch a sexually explicit video featuring a woman's body—they struck me as different from any other group of men, off to a night out at, say, Hooters. They seemed—I don't know how to say this any other way—as if they were heading off to approach the female body in a way that was, yes, sexual, but also *respectful*.

After the men exited, Caroline Muir took the stage. She is a surreally juicy-looking, witty blond woman who appears to be about forty-three, but who is, in fact, in her early sixties—a fact that when revealed, elicited gasps from the now woman-only crowd. That night her hair was curled in wild tendrils, and she wore a loose salmon-pink top, slim white jeans, and delicate sandals; her toes were painted shell pink.

"Yes, we pamper the Goddess," Caroline Muir began, and she

then segued into a discussion of "female ejaculate," that awful phrase for the liquid that emerges during orgasm in jets from the urethras of many women, which is called *amrita* in Sanskrit. "Amrita comes through heavenly realms," she explained, according to Tantric tradition, and "comes through us into the vagina. Energy comes down and down. You can let go—if there are towels with you. You want to put it on your own face. He can drink it and become very awake—oral sex is not the best thing for him to do late at night—he'll be walking the halls while you are sleeping like a baby."

"Why?" asked a woman in yellow. "Does it have caffeine?"

"It's your life force. Porn films have reduced it from being a sacred experience to: 'I hear you squirt.' I have never 'squirted,' " she said with some hauteur. "I have released lots of *amrita*. The nectar of the Goddess." I sat down and wondered if it would get less weird, and it did.

"Tantra," she explained, "says that you miss the boat of love if you're living in the left hemisphere of the brain—that love is a mystical experience that only happens in the right hemisphere. We'll do a [*niyasa*] at a point in the body called 'yoni-nadi.' It gives access to the core of the second chakra's energy—it is the point that male Tantrists press for ejaculatory control. I proposed that women had this same area; I had met some triple-Scorpio women in the swinging sixties; I met my first multiorgasmic, ejaculating women at that time.

"I watched my girlfriends wake up! I watched women come alive, and crazy emotions emerge. I watched them go from numbness to awakening or orgasms to living orgasms—to dancing in the sky. When they release that second-chakra energy, that passion for life emerges: for your kids, for your job; you become able to live all of your life with that passion."

Now that there were only women in the room, an intimate atmosphere of female secrets shared started to prevail. "Sacred spot massage will begin to awaken what's dormant," Caroline Muir said to the women, now gathered closely around her on pillows, like an all-ages sleepover. "Clitoral is what people usually do; but with this G-spot or sacred spot area—which is, again, closely connected to the clitoris—we are going into that deeper soul of your sexuality." Sacred spot massage, she went on, "is an activation of the second chakra and a banishing of the sexual residue of the past. All of the good reasons to be shut down—guilt, fear, shame—go into this chakra. And you learn to make love from men who never learn to make love. With this massage the question is: What part of the *psyche* are we going to touch?

"Twenty-five percent of men at the sacred spot massage retreat, when they touch the vagina for the first time—nothing. The labia— it's like visiting Utah: 'Nothing's happening here.' It's numb; it's asleep. Thirty minutes later, same yoni: It's Rio de Janeiro! Mardi Gras!

"These [vaginas, labia] are places of paranoia and mistrust. You are not told, as a girl, when you touch yourself, 'Put love into your yoni.' This [sacred spot massage] practice resolves the sludge that you have picked up in your yoni for as long as you've been living." I was hearing the neuroscience that Dr. Coady had introduced to me; the studies of multisystem dysregulation in the experience of vaginal pain; the dysregulation in the systems of the rest of the body caused by sexual trauma; the studies showing that stress affects the actual vaginal tissue of female rats; Dr. Burke Richmond's clinical experience that sexual trauma can cause perceptual dysregulation— underneath the gentle Tantric descriptions of what sounded like the same phenomenon. The idea that the vagina has a rich, nuanced memory bank and, yes, a physical and emotional biography of its own, was being confirmed at once, by two separate cultural para- digms.

Caroline Muir went on: "The clitoris has analogies to the penis. It wants release. You feel better after release. We've learned to burn it up and hopefully get it over with before a man is done with his pleasure. I was only successful in terms of clitoral orgasm. Vaginal orgasms were a mystery to me. Other girlfriends said, 'Whoa, it's like the Fourth of July in there.'

"We discover our sexual pleasure under the sheets 'cause it's warm and juicy down there—it feels good. But your mom, or religion, made you feel ashamed. Not a lot of good press and PR on female pleasure, owning it and knowing you deserve it and learning enough about your own pleasure to teach a man to give it to you.

"When you start to awaken inside, the sacred spot area—it reveals to you more of the truth about your divinely feminine nature. When you fall in love with your divinely feminine self, nothing will be more precious to you. She will never leave you, 'she' being the essence of who you are. As this spot and the clitoris awaken to your potential, it is like a roller coaster. You're not just expected to orgasm; that's a support along the way that shows that something is working well. Many women experience a lot more vaginal pleasure with this massage; women wake up. You see light more clearly when you clean the window. This is not taught in Sex Ed 101: 'You have a yoni, you know, it's not just a pussy.' "

Caroline Muir demonstrated sacred spot massage technique by curling forward the index and middle fingers of her left hand. She demonstrated that the right hand goes on the clitoris while the left hand curls under for the "sacred spot."

"Penises like it a little rougher than yonis do; we are more delicate, like the petals of these roses." She gestured at the blooms in front of her. "You don't want to rip the petals open to put it in.

"If we're heterosexual women we haven't actually explored other women. If you have a chance with a friend to explore what a yoni looks like and feels like other than your own, it is one of the great rites of passage. 'Wow, yours is really tiny, I can hardly find your inner labia.' 'Wow, your inner labia are so voluptuous.' We need to bless the yoni, from a female perspective.

"Here are the stories we tell ourselves:

1. 'I know I won't come.'
2. 'I know I won't get wet.'
3. 'I'm sure he's getting bored.'
4. 'I'm sure he wants to get on with it.'
5. 'I'm sure I must smell.'
6. 'I'm sure he must think my yoni's ugly.'

"All of these things we do to convince ourselves that we are not beautiful, not desirable.

"The men tonight do not take their clothes off or become naked. They must leave after one and a half hours. This is all about you."

Caroline Muir opened the floor to questions.

A woman with tattooed biceps and a red bandanna around her neck spoke up: "My orgasms aren't as intense. I have different types now—not contracting, but whole body orgasms, waves of pulsation—not the traditional thing." She held up her hand and squeezed it into a fist, as if to demonstrate "the traditional thing."

Caroline Muir responded, "They are waves of orgasmic energy. When you are twenty, you have hot, fast orgasms. When you are older, they soften and get more intense. The pathways between genitals and brain have had more years to wake up. There are more pathways, so it feels different from fast, hot clitoral orgasms."

"I feel a loss," the tattooed woman said, "because I want both."

"That's very normal," Caroline said. "And women in their twenties, if they don't have children, just don't have all their energy going to children."

A tanned woman in expensive sweats, wearing a long sleek braid, said: "I'm thirty-four. In my late twenties I stopped having powerful orgasms. I was with a sex addict . . . I used vibrators constantly for years; every day. Did I damage myself? It's been years. I can't get it back." She started to cry.

I was startled—I had just started getting e-mails from informants who knew I was writing about the issue of desensitization through porn and vibrators.

Caroline Muir replied gently: "Every time we get used to vibrator speed and then we try fingers, it is an adjustment." A tall blond woman stroked the arm of the woman who was weeping. "The vibrator is that young, hot, fast energy. Yonis don't love that."

"You don't think I caused myself damage?" asked the woman, the tears still in her eyes.

"No," said Caroline.

"I'm fifty-five," said a short-haired matronly-looking woman in a bright floral print top. All my stereotypes were collapsing: this woman, who had a Southern accent, would have looked perfectly at home at a Baptist church picnic. "I'm not able to use a vibrator anymore," she said. "Every time I try, it's like going to McDonald's. I don't want to eat there." After having sacred spot massage and starting Tantra practice, she said, "The quality and difference in my orgasms is like: 'What's *that*?' I don't even recognize what that was . . . these orgasms are so different from what I was used to. My libido was much dampened when I was younger; but now it just went straight up. I've had to practice a lot by myself. My hands are small, but I use this; it works." Out of her well-organized black purse, the woman whipped a nearly foot-long vibrator—or rather, a masturbatory device. It was clear Lucite, not electronic, and shaped like an S-curve with a knob at the end. All the women began asking for details about it, and its owner passed it around.

A woman who was dressed like a trophy wife from Westchester—cardigan sweater, pearls, pageboy haircut—asked Caroline Muir if she could be hired to do personal yoni massage. "I do indeed do yoni massage with women. It costs $250 an hour for two hours. I am not bisexual; arousal happens, but that is not my goal. There is crying, emotion: 'Oh God, this is so tender!' The tenderness is what we lack."

Caroline Muir continued: "The massage awakens a lot of memory. When I had it for the first time, I could smell the ether of the hysterectomy that I had undergone at the age of twenty-six; I could remember childhood transgressions—a finger poked in. Sacred spot massage awakens memories."

(As an aside, Caroline Muir noted that men's "sacred spot" is in the anus, against the prostate—which, if the connection of sacred spot anatomy to defenses, emotional vulnerability, and release is true, raises very interesting questions about why heterosexual men are often so hyperaverse to the thought of homosexuality; why they often see receptive homosexuality as feminizing; and why the masculine language of being anally penetrated is synonymous with a loss of mastery. Could the idea of penetration—of male "sacred spot" release—threaten heterosexual men with a potential loss of *emotional* mastery?)

"The awakening of the unconscious and the releasing of energies through scared spot massage makes room for a new life of pleasure and love. We have given this workshop for twenty-five years, and the success of it is not 'better sex,' but sexual healing."

I raised my hand and put to Caroline Muir the connections I was hearing about regarding blocks in the vagina, or release in the vagina, and female creativity.

"Yes," she said emphatically. Indeed, in her explanation, female sexual energy doesn't *spark* creative energy; it actually *is* creative energy: "Shakti, or feminine, sexual energy is transferable energy. Shakti *is* the creative force. In the right combination, it creates life. Meaning: here is the creative life force, feminine in nature, and I've deepened my ability to breathe this yoni energy into my brain. The more vaginal—not clitoral—releases in a woman, the more she is going to want to save the world, save her grandchildren, paint paintings, make a difference on the planet.

"The energy awakening doesn't have to be orgasmic. Every time you receive loving touch of an awakening nature to your vaginal tissue, you will in increments wake up. You may not notice it the first twelve times. Then, Whoa!"

———

Night was falling outside. I looked around the room one last time: I was skeptical still that a night in the hands of a stranger could be so life-changing—I couldn't imagine doing it myself—yet I hoped that all those women, in their poignant and brave journeys, would find what they needed to find. Each of them, in her own way, was telling a compelling and fundamental truth: what she knew she had been given, sexually, by our culture, was not enough to reflect who she truly was.

As I plunged into the lighted chaos of Broadway, Caroline Muir's words to the searching women stayed with me:

"Most of the journey is shedding those layers of 'I'm not enough.' The Beloved is not the husband or the lover. The Beloved is in *me. The Beloved is me.*"

I had became convinced that Tantra had some answers to the question of how female sexuality was best understood. But even with my glimpse at the sacred-spot-massage retreat, Tantra still intimidated me.

I interviewed several Tantric "dakinis"—women from all kinds of backgrounds who had trained at Tantra workshops and practiced Tantra in their daily lives. From their own descriptions, these dakinis were much more orgasmic than groups of comparable women from whom I had also heard about their sexual lives. They also seemed unusually happy and energetic, and no matter what they looked like—and, as in any group of women, few of them looked like fashion models or conventional beauties. Unlike a theoretical control group, they seemed very satisfied with their own femininity, and had a kind of assurance about their sexuality.

The more I learned about Tantra, the more something else emerged: I saw that Tantric practices regarding female sexuality matched up in interesting ways with emerging new science on the brain and endocrinology. The Tantric masters of centuries ago seemed to have identified key points on the female body that corresponded to important neural pathways: the "sacred spot" matched the G-spot. The Taoist texts of ancient China encouraged men to suck on women's nipples, explaining that doing so causes women's bodies *and their minds* to relax; science has shown us that sucking on a woman's nipples releases oxytocin, the relaxing hormone. The Tantric and Taoist masters had identified significant fluids in women's vaginas that, though they were esoterically named, seemed to correspond to what the latest science was discovering about trace chemicals and hormones in body fluids. Tantric masters had identified female ejaculation, which is only now being studied by Western science. And Tantra simply got outstanding empirical sexual results for women who took these workshops.

My interest in divining Tantra's "secrets" is what led me to Mike Lousada, the man whom I would come to think of as "my resident adviser for all things yoni," and whose conversations would have such a lasting impact on me. His website, Heartdaka.com, is intriguing. The top of the home page reads "Mike Lousada's Sacred Sexual Healing in London," and beneath that runs a Rumi quotation, "Your task is not to seek love, but to merely seek and find all the barriers within yourself that you have built against it."

A series of intimate questions confronts the site's visitor: "Do you hold back from being in a relationship?"; "Do you feel there is more to sex but aren't sure what it is?"; "Do you feel unable to enjoy sex?"; "Do you have difficulty experiencing orgasm?"; "Do you want to reclaim the innocence of your sexuality?" But the ecstatic testimonials—all from women—quickly neutralize any potential threat.[5] "Thank you for holding me so skillfully in my vulnerability," Ms. D; "After seeing you, I hear my heart beat, I feel so alive—a real woman . . . Thank you," Ms. S; "Thanks, Mike. I feel grace and courage, feminine, protected, clarity, focused . . . a serene smile on my face," and so on. And there at the bottom of the page, as if Heartdaka.com were any old business, was a link to Lousada's Facebook profile, complete with his photo: a handsome man with a beard, seated on a rock, gazing out into the middle distance, and wearing hippieish trousers.

So, after some hesitation, I called Lousada and made an appointment. I learned that he charged a hundred pounds an hour (about $150).

He explained that his mission was to empower women sexually, and that he also focused on healing women sexually—via yoni massage—who had been erotically traumatized. His client base included women from all backgrounds and of all ages. His track record is impressive, to say the least: he has restored the orgasmic potential in hundreds of women.

Wow, I thought, this was a lot more explicit than the vague "workshop" and nebulous "massage" I had anticipated. I explained that since I was in a relationship I would not be open to actual yoni work, and he soothingly assured me that he would respect my boundaries.

The fact that I was going to interview a male sexual healer/yoni guru also wreaked havoc on my judgmental feminist reflexes about the sex trade and its morality.

I was fascinated by my own reaction and the reactions of my women friends and colleagues after I committed to seeing Lousada. Not a single female friend expressed horror or aversion; they were either totally captivated, or annoyed that they couldn't go too. E., a happily married mother of two, kept e-mailing me: "Well? Have you gone yet? What was it like?" We did not maturely consider this notion; our responses were not enlightened or politically correct. Rather, we all regressed to an almost adolescent state, with the feminine equivalent of locker-room chatter flying back and forth among us.

And yet, Lousada did not seem like anyone's victim or predator; with what intellectual cudgel could I beat his decision to enter an aspect of his sexuality into a market economy? I was brought to a standstill, in relationship to the issue of prostitution, by the very fact of him.

"Do you consider yourself a sex worker?" I asked, in our initial conversation.

He said that he preferred the term *sexual healer* (though now, a year later, as he has started to address a more mainstream and medical audience about his successful techniques, he identifies himself as a "somatic therapist"). He went on to say that he works clothed or unclothed, as the client wishes, and that the client can be dressed or undressed, as she likes, as well. Images flashed through my head—I couldn't quite believe that I was about to encounter my first yoni empowerer or, as I mistakenly saw it then, male sex worker catering to women. Did women seeking out someone like Lousada mean that women are just as "horny"—awful word, but there aren't a lot of good substitutes—as men have been so long portrayed? Or did it, rather, testify in a small way to a widespread sexual sorrow among Western women? Were women who could afford to, really seeking sexual encounters with hired men regardless of how the men described themselves—encounters that they could guide, and for which they could set the pacing—because their sexual lives with their own partners were not working well?

Lousada's "studio" is actually a charming renovated cottage near Chalk Farm, an area of north London. He opened the door. As in his photo, he was a fit, golden-skinned, curly-haired man who, alarmingly, immediately offered me a hug. Tantra must do wonders for the system, since he was forty-three, but looked a decade younger. I nervously sat on the floor, as he indicated, and looked around: we were in a warm sitting room with piles of red and orange pillows, a shrine to the Hindu goddess Kali on a low table, and candles and incense burning around us. To my horror, a male photographer was there.

I had arranged with the *Sunday Times* to write an article about my visit to Lousada. A photographer from the paper was supposed to arrive at the end of the session. But Lousada explained that he had asked him to come at the beginning, to spare me from revealing myself too much. "I was thinking of your well-being," he explained. "Things happen in a session," he continued. "It can be overwhelming. You may have awakened trauma; you could become ecstatic, or shout—or you might have been crying." I felt taken aback, and a bit stage-managed. Wasn't one's personal sexual healer supposed to keep one calm, rather than stress one out by upending one's professional arrangements?

Lousada then consulted with the photographer about possible shots, and suggested that I get into the "yab-yum" position with him. He gestured toward a statue that showed Shiva ecstatically entwined with a goddess, her thighs wrapped around his waist, their groins touching. "I'm not going to do *that!*" I burst out. As a compromise, the photos ended up being Lousada and me simply seated in the lotus position, face-to-face.

Before we began the session, Lousada explained that many of his clients had been sexually abused as girls, and as a result experienced aftereffects ranging from a deep rage against men, which manifested sexually, to an inability to feel deeply or to be orgasmic. Sex with him—he used his hand, for the most part—helped them, he claimed, heal their rage and depression.

Lousada soon began to guide me in Tantra 101. He had me sit before him on a cushion and engage in breathing exercises. We faced each other, inches apart. He had me visualize each chakra, from my head to my "root chakra," which in Tantra is the sex center (and which, I now know, corresponds to one of the three branches in the female pelvic nerve): "Feel your root chakra extend into the earth. . . . Feel it growing strong. . . . Your yoni is extending roots into the earth . . . now the roots are splitting rock."

I burst out laughing. The photographer snapped away.

"Nervous?" Lousada asked. "That's okay."

"No," I said, barely able to contain myself. "It's just funny."

But somehow the thought of a mighty earth-splitting yoni—in a generally yoni-hating and yoni-insulting culture—was . . . not unpleasant funny, but nice funny; still laughing, I pictured, as if in an animated movie, a mighty yoni superhero—a yoni avenger.

Then Lousada had me stare deeply into his eyes while we breathed in unison. At this point, I was checking my gut to see if he was a cad, a predator, or just a poseur. But in fact he met my gaze levelly and I had to admit, I trusted his motivations. My judgments were flying out the window, and when I considered his repeated mission statement—that his life work was to heal women who had been sexually harmed—it was very difficult to find a reason to dismiss or deride his work.

At the end of the breathing session, he smiled and said, "Welcome, Goddess."

And I couldn't help smiling, too. I thought of all the women in loveless marriages, women who were verbally ground down daily with disrespect or simple disregard. I thought, too, of the "whore with the heart of gold" stereotype, and the frequent report that many men visit female prostitutes just for the experience of someone listening to them or praising them. For many women, Lousada's acknowledgment of the sacred feminine in every woman could alone be worth the price of admission. How many exhausted moms, or taken-for-granted wives, wouldn't be at least as tempted by an apparently sincere "Welcome, Goddess" for only a hundred pounds, as they might be by a great new outfit or hairstyle?

"How exactly," I asked him, "do you heal women sexually?"

"I engage in 'yoni-tapping,' " he said, to address the trauma stored in the genitals. For various reasons—including the fact that a body worker can't get a license to touch the genitals—body workers don't usually look at trauma in this part of the body, he explained. "But I start with massaging the body. . . . Then I move into working on the yoni. First I work externally. When it's appropriate I ask if it's okay to enter [the client] with my fingers. The yoni is a sacred space. It is the holy of holies of your body. No one may enter without your permission. I ask: 'Goddess, may I enter?' If I get the consent, I check with the yoni to see. I place my fingers at the entrance to the yoni. If the yoni is ready to receive me, it will draw me in. There is no need for me to push my fingers, or 'insert'—it will actually draw me in, with a kind of reaching out or suction, if a woman is ready to receive.

"If this [reaching-out action] doesn't happen when a woman is having sex, she is actually dishonoring her own yoni." He went on to say that he advises men never to go with what a woman says verbally about her readiness—never to enter "if the yoni doesn't say yes, too." I thought that would be good advice to give to young men, as part of their basic sexual education.

Does he ever have intercourse with his clients? "I don't generally have intercourse with my clients unless it is extremely therapeutic." He restated that he generally worked with his hands. I asked if his clients ever became addicted to him; he replied that he is careful to keep appropriate boundaries, and that his intention is to free the client from addictions. He admitted that they could develop emotional attachments, but that he handled that situation as any therapist would handle transference. He added that he had a girlfriend, who also does sexual healing work, sometimes in concert with him.

"Do your clients have orgasms?" I asked.

"Generally," he replied, "but that's not the goal. I have three types of clients. Women who come to me because they are not happy with their relationships, with their own masculine or feminine. They yearn for a masculine man but they're not attracting that because they are 'in their masculine' [forced to live in an unbalanced way and drawing too much on the masculine side of their personalities] themselves." He spoke about the pressures of modern work life on women—how it rewards them for becoming unbalanced in this way and discourages their drawing on the feminine within them. When they see him, he claimed, they restore a feminine balance and start to attract grounded, responsible, protective, masculine men. I was skeptical, and he offered to put me in touch with some of them. Lousada said that a man's task in relation to a woman is to "hold her" as a wineglass holds wine. By now I had heard variants on this Tantric idea that a man's role in sex is to hold and support the wildness of the woman. "The true state of women is oceanic bliss," he said; a man needs to let a woman "move and breathe" so that she may enter "her flow."

This was getting a bit oceanic for me, so I asked him about the second category of client. Category number two, he said, "Are women who have suffered severe abuse or trauma. And they want to deal with it because it is ruining their lives."

Category three? "Sometimes my clients are women who just want to experience pleasure."

"What if you don't find them attractive?" I asked.

"There is always something beautiful about a woman," he said, rather endearingly. He explained that some of these clients are in their fifties or sixties; some are physically challenged in various ways, or disabled; many are alone in their lives. "In a session," he said, "I can always see something."

He says that he typically takes two or three hours for the yoni massage; he wants the woman to feel that there is no rush.

This timetable struck me profoundly, as did the descriptions I had heard from the Muirs' workshops' time allotment (an hour and a half) for "yoni massage" alone. This was obviously a completely different idea of the relationship of female pleasure to the allotment of time than the one we inherit in the West. "Isn't that a little long?" I asked. "I can imagine that if you tell an average man that he needs to take two or three hours to pay attention to the woman in that way, he will immediately look around for the remote control," I joked.

"That's why I need to teach men," Lousada responded seriously.

I was sold, at least on Lousada's sincerity. On to the massage—or the amount of it I was comfortable with.

He led me upstairs, into a seductive little bedroom. The photographer had left by then. The bedroom was lit with candles and fragrant with more incense. There, once again, we got into a negotiation: he was intent on a yoni massage. It was such a frankly sexual situation, with none of the lotus-y deniability I had imagined when I first looked at his website and thought it would involve some vaguely sensual massage—I couldn't go there. I was in bed with an attractive stranger and there was no way to pretend that what he was proposing would not be a form of sex. The nice monogamous Jewish girl in me once again drew a line.

"Can't we do some . . . body work?" I asked. He also had a Reiki qualification. "Reiki?" I added, hopefully.

He looked insulted. "Yoni work is what I *do*," he said, with professional pride.

Finally we agreed: he would work with me nonsexually and I would keep my shirt and sarong on. Well, within thirty seconds I was in a state of—yes—oceanic bliss. Within five minutes I was laughing, and within ten minutes I was in an altered state.

What was he doing?

"What are you *doing*?" I asked. Lousada explained that through a great deal of training he could project his Shakti (male) energy into every part of his body—including his hands, his fingers—and that that was what caused the effect of his touch. He was tracing, he explained, the meridian lines of my body—lines of energy, or *chi,* that Eastern medicine believes form a network between chakra points—with the tips of his fingers. There was some inexplicable kinetic charge. Our session lasted for an hour, and, yes, even though it was not a sexual exchange, there was something electrifying and life-enhancing about physically "receiving" in that leisurely, agenda-less way, for an hour.

When I left Lousada's studio, I was on what I now knew to be a dopamine high. Colors looked brighter, the world seemed full of joy and sensuality, and the friend who in fact met me afterward said—if grumpily—that I looked flushed and beaming.

I went back to Lousada by phone to try to tease out how his method actually worked—I especially wanted to understand what he saw as the link between a woman's healing from vaginal massage, and her emergence in areas of her life beyond the sexual.

"When a woman feels safe, she allows herself *to* herself—not to me—and to her orgasmic pleasure. A man takes four minutes to reach orgasm on average," Lousada noted again, "a woman, sixteen minutes. Unless he is patient, he is going to come more quickly than she will. So when we talk about 'normal sex,' the man ejaculates just when the woman's body is just beginning to soften, open, relax into that beautiful . . . it's over. A lot of women have given up on that kind of sex. Women are withdrawing from that kind of sex and conclud-ing it's not satisfying.

"Many men are not spending the time with their lovers that is necessary. Women experience that kind of sex and think that is 'sex.' It is partly due to a lack of knowledge, for both men and women. Women's true sexuality is suppressed in society. Our culture doesn't allow the same kinds of response to women that it does to men. Stud-ies show that twenty-nine percent of women never have orgasm in intercourse. Fifteen percent of women do so only rarely. Compared to point six percent of men. Tests on women have shown that there is no physiological reason why all women can't have orgasms. That tells me that preorgasmia is a psychological condition.

"We [men] need to make women feel safe if we want them to re-spond orgasmically. We need some rudimentary knowledge of where to touch and how—simple anatomy, and sensitivity. Actually one of the most important things for men to remember is that we all take actions based on our own sexual experiences, so men are doing to their wives and lovers what they think feels good based on their own sexual makeup, and women are not telling them that there is another way. So when a woman comes to me and says, 'My lovers aren't giving me orgasms'—she has often not been taking responsibility. Very few of my clients express their own sexual desires. I've had clients say to me, 'I wish I could have an orgasm, it would be a beautiful gift for him,' or 'Damned if I'm giving him my orgasm.' So yes, there are things men can do, but it is women who need to be healed. Women get in touch with their sexual selves and become more creative; spiritual; artistic. They get different jobs! It's about releasing their life force."

Well, that was a strong assertion, and I needed independent corroboration. So I asked him to connect me to a client of his who would confirm this far-reaching claim.

He put me in touch with an articulate, thoughtful woman in her thirties, whom I will call "Angela."

"I read your article in the *Sunday Times* and made an appointment," said Angela. "I had felt completely disconnected from men, and experienced a long period of celibacy. My romantic relationships were not positive; I had a problem with sexual harassment as well. I had a boyfriend, but it wasn't a deep relationship; I couldn't open up to him physically. I wasn't ready to open up sexually. It had been a while.

"Seeing Mike affected my creativity completely. I needed healing from a man. I had five sessions around that time, and still have sessions with him every few months. The first two sessions were mainly talking—quite therapeutic. Since the third session I have had yoni work. The first session was talking, holding, and me weeping. Acknowledging how I felt. The second session was profound—acknowledging how angry I was. Mike had me shouting, "FUCK OFF!" at him to release my rage. It was big for me to bring this up in front of a man. . . . I was sure that if I was angry in relationship to a man I would be sent away.

"After that experience, I started to write short stories—I was being more myself. The third session was yoni work: I had ejaculated when I was younger—it was very moving to have that occur again.

It was about me, he was interested in me, my pleasure—that was a big thing. I had enough time. In my previous sexual experiences, I had often felt rushed—and often felt quite nervous about what men want. I found it very difficult to relax during sex, though I was able to have orgasms, and had experienced multiple orgasms. Previously, though, I'd often sort of disappeared when I'd had an orgasm—not in a good way, for sure. To stay in my body when I had an orgasm was a big thing. A lot of emotion came up: past trauma. It felt safe: because of the emotional safety I was able to relax more: he knew what to do.

"I'd never had a vaginal orgasm before—they had all been from my clitoris—but I did with him. He found some sort of spot that totally worked. I was able to get into my sexuality very deeply, flow very intensely—I was angry, crying. . . . He's an example of what a respectful man is. I wanted respect but didn't know what that looked like, felt like. This helps me to feel more confident in my ability to judge a man's integrity.

"I have had multiple orgasms before—about two or three in a row . . . with Mike, I had a dozen: I was able to be passionate. I'd had an 'energy blockage' previously—here I'd be able to have a good scream. In previous relationships, men didn't allow me to be emotional. In my family you couldn't express feelings. To be allowed to be emotional with a man . . . I am now much more able to speak up for myself.

I stood up to my manager. I argue my point more in general—I would not have done that before. I started realizing that I'd always assumed that others were right and I was wrong—I started realizing I didn't need to parrot people. I could be myself more. I felt more self-confidence. I was feeling better when I looked in the mirror. I had been told I was ugly. [After working with Lousada] I liked my face a lot more. I am accepting that I am a volatile and passionate person. It comes out a lot more. During masturbation, I was able to give myself better orgasms. My sexual fantasies changed. . . . I was always being dominated [in my fantasies previously]. There had always been a warped vision of a father figure. Now I could give myself orgasms without even thinking of a man—now my whole body is having an orgasm. So physical changes are simultaneous with psychological changes for me.

"Another thing—I had always wanted to go into opinion-based writing; but I had moved back in with my parents and was working in an office. After working with Lousada, I got a more creative job. I knew the whole time I would get it.

"Creativity? This time, creatively, it was like I had melted into everything. I was there. My brain wasn't chattering—I trusted my body to take over; I felt free, with a feeling of integrity. My goals are more physical. I have a sense of being held and knowing I won't be dropped. Mike talks a lot about women being Goddesses; I definitely feel like a Goddess. I have been writing stories about the Goddess Persephone. Her husband brings her underground but it's a good thing. . . . She chooses it. It's all about connecting with the darkness. I'm seeing the Goddess in myself; seeing the Goddess in other people—seeing the God in Mike—I am more compassionate. I can see myself in others.

"After these sessions with Mike, all this was unblocked. It's like a rocket going off. I'm attracting much more positive men in my life. I feel capable of having a romantic relationship. I have a safe sexual space."

"Do you feel your emergent sexuality equals emergent aspects of your self?" I asked.

"Yes," she replied. Then she added: "Some wounds women have can only be healed by a man."

---

Lousada's description of the vagina "reaching out" when it was ready, so odd to me at first, made more and more sense as I did further research into Tantric tradition and its Taoist counterpart. The Eastern traditions see the vagina as alive—that is, as expressing its own kind of will, preferences, influence, and agency—a way of seeing that is fundamentally alien to us, and that is so very different from the passive, receptive, personality-less, and effectively *voiceless* way the vagina is portrayed in our own culture.

The very definition of what it means for a vagina to "open," though it is the same word, has two completely different interpretations in Eastern and Western cultures. In the Eastern traditions such as the Tantra and the Tao, the man addresses, with caresses and care, the "gatekeeper," the outer vagina and labia, and awaits permission for further entry, whether by hand, tongue, or penis; and the subsequent opening of the vagina is itself a complex, gradual, and graduated process, which develops over time and under the influence of various attentions and entreaties. In the West, the "opening" of the vagina is understood to be subject simply to a woman parting her legs, or a man's penetration of it with his penis; the vagina opens, in the West, like a mechanism, or like a door, a curtain, or a box. The Eastern model of vaginal opening, in contrast, is more akin to an "unfolding" or an "unfurling," a "coming alive" or an "expansion"—more like a time-lapse photograph, like a lotus expanding in the sun.

And I took away from my Tantric explorations a wonderful phrase. As my friends and I now sometimes joke—or half joke—to one another, when narrating a romantic adventure, "But what did the *yoni* have to say?"

# Radical Pleasure, Radical Awakening:
# The Vagina as Liberator

*Today I want to paint nakedness . . . I wish you . . . would take me out into the night—way out there into the dark blueness— and that the day would never come . . .*

—Georgia O'Keeffe

The more I learned about both the latest brain science around female arousal, and about the ancient practice of Tantra, the more it seemed that a group of Hindu spiritual seekers centuries ago had figured out pretty fully a set of insights about the mind-body connection in sexuality with which Western science was only now beginning to catch up.

Indeed, these two traditions, the Western medical/sexological and the Eastern Tantric, are starting to inform each other. Since I first met with Lousada, he has further developed a prominent practice consulting with, and presenting methodological papers to, mainstream physicians' groups focused on sexual health and dysfunction in women.

When Lousada was gazing deeply into a client's eyes, he was stimulating the neurobiological response prepared in women by eye gazing as they instinctively seek, as both genders do, to gauge from dilated pupils a possible partner's health and arousal levels.[1] When he said, "Welcome, Goddess," he was destressing her, reassuring her on the level of her autonomic nervous system (ANS) that she was sexually safe—respected and valued, and seen as uniquely lovely by a potential partner. This allowed her system to become ready: her nipples to engorge, her skin to flush, and her vagina to lubricate. Because of the stronger connections between the hemispheres in the female brain than in the male's, when Lousada verbalized positive imagery about her vagina, her mind and body were both better prepared to start processing sexual images and thoughts.[2] Because women react with a far more pronounced relaxation response to being stroked, Lousada's non-goal-oriented, nonpressured stroking boosts the positive female cycle of heightened relaxation to heightened arousal. Tantra, seen in this light, is really not something so mysterious at all, but rather a form of applied neuroscience, intentionally activating the brain's connection to the sex organs.

The mysticism-inducing ANS in women—along with all of a woman's sexual and other body systems working together in ways that go far beyond what we in the West identify as "sex" but that are nonetheless vital to women's sexual and emotional happiness—I will call "the Goddess Network." The things that men need to do to women to engage the Goddess Network—what sex educator Liz Topp called "the things women need that men don't need," and for which we, revealingly, don't have a single name—I call "the Goddess Array." I am especially likely to identify as part of the Goddess Array an act or gesture or caress that is confirmed by the intersection of both basic Tantric practice and recent or established scientific research, though there are no doubt countless additions and variations to this brief summary of the Goddess Array.

The data from both the Eastern and the Western traditions reveal that any man or woman can give the kind of attention the Goddess Array requires to all those areas in women that should, ideally, be reached and caressed. As Lousada put it, "patience and compassion" from men in particular, in attending to women's sexual responses are much more important in bringing women to a high state of physical ecstasy and emotional release than is any more superficial measure of physical endowment.

Before we go through "the Goddess Array," though, I just want to note a caveat: women are often encouraged to see public discussion of their sexuality as setting some new goal, or as being proscriptive or prescriptive. This is not my intention at all. I cannot stress enough: every woman is different. I wish to make clear that I offer these only as information—based on what works in Tantric practice, and specifically on what works in that practice that turns out to have a basis in recent science.

Some women may like all aspects of "the Goddess Array" all the time. Some will want a little of what follows, some may want a great deal; or what the same woman wants will vary at different times (including, neurobiologically, at different times of the month). Other women will never respond to this set of gestures and approaches. Still others may like these gestures and approaches often but, at other times, will prefer fast anonymous sex in dark alleyways. These gestures and approaches are points of exploration, and my discussion of them is to elucidate the mind-body connection in female sexual response.

## FIRST, VALUE HER AND HELP HER

Dr. Helen Fisher pointed out, in *The Anatomy of Love,* that women's evolutionary need to have a partner to help her during the vulnerable first two years of a child's life predisposes women to value behavior from men that indicates that they are cherished and being committed to. I call this "investment behavior." This is different, as Dr. Fisher herself points out, from the old canard of evolutionary biologists who insist that fertile young women will respond sexually to older men with money and power.[3]

Dr. Fisher's persuasive theory about women benefiting in evolutionary terms by responding sexually to men who demonstrate that they can partner effectively for the baby's vulnerable years, and who show that they can keep mother and baby safe, led me to wonder—given that this was so valuable evolutionarily to women, their bodies, indeed their vaginas—if it might prompt them to "notice" or register such actions in potential mates before their minds had paid attention, in the same way that recent science has established a biological basis for the "gut response" to others.

Both Tantra and contemporary science confirm that there is a pulse in the vagina. Indeed, several recent Western studies of female sexual response measure it. Most women are raised to pay no attention at all to this pulse outside of a sexual context. When you draw women's attention to the delicate, ever-present, distinctive pulse in the vagina, they can note it in most circumstances, and certainly often in nonsexual contexts as well.

It seems plausible that this pulse tells a woman a great deal about how safe her emotional setting is, and how valued and safe she is sexually within it.

No one with whom I spoke, either in person or online, had ever heard of the concept of the vaginal pulse. (Neither had I before I did the research for this book.) Researchers of female sexual response actually measure it now in standardized units, in a unit of measurement called "VPA"—vaginal pulse amplitude—which is measured in turn by a "vaginal photometer," a device that sends a light signal to track vaginal blood flow. Researchers are finding important connections between the VPA and female sexual response.[4] But once women did hear the concept, and I had told them about the brain-vagina connection, none of the women with whom I spoke had any trouble at all identifying her own vaginal pulse and answering my questions.

I asked women respondents to my online survey to note when the vaginal pulse gave a particularly noticeable thump or beat in a nonsexual context. What was happening?

Some women confirmed that the "thump" or "stronger than usual beat" of the vaginal pulse, as two respondents put it, resulted from some behavior by a partner or husband that was kind, or that showed an ability to protect effectively, or that demonstrated "investment behavior." (Unfortunately, I did not receive answers from women who identified themselves as lesbian or bisexual to this informal survey; a quantitative study that would show whether women of all sexualities experience the pulse in the same ways when their lovers do similar things, or whether different things trigger the pulse in women of different sexualities, would be fascinating, of course.)

"I felt the vaginal pulse when my boyfriend and I were grocery shopping in a supermarket and he remembered—I had forgotten—that we needed cat food for my cat."

"I felt the pulse when my husband took me out to dinner on my birthday and he drew out my chair for me."

"We were camping and I realized my pillow smelled moldy. My husband gave me his pillow, so he didn't have one; he used his coat. I felt it then. Sometimes the pulse is so hard it is almost uncomfortable. I definitely wanted to make love then, to relieve the tension."

"My husband was teaching our son to fix his bike. I felt it."

Some women reported feeling a vaginal pulse when their partner showed physical strength, artistic creativity, or certain kinds of skill or self-mastery or emotional openness:

"I felt it when we were at the dump! He knelt and lifted up an old couch we were getting rid of, and threw it off the back of the truck."

"When we were at a family event, and I noticed him spending time talking to my elderly grandmother, which takes a lot of patience."

"When we were first dating, and I watched him drive really skillfully on a rainy road."

"When I heard him sing for the first time."

"When he cooked breakfast for me."

Many of the women's responses to these questions showed that while a man's ability to offer emotional security and caring can have erotic effects on straight women, so, too, can the promise of a man's capacity for creativity and for adventure or risk. Dr. Pfaus explains this seeming contradiction with the dual nature of the female ANS—it likes to be relaxed and then it likes to be activated. This certainly helps explain why in generation after generation, adolescent girls and young women scream with sexual excitement after being sung to by male rock stars and balladeers; the singing activates the ANS. He also noted that the female ANS relaxes best when free from "bad stress," but that "good stress," like dangerously exciting scenarios that the woman still controls, can be sexually compelling, especially to those women with low baseline ANS activation.

But what I certainly did not expect to see were answers revealing that women experienced the vaginal beat more strongly in entirely nonsexual and even nonrelationship contexts—settings in which they encountered aesthetic beauty or natural beauty, in which they were being creative, or in which they asserted their own power or identity. This would suggest that a woman's relationship to her own mind and body is erotic *first;* that her existential excitement at being alive and responsive to the world around her is erotic *first;* and that this eros comes before any erotic awakening triggered by an "other":

"I felt it beat one night when I was filling my car at a gas station. I was facing a state park mountain range, and I noticed a mass of fog coming in over the tops of the mountains. I felt the thump when I realized how beautiful and majestic the scene was."

"I was listening to a Mozart Requiem, and in a section with cascading notes, I felt the pulse."

And a man reported: "I had a female friend who had an orgasm while we were hiking, just from the beauty of the trees and the riverbank on which we were standing."

The vaginal beat even showed up stronger in contexts of competition, winning, or ego validation: "I felt the pulse when a coworker who had done something unethical—which I had known about, but no one had believed me—was found out. I am not proud of that but it is true. I felt powerful."

"I felt it when I crossed the finish line in a marathon."

"I felt the pulse at my first art show when I listened to people praising my work."

"At the racetrack."

The vaginal pulse is evidently not just a way for a woman to discern her own sexual arousal: it also seems to be a way for the vagina continually to inform the woman about herself on many other levels.

## BRING HER FLOWERS; DIM THE LIGHTS; RELAX HER

In Spike Lee's 1986 film *She's Gotta Have It,* the following dialogue takes place between a man and a woman who have just begun kissing.

"Where are you going?" the man asks, surprised, as the young woman, Nola, gets up out of bed.

"To get the candles," she replies seductively.

"Are you sure you have enough?" He gestures at the dozens of candles behind them, sarcastically.

"Don't you smell them? The candles, they're scented," she replies, still low-voiced.

"Yeah, they smell good," he replies abruptly. "Now, why don't you undress?"

This is a classic gender miscommunication. Nola isn't just trying to "get the candles"; she is trying to get into an altered, heightened ANS state that will affect the intensity of her orgasm. But her male lover thinks she is just wasting time on pointless atmospherics that could be better spent cutting to the chase.

For Nola's brain, the candlelight *is* part of her physical desire, not just some random decor. In Louann Brizendine's *The Female Brain,* she explains the neurochemistry of this:

> *Finally, everything was in place. Her mind was calm. The massage did the trick. Vacation was always the best place. No work, no worries, no phone, no email. No place else for Marcie's brain to run. . . . She could let go and let it happen. Her brain's anxiety center was shutting down. The area for conscious decision making wasn't lighting up so intensely. The neurochemical and neurological constellations were aligning for orgasm. . . . Female sexual turn-on begins, ironically, with a brain turn-off. The impulses can rush to the pleasure centers and trigger an orgasm only if the amygdala—the fear and anxiety center of the brain—has been deactivated. Before the amygdala has been turned off, any last-minute worry . . . can interrupt the march*

*toward orgasm. The fact that a woman requires this extra neu-*
*rologiocal step may account for why it takes her an average three*
*to ten times longer than the typical man to reach orgasm. . . .*
*Nerves in the tip of the clitoris connect straight to the pleasure*
*center in the female brain . . . if fear, stress or guilt interfere*
*with stimulation, the clitoris is stopped dead in its tracks. . . .*
*The clitoris really is the brain below the waist.*[5]

The quality of women's orgasms is measurably affected by light-ing and by the "coziness" and beauty of the surroundings in which they are making love. Lousada had started his session by seating the "Goddess," whomever she might be, next to an altar filled with flow-ers, and before a beautiful *tangka*, or embroidered sacred tapestry. He also lit candles. In Charles and Caroline Muir's Tantric "sacred spot" weekend workshops, the men are carefully instructed to pre-pare by drawing a bath in the hotel suite for the woman in the couple. Tantric texts always advise couples to make certain that lovemaking takes place in a setting in which there is beauty and order: to put a lo-tus or other flowers in water near the bed, and burn incense in front of an elegantly appointed shrine full of lovely pictures or statues. The ancient goddesses of female sexuality and fertility, from Inanna to Astarte to Aphrodite, were associated not just with sex but also with flowers, the decorative arts, adornment, and aesthetic beauty.

While this kind of aesthetic preparation may seem extreme and cumbersomely lengthy to a Western reader, and is certainly not practicable at an hour-and-a-half minimum on an everyday ba-sis, it should never be dismissed as trivial. This Tantric advice is grounded in neuroscience: soft lights, flowers, preparation gestures in tribute to her comfort such as running her a bath, are all far more likely to put a woman into the state of deep relaxation that will pre-pare her ANS for much higher levels of arousal than sex without these preparatory gestures.

This set of preparation gestures is also often erotic to women even when they engage in them alone. When a woman puts on soft lingerie and perfume or lights candles and fills her room with flowers, it often makes her feel aroused and capable of arousing. This transitional preparation changes a woman's body's responses, and her relaxation allows for the play of her imagination.

Is the Tantric (and Sumerian, Phoenician, Cretan, Hellenic, and so on) association of female sexuality with flowers and adornment, in this hard-core age of ours, a kind of Ganges-via-Northern-California hooey? Or is there in fact something deep in feminine neurobiology that these ancients clearly understood? Why do men who are courting bring flowers—especially lushly petalled, vulval flowers such as red roses—and why will any control group of heterosexual women instinctively agree that they don't want the guy who brings chrysanthemums, or carnations? Why does it seem to matter, erotically, if the flowers were ordered thoughtfully in advance, or picked up hastily at the deli down the street, and offered in their plastic wrapping?

Why does it come to really matter to many women who have been in long relationships if their husbands stop bringing flowers altogether—and certainly if they forget to send flowers on Valentine's Day? Why are women so sensitive—*why is it such a big deal?*

Could it be because there is something about this thing—so often forgotten, or overlooked—that women need, in order to protect and maintain a strong sexual response to their mates? The answer is yes. Not every woman will want candles, flowers, or music; some will want other kinds of more provocative focus, but virtually every woman will want some unique preparatory tributes or gestures. Even if she just wants a hot fast physical encounter, she will want it more if he has made some gesture that she experiences as romantic, or as communicating his desire, at another point in the day. When men over time "forget" to do these things or think that they don't matter anymore—the woman is married to him now, for instance, so why actually "seduce" her each time sex is on the agenda?—they inadvertently virtually guarantee that their wives will have more trouble wanting them passionately, over a period of time.

We saw how powerful the role of the sympathetic nervous system (SNS) is—that is, relaxation—in preparing a woman's body for arousal. Buried within a study of an unrelated phenomenon—the famous 1981 study by John Delbert Perry and Beverly Whipple of the G-spot and female ejaculation—the researchers shared some important asides about the environment in which they tested their female subjects' vaginal sensations.[6] Perry and Whipple discovered a difference, in their terms, between uterine and vulval (clitoral) orgasms. They measured women's responses when the G-spot was touched, they measured the women's uterine contractions during orgasm, and they recorded whether or not they "ejaculated"—that is, emitted from their urethras a clear fluid. (Researchers are still debating whether or not female ejaculation has been proved, and are not completely certain what the urethral liquid consists of.)

In this aside, Perry and Whipple cautioned other scientists to take into account the role that the environmental setting was likely to play on the orgasmic outcomes they measured. In other words, Perry and Whipple had sought to look at G-spot sensation versus other kinds of vaginal and clitoral sensation; but in the process they were finding that the comfort and lighting of the setting affected the intensity of the orgasms that they were measuring, and even affected whether or not their female subjects could ejaculate.

In one case, the researchers tested a subject in a sterile, bright doctor's office—a setting many people associate with pain, illness, and disease. The subject, disappointed in her "poor showing" in that environment, requested that the test be redone. "Propitiously," the authors wrote, "the physician's office [that had been used previously for the test] was not available for the re-evaluation procedure, which was carried out in the subject's own living room, in the presence of her sexual partner. In this setting, her vaginal myograph measurement was 26 microvolts (compared with 11.8 in the office), and her uterine myograph measurement was 36 microvolts (compared with 6.88 a few days earlier). The subject was greatly relieved at the new data thus obtained, which she felt better reflected her self-understanding of her state of sexual health."[7]

Then another group confirmed this first subject's dramatically different results in a more cozy setting. Because of a scheduling glitch, a whole group of test subjects also had to shift their second test locations. This second location was also a doctor's office, as the first one had been. But this office, in contrast, was one in which biofeedback was done. Biofeedback requires a relaxation response in the subject, in order to be successful. The second office was soothingly lighted, comfortably furnished, and appealingly decorated.

In the lower-lit, more aesthetically pleasing settings, the same women's orgasm intensity measurements jumped. The same group of women even ejaculated more often in the more pleasant, more relaxing second setting than in the clinical first setting.

If you read the researchers' careful scientific language, you can see that they are saying that the more "seductive" physical setting led women who ejaculated to have almost twice as many "microvolts" in the measurements of their vaginal contractions and almost four times as many in their uterine contractions during orgasm than women had had in the brightly lit, clinical setting—and what girl doesn't want *that:*

> *The substantial difference between these two measurements on the same subject suggested a variety of post hoc explanations such as partner presence, fatigue, menstrual cycle position, experimental environment, and practice effects. The only variable for which data were available was experimental environment. Subjects were retrospectively divided into two groups; one consisted of those women who had been measured while on a standard gynecological examining table in a physician's office or clinic, and the second group was comprised of women who were measured while in a reclining chair or upon a sofa in a biofeedback therapist's office.*
>
> *The results of this post hoc analysis suggest that the environment of the examination may have been important. There were only slight differences in the case of non-ejaculators, who tend to have weaker muscles. But for ejaculators, the differences were substantial: the 6 ejaculatory women measured on a gynecological table averaged 8.32 uV (SD = 3.44) with the vaginal myograph, compared with 12.95 uV (SD = 6.15) for the remaining*

*19 women, t (16) = 2.33, p = .05. Uterine myograph differences were also noted. The 5 ejaculatory women on the gynecological table group averaged 7.38 uV (SD = 3.51) compared with 15.88 uV (SD = 4.42) for the 11 other ejaculatory women, t (10) = 4.13, p < .01.*[8]

Beverly Whipple has found an even more groundbreaking connection between the differences in how vaginal, clitoral, and G-spot orgasms are experienced by women, and different parts of the female brain. In a 2011 presentation, Whipple and her coauthors showed that indeed clitoral, vaginal, and G-spot sensations and orgasms appear in different—that is, separable—but related parts of the female brain; not only that, but they found that women use different emotional and sensory descriptors for clitoral, vaginal, G-spot, and "blended" orgasms (with most women preferring "blended"). These differences are so well documented by Whipple's work that she calls cervical or G-spot orgasm "deep orgasm" and designed a vibrator specifically to activate it.[9]

The conclusion that Whipple and Perry drew from their earlier, 1981, study is clear, and potentially very exciting: "this post hoc analysis . . . does suggest that careful attention to the experimental environment and its 'sexual' (or antisexual) mood is necessary in future research into sexual functioning."[10]

Many women have spoken to me about what they feel they have lost, sexually, in long-term relationships. I have noticed that many women speak with great bitterness about having to be the one to make reservations for "date night," or to hire the babysitter on Valentine's Day. This bitterness is intensified if the women remember a courtship period in which they did not have to do this kind of work. There seems, in their narratives, to be something about "having to be the one" to do this labor—it is described as labor—that is connected to sexual flatness; their resentment seems linked to some sense that if they make the reservation for date night, the night won't be arousing to them; they will be, romantically, going through the motions somehow.

When they have to do all the romantic "work," they are angry because they are rightly perceiving that their men have abdicated their role of tending to the absolutely minimally necessary tasks that continually reignite their wives' desire for them. They are angry because they know the men will want sex later, but they feel that the men have stopped valuing the wives' own arousal.

(They are also angry because they probably are starting to get tense and uncomfortable, anticipating, as Dr. Pfaus's sexually frustrated female rats eventually did, bad sex; arousal without good release—negatively activated dopamine—is, as Dr. Pfaus explained earlier, an extremely physically negative experience for female mammals, whether they are in a laboratory cage, or in a suburban bedroom.)

Straight men would do well to ask themselves: "Do I want to be married to a Goddess—or a bitch?" Unfortunately, there is not, physiologically, much middle ground available for women. Either they are extremely well treated sexually, or, if solo, treat themselves well sexually—or else they are at risk of becoming physically uncomfortable and emotionally irritable. As Dr. Pfaus's studies on female sexual stress reveal, the stress levels caused by sexual frustration are not something female mammals can control. Tantra and neuroscience strongly suggests to men in that situation, even if they think their wives or girlfriends are temporarily insane: Bring home a rose. Make the restaurant reservation. Tidy the bedroom. Light the candle.

## HELP HER GO INTO AN
## ORGASMIC TRANCE STATE

Relaxation and disinhibition go together. The SNS, when it is really activated, is a female sexual trance state's best friend.

Recent neuroscience is confirming what Tantra has always maintained—and what the loss-of-self scenes in women's greatest fictions hint at: climaxing women go into a trance state that is different from what men experience in orgasm. In "Regional Cerebral

Blood Flow Changes Associated with Clitorally Induced Orgasm in Healthy Women," Janniko R. Georgiadis and others looked at MRI images of the brains of women subjects who had been asked, first, rather awkwardly, to imitate the body contractions of arousal and orgasm but try *not* to become aroused—this was to control for movement showing up on the MRI—and then, having done that, they were asked to go ahead and masturbate, or be masturbated by their partners, to orgasm. The MRI images of the women's brains exploding in rainbow spots of color at the moment of orgasm—in different places in the brain than the researchers had expected—was an image of breakthrough science: "the first account of brain regions involved in experience of clitoral stimulation."[11]

The findings could be read as hinting—not by any means confirming—that the ages-old fear that sex makes women into something like witches, or into maenads who have no moral boundaries at the moment of orgasm, may have a bit of truth to it. The researchers found "significant deactivation of dorsomedial prefrontal cortex," which is the location of the brain's engagement with "moral reasoning and social judgment." This finding "implies absence of moral judgment and self-referential thought" in just that part of the brain that usually takes care of those functions, at the moment of orgasm. This suggests that when women are climaxing they lose an awareness of a separate self, lose self-consciousness, find it hard to self-censor—as when a woman can't help vocalizing, for instance, in a hotel room with thin walls, even if she will be embarrassed after lovemaking that she has caused a ruckus. The Georgiadis group found "increasing RCBF during stimulation for inhibition," which means that the women's brains were showing less activity in the area where behavior can be inhibited. This confirmed an earlier finding by Mah and Binik, in 2001, which showed engagement in the area of the female brain during orgasm that regulated "loss of conscious control."[12] The later researchers also found that female orgasm was experienced in the "ventral midbrain"—which is exactly where the Tantric "third eye" is supposed to extend into. (Dopamine is active here: the ventral midbrain is where the "dopaminergic cell" group is located.)

But the finding of this group of scientists, that women go into a disinhibited, out-of-conscious-control trance state, is important to understand for other reasons as well. Indeed, when Janniko Georgiadis and his colleagues found that clitoral orgasm creates activity in a part of the brain related to behavioral disinhibition and deregulation, they explained, quite poetically for a journal of neuroscience, why the French refer to female orgasm as "*le petit mort*" (the little death). They made the point that for women, unlike for men, orgasm leads to a state that feels like a loss of a certain kind of regulated consciousness, or a loss of a certain kind of self. I think this finding is extraordinarily important in our understanding that sex has radically different meanings and associations for women than for men. We should realize that in terms of certain aspects of pleasure, there are similarities in sex for women and men; but we err if we stop there. In some senses having to do with consciousness—and not with pleasure—sex for women is a different thing altogether than sex is for men.

I believe that this neurological activation of an experience of a lost self, a submersion in a tide of a force beyond one's own control, an overtakenness with disinhibition against all of one's conscious will, has powerfully influenced women's fiction. Images of awakened sexuality leading to the dissolution of a limited sense of self abound in women's novels. Edna Pontellier, the heroine of Kate Chopin's *The Awakening*, once she is sexually awakened, swims out naked to sea, and to a possible death. Maggie Tulliver in George Eliot's *The Mill on the Floss*, once sexually awakened, as we saw, is swept out to her death in a flood. Christina Rossetti's Laura and Lizzie, in "Goblin Market," once they taste the erotic fruits of "goblin men," are nearly torn apart and annihilated. Charlotte Brontë's Jane Eyre, in the novel of that title, once sexually awakened, loses consciousness, nearly starving to death on a heath after a storm. Perhaps these scenes are not about sexual punishment, but rather reflect glimpses of altered states related to sexual fulfillment, and perhaps, too, they reflect the understandable anxiety caused in women writers and subjects who value self-control over the disinhibition of the female brain in a state of sexual transcendence. So many women writers, from Charlotte Brontë to Christina Rossetti to Edith Wharton, express both an attraction to and a fear of an erotic loss of self or loss of control. If you understand the science, this fear of and attraction to the female orgasmic experience—because it involves the sense of a dissolved self and a loss of conscious control—are both very reasonable reactions on the part of women writers and artists, and indeed, women in general.

Neuroscientists are identifying parts of the brain that may be connected to some people's self-reported experiences of "oneness" or the dissolution of a sense of self, even if that experience is very brief. Kevin Nelson, M.D., in his book, *The Spiritual Doorway in the Brain: A Neurologist's Search for the God Experience,* speculates that the sense of a "loss of self" in the mystical experience may be related to the shutting down in certain moments of "the temporoparietal brain"; he notes that "important parts of the neurological self are within the temporoparietal brain," and that when the brain centers that construct a "neurological self" are quieted, people can have the sense of "oneness with something larger."[13] Could this be useful in reading the possible implications of the Georgiadis study? Could it be useful in understanding the attraction and dread that recurs in women's fiction toward scenes of sexual awakening that are followed with scenes that seem to threaten erasure of the self?

Edith Wharton writes to her lover Morton Fullerton about the "golden blur" that her thoughts and words—her conscious identity—become at his touch, and she uses a vaginal metaphor of a chest or box full of treasures to enter and describe this mind-state:

> *I'm so afraid that the treasures I long to unpack for you, that have come to me in magic ships from enchanted islands, are only, to you, the old familiar calico and beads of the clever trader. . . . I'm so afraid of this, that often & often I stuff my shining treasures back into their box, lest I should see you smiling at them!*

> *Well! And if you do . . . And if you can't come into a room*
> *without my feeling all over a ripple of flame, &, wherever you*
> *touch me, a heart beats under your touch, & if, when you hold*
> *me, & I don't speak, it's because all the words seem to me to have*
> *become throbbing pulses, & all my thoughts are a great golden*
> *blur—why should I be afraid of your smiling at me, when I can*
> *turn the beads and calico into such beauty?*[14]

In *The House of Mirth* (1905), Wharton also seeks to describe the loss of self that realized sexual passion threatens, or proposes, to women as she describes her heroine, Lily Bart's, sexual temptation: "The mortal maid on the shore is helpless against the siren who loves her prey: such victims are floated back dead from their adventure."[15]

This activation of the part of the brain involved with a loss of all conscious boundaries poses an incredible challenge to the female writer or female philosopher because it means that women's experiences of the boundaries of the self—if these women are orgasmic—are regularly *different* from men's experiences of the boundaries of self. The self has been constructed in masculine, Western philosophy as rational, conscious, guided by will, and master of discrete boundaries and of autonomy; but orgasmic women's brains regularly have a subjective experience of the self as unbounded, flowing into or overtaken by a greater force, limitless, not subject to conscious control. The uncanniness of that orgasmic loss of control certainly could be why men have portrayed women sexually as irrational, as maenads and witches.

That wild cell group in that crazy, out-of-control female ventral midbrain? It responds ecstatically to a whole range of stimuli: "this cell group plays a crucial role in a wide range of rewarding behaviors [Macbride et al. 1997, Sell et al. 1999], including euphoric states induced by drugs [Breite et al. 1997, Sell et al. 1999], pleasurable music [Blood and Zotorre 2001] and eating chocolate [Small et al. 2001]."[16] These researchers found the physical mechanism for why orgasm was reinforcing in women—how it led them to seek out those ecstatic feelings, those heroin-like feelings, again and again:

"PSA correlated positively with RCBF in ventral midbrain" which explained "the reinforcing nature of orgasm in women." That is, they found the science that underlies millennia of patriarchal fear of female sexuality: when women have orgasms they are indeed biologically designed to find them reinforcing—to want more and more and more.

The Georgiadis researchers cited other studies that showed— feminists may not like this—that "cervical stimulation was more important than clitoral in activating the female hypothalamus [Komisaruk et al 2004]." Why does this matter at all? The hypothalamus is "well known for its role in female reproductive behavior [Dr. Pfaus 1999]" and "during female orgasm it may release oxytocin [Carmichael 1999]." [17] If you are a heterosexual couple, a vaginal or blended orgasm is more likely to get you pregnant because of the role of what is unpoetically called "upsuck" in vaginal contractions. This is not to advocate any one approach over any other or to suggest that you should try to like something, sexually, that you may not like. It is just to disclose what scientists are beginning to know about the different kinds of female orgasms that are more or less likely to get you pregnant, and more or less likely to make you fall in love and stay in love.

(One young female scientist I met, who had done research with Dr. Pfaus, explained one of these studies to me while we were at a reception in an imposing academic building. She is a charming and well-bred twentysomething who was wearing, for that occasion, a summery batik maxidress. Holding a glass of white wine with slender fingers, her bearing impeccably ladylike, she remarked, "This finding is why farmers are paying people to fist their cows.")

Women know that they go into something like a trance state during really powerful sex, and this trance state is an encounter with the self on another, higher level. We misunderstand women if we see their interest in romance as being only about the "other"; if a male or female lover can help a woman get to this trance state, that love is not just compelling to her because of the "other": it is compelling to her because, through this sexual experience, she is awakening and engaging with profoundly important dimensions of her own self.

## HUG HER, CUDDLE HER, TAKE HER SLOW DANCING: THE SECRET LIFE OF THE MALE ARMPIT

*I think about going through his bureau drawers, pull one open and bring a folded t-shirt to my nose. I can still smell him in so many places, and wonder what it will be like when that, too, is gone.*

—Sally Ryder Brady, *A Box of Darkness*[18]

When you really listen to what many heterosexual women feel they are missing sexually, you often hear them speak about sexual longing in metaphors involving scent. One woman with whom I spoke, a vibrant Portuguese literature professor in her thirties, spent years in a relationship with a supportive, "safe" man who was perfect for her on paper; but she returned obsessively to the fact that they did not "match" as physical types. She fixated on the sense that there was something about his smell that was wrong for her. "I once read a novel in which the hero said, 'She perfumes my days.' I want that; I want to feel that a man 'perfumes my days' and that I do his."

The smell of men has powerful effects on the mood, hormonal levels, and even fertility of heterosexual women. Ivanka Savic of the Carolinska Institute in Stockholm, Sweden, found that when women and gay men inhaled a hormonal component in men's sweat, a PET brain scan showed lit-up areas around the hypothalamus, suggesting that the female and gay male brains had a sexual rather than an olfactory response to the stimulus.[19]

Denise Chen, a psychologist at Rice University in Houston, and her colleagues, speculated that if humans do produce and respond to sweat pheromones, then a woman should respond to male "sexual sweat" more than to the control sweat.

Chen and her team asked twenty heterosexual men to stop wearing deodorant and other scented grooming products for several days. The researchers then put pads under the men's armpits, and wired the men to electrodes, as the men watched pornographic videos. The researchers analyzed the "aroused" male sweat and also analyzed pads collected from under the arms of the same men when they were not sexually aroused.

Then, nineteen heterosexual women smelled the men's "aroused" and "unaroused" sweat pads, while they themselves underwent brain scans. The women's brains reacted very differently in response to the "aroused" male sweat.

The "sexual sweat" activated the women's right orbitofrontal cortex and the right fusiform cortex, but the "unaroused" sweat did nothing for them. These are the brain areas that help us recognize emotions and engage in perception. Both areas are in the right hemisphere, where smell, social response, and emotion are mediated.

Chen concluded that her findings bolster the idea that humans do communicate via subconscious chemical signals.[20] To me this finding also suggests that women's bodies know categorically and uncompromisingly when a man is or is not sexually interested in them, even if everyone in the couple is saying the "right" things. This may have been what my friend, who has a strong sex drive, and whose partner did not "perfume her days," may have been experiencing: his sexual interest in her was not strong enough for her. This finding suggests that she could not will that relationship to be a success if she had tried to forever. She couldn't smell enough of his arousal—a scent that would in turn have aroused her.

Specific scents have been found to boost vaginal blood engorgement: cucumbers and Good & Plenty candies both are at the top of vaginal-engorgement-activating scents, according to one study (and both are phallic in shape).[21]

It is not just men's arousal levels that women can subconsciously smell. Another study shows that women are attracted to the underarm sweat of men whose DNA is unlike theirs, and repelled by the smell of men whose DNA is too much like theirs. There is an important exception to this preference—when women are pregnant, they prefer the smell of men whose DNA is like theirs; researchers suggest that this finding may be the result of pregnancy being a time when women wish to be near kin.

A study, by Virpi Lummaa and Alexandra Alvergne, "Does the Contraceptive Pill Alter Mate Choice in Humans?," should give us pause and lead us to take very seriously the impact of the Pill in terms of men's smell and its effect on female mate selection. "Female and male mate choice preferences in humans both vary according to the menstrual cycle. Women prefer more masculine, symmetrical and genetically unrelated men during ovulation compared with other phases of their cycle, and recent evidence suggests that men prefer ovulating women to others. Such monthly shifts in mate preference have been suggested to bring evolutionary benefits in terms of reproductive success. New evidence is now emerging that taking the oral contraceptive pill might significantly alter both female and male mate choice by removing the mid-cycle change in preferences," they write.[22] This study suggests that when women are on contraceptive pills, they smell men in a different way than they do when they aren't, because the Pill tricks women's bodies into believing that they are already pregnant. So while they are "on the Pill"—and hormonally pregnant—but dating, these young women prefer men who smell like their own kin. Then—married—they go off the Pill in order to start their families. Hormonally not pregnant again, they get their normal scent responses back—and the young marriages are suddenly in terrible trouble. The women find themselves to be sexually repelled by their husbands—saying things like, "I can't stand for him to touch me"—at just the moment when the new couple wishes to conceive. Anecdotally, many therapists say these young wives tell them identical stories: they feel suddenly that they have married the wrong man; specifically, the young wives report that they can't bear their husbands' smell.

Not only can women's bodies tell by scent if men are into them sexually, and if a mate is a good match, but male armpit sweat and its pheromones can also relax women. George Preti, of the Monell Chemical Senses Center in Philadelphia, and his colleagues found that male pheromones affect both a woman's serenity levels and her fertility levels.[23] Researchers in the study, reported in the journal *Biology of Reproduction,* placed pads under the armpits of male subjects. The team collected the sweat on pads from under the armpits of a group of male donors. They then extracted the concentrated chemical compounds from it, masked this compound with a fragrance, and whisked it systematically under the noses of women volunteers. After six hours of exposure, all the women reported feeling more relaxed and less tense.

When women who have long been married say that the romance has gone out of their marriages, they often use the phrase "He never takes me dancing anymore." An ad for British railway sleeper cars shows an affluent, middle-aged man on one side of the page and his wife on the other. Under the man the caption reads: "Room service. Snoozing. Golf." Under hers, it reads: "Candlelight dinner. Flirting. Dancing under the stars." If the hypothetical couple's weekend away turns out to revert to his side of the wish list at the expense of hers, the marriage will suffer, even though no one clearly sees why. She won't be able to really relax and get deeply aroused, because she won't have had the chance to really smell her mate, who has been out on the golf links all day—among the other aspects of the Goddess Array she needs to experience.

For if we tease out this female-romance cliché—"dancing under the stars"—a bit further, the kind of dancing this hypothetical woman misses is not, generally, rock and roll or hip-hop dancing, in which the partners dance at a pheromonal remove from each other. Rather, the feminine romantic image is of some version of a touching couple's dance with a frontal embrace, such as the waltzing scenes that signal romance in pop culture landmarks such as *Gone with the Wind,* or Disney's *Beauty and the Beast* and *Anastasia.* Indeed, in many classic love stories, the heroine realizes she is in love with the hero after she has danced with him in this frontal-embrace way—that is, gotten a good long inhalation of his intoxicating pheromones, to a rhythmic melody that is activating her ANS, and secured a sense of his familiar or, better, excitingly unfamiliar, DNA.

"We never cuddle anymore" is another refrain from women in sexually and romantically frustrating marriages; and again, when we tease this out, a cuddle on the couch typically nestles the woman's head against the man's shoulder or chest; in bed, a cuddle often positions the woman's head on the chest of her husband or lover. Female cuddling often means scent inhalation.

What is the unifying element for dancing, cuddling, and hugging, and why are they all vital for heterosexual women? They all have to do with activating the secret life of the male armpit, and its relationship to heterosexual female desire.

People have extraordinarily strong emotions about this. I posted an informal questionnaire about male sweat (hugs, embraces, and dancing) online, and within forty-five minutes received eighty-seven extensive answers, from both women and men. Everyone, it seemed, wanted to tell me about the male armpit.

"When I am stressed and I get a hug from my husband, it calms me down right away but it helps if I get a strong whiff of his scent," wrote one woman.

"I sleep with my boyfriend's T-shirt when he is away because I can't sleep otherwise," wrote another.

"I left a man who was perfect for me in every way because he didn't smell right, and it was a tragedy but there was absolutely nothing I could do about it," wrote a third.

Men, too, were amazed at the effect of this unglamorous signaling system in their armpits. "When it is winter and I don't get as sweaty, I skip using deodorant and I notice I get far more interest from women," wrote one man.

George Preti and his team, mentioned above, found that male sweat not only affects women's levels of calmness and women's fertility levels.[24] That was not all—the women, after sniffing the chemicals in male sweat, would also, though the study did not highlight this, have felt much more readily aroused, for the scientists found surges of luteinizing hormones in their brains—far greater surges than in the nonsniffing control group.

Luteinizing hormone is a key building block of female sexual desire and plays an important role in triggering ovulation. What teachers usually fail to mention to eager teenage girls in eighth-grade sex education is that this hormone is also key to triggering and amplifying the female sex drive. As women approach ovulation, pulses of this hormone increase in size and frequency in the female brain, which is why you are more lustful in mid-cycle. So in the Preti experiment, when women smelled the male sweat extract, they also experienced a surge of the female-sexual-desire hormone.

But if women are away from their men all day and smell their partners mostly when they are not aroused—because both members of the couple are exhausted from work and parenting—she may "hear" him on an intellectual level say "I love you" or even "I want you"; but on a visceral level, she will have a more difficult time feeling it. So many young couples in our culture transition from courtship—when they could spend weekends in bed together, and, fully sated with scent, feel deeply in love—to dual-career work and young parenthood, when they can barely spend twenty minutes in each other's arms in a forty-eight-hour period. At that point, it is often the women rather than the men who start to feel disenchanted, trapped, and haunted by a sense of the terrible prosaicness of life, a sense that something is missing.

So let us go back to our starting template—the numbers that show such drastically low libido among a third of Western women. The women whose libidos are dropping, whose marriages now seem tedious, and who are feeling that the world is colorless and flat, may believe that this is due to the stresses of adult life and all their responsibilities. But what if the hardworking women in our culture are also neurologically starved of worlds of scent—along with the worlds of touch, gazing, stroking, pleasure, and so on—that their very natures minimally require in order for them to feel connected, excited, hopeful, and "in love"?

Why are vacations so relaxing and so sexualizing for these same overscheduled couples? Why do so many couples who are struggling with infertility become pregnant on vacation? Is it partly because she finally has time to get to know him again—on an olfactory level? Is it because she is getting enough of the arousing and calming scent from him that reminds her that, even if he sometimes repeats his stories, or he sometimes drops his laundry on the floor, or even if his hairline may be receding, on another, entirely animal level, he can make her calm, aroused, and happy?

It is heterosexual women, not men, who are calmed by the opposite sex's pheromones. So today, if straight men can't smell women often or closely enough, they may not become as aroused, but this does not stress them. However, if straight women can't smell men often or closely enough, they are both more sexually apathetic and more stressed. And you recall what stress does in turn to the female libido—further depresses it.

We have an epidemic of infertility in the United States and Western Europe: straight women are not smelling men closely or often enough, perhaps, to boost the levels of luteinizing hormone they require for optimal fertility. Marital counselors tell women and men to talk though their problems; fertility doctors send men into rooms to masturbate and then they inject the semen themselves into the vaginas of women who are suffering from irregular periods or with low fertility levels. Again, if you understand the profound nature of the animality of women, you see that these practices are incomplete. Marital counselors should start by telling men to hug women; to stroke if the women are open to that; to take women, if they are willing, ballroom dancing. Fertility specialists should make sure, before anything else, that women are getting well and regularly cuddled, and brought to orgasm, by their men.

Bob Beale, in *ABC Science Online,* reported on the Preti study and cited speculation by another member of the research team, Dr. Charles Wysocki, that women may have evolved to have men's smell trigger their ovulation.[25] That is, the smell of a male partner may help to trigger ovulation at the ideal time while making women more relaxed, so that they will be receptive to sex at the right time of the month for them to conceive.

I would have to argue that the phrasing of Dr. Wysocki's conclusion shows how profoundly even scientists at the cutting edge of sexual-response research are missing something crucial about female desire—including a possibly more accurate reading of the cause and effect in the data—by having unconscious male-centered models of what sex *is*. In Dr. Wysocki's conclusion, an otherwise mostly uninterested woman smells a guy, it triggers her ovulation, and then, now that she is fertile, she is also relaxed and "receptive" to his sexual approach. What if this reading is missing her sexual agency? What if she smells him; she gets a surge of luteinizing hormone; she becomes relaxed and aroused. This relaxation and arousal makes her wish actively (not "receptively") to seek out more sex and orgasm, further smelling her man—women get lots of male armpit scent in missionary-position heterosexual sex. This additional man-smelling in turn regulates her cycle further, thus supporting her continued fertility. In other words, his smell drives her to ovulate, which drives her to seek sex, which leads her to smell him more, which further boosts her fertility. In this reading, which is more aligned with Dr. Pfaus's more progressive, female-agency-centric view of mammalian desire, males don't "make females fertile"; males may make females want to have sex, but it is the female wanting-to-have sex that *keeps* females optimally fertile. The traditional and somewhat sexist male view of evolutionary biology is that sexy-looking females are fertile females (a hard prospect to apply practically to a lab rat, for instance); but we have to add a dimension from the latest neuroscience: it seems that *lustful* females who continually choose sexual agency and sexual engagement are the more fertile, and thus the more evolutionarily successful females. It is not, based on this model, how conventionally pretty you are, but how sexually questing and driven you are, as a woman, that will help you optimize the reproduction of your DNA.

One continued problem with really understanding female sexuality in our culture is that all of our language about the vagina positions women in a state of sexual passivity and casts the man in the drama as the sexual pursuer—instead of understanding that the vagina, too, is on a quest. In this model—in my version of the same story and reading of the same data—the woman's arousal is the center of the narrative. It is not a side effect of the drama, or a momentary carrot on a stick briefly waved about by Mother Nature to allow the central player, the inseminating male, a moment's handily timed ingress. In this interpretation of the same data, which is a more natural evolutionary interpretation, it is the woman's needs that drive the sexual quest. In my reading of this data, the vagina is, in evolutionary terms, as many have called it in other contexts, "the Center of the Universe."

## GAZE INTO HER EYES

When Lousada begins a Tantra session, he spends many minutes—perhaps ten; it felt like an eternity to me—face-to-face with his client, gazing directly and searchingly into her eyes. Many of his clients have trouble at first tolerating this gaze, or start laughing, or must look away. But all his clients whom I interviewed—and I myself—sooner or later found this deep exchange of gazing very profound in creating an atmosphere that supported the feminine.

Why is this? Dr. Daniel Amen, in his book *The Brain in Love,* shows that eye-to-eye gazing reveals clues about sexual arousal and that the gaze is involved in mirror neuron behavior, which gives people signals about how others feel about them.[26] Daniel Goleman, in *Social Intelligence: The Revolutionary New Science of Human Relationships,* discusses the neuroscience of the importance of gazing into one another's eyes in intimate contexts: "Those long gazes may have been a necessary neural prelude to [a couple's] kiss. . . . The eyes contain nerve projections that lead directly to a key brain structure for empathy and matching emotions, the orbitofrontal (or OFC) area of the prefrontal cortex. Locking eyes loops us. . . . This tight connection [of the OFC with the cortex, amygdala and brain stem] . . . facilitates instantaneous coordination of thought, feeling and action. . . . [T]he OFC performs an instant social calculus, one that tells us how we feel about the person we are with, how she feels about us, and what to do next in accord with how she responds."[27]

Is it surprising, given the power of the OFC, that women long for eye-to-eye gazing as a form of connection? It is actually, neurologically, a medium of connection. Women can often crave "the gaze"—the direct eye contact that other women and small children give them continually. They read this as a strengthening connection. In contrast to this, men have a natural aversion to a deep face-to-face gaze. Men prefer interacting side by side—they interpret a direct gaze as threatening. For the first two years of courtship, when studies show that men's neurochemicals become more like women's, and vice versa, men will provide women with this kind of face-to-face gazing; this gazing tends to diminish significantly after that initial courtship period.[28] (Female rats gaze deeply before they are ready to have sex: they engage, as you recall, in "headwise orientation"—they will gaze intently face-to-face with the male rat, and then run away, to initiate sex.)

In humans, direct eye contact requires trust. In a sexual context, eye gazing paired with pupil dilation means that you can read what your partner feels about you, since pupil dilation means sexual arousal. Romantic restaurants are dimly lit to support pupil dilation, which then reads as arousal.

But the female craving for a deep gaze with a male lover does not subside: most romance scenes in films and in novels involve descriptions of the man "gazing deeply into her eyes." In the wild, courtship and sex between primates involves deep eye-to-eye gazing. This deep feminine hunger for what I have to call "gaze contact" or perhaps even better, "gaze communication," may help explain many mysteries about some of the stresses of married life and long-term heterosexual relationships.

Many women read deep eye-to-eye gazing from a man as sexy. Gaze communication is part of the Goddess Array. How many women are "gaze starved" and seek unconsciously to provoke their male partners—just because they wish his full eye-to-eye attention? How many women feel that their partners rarely gaze deeply into their eyes unless they are angry? A familiar and frustrating experience to many women is the feeling that their husband or male partner is going about his business with her, day after day, without ever really *looking* at her. This building frustration in her can lead to those provocative, "bitchy" interactions from her that, to the man, will feel as if they have come out of the blue. She herself may not fully understand why she is suddenly so irritated with him. He hasn't said anything awful, done anything terrible—he has just gone for three or four days not really, from her perspective, *looking at* her. Poor woman—she is not conscious of being deprived of the deep interactive gaze she craves, because this is not information that is widely understood or available. Poor man—he may feel perfectly companionable, while she begins to seethe, because side-by-side activity with eyes averted from each other is how men happily spend time with male friends and colleagues.

Data show a marked drop in marital satisfaction after the birth of a first child—and babies are evolutionarily programmed to seek the caregiver's gaze and lock in on it.[29] Might it be that some new mothers—starved of deep gazing from their husbands—are more at risk of being drawn into a charmed circle of mutual gazing with their babies, which leaves out the man? How many new mothers are seduced by the baby's deep interest in gazing into their eyes, into a relationship with the baby that becomes primary, one that leaves the father sidelined as a romantic partner? This unhappy triangulation after the birth of a new baby, and the subsequent complaints of a low-libido or even sexless marriage, are extremely common in our culture. How much of that trigger is the gaze-starved mom?

A man who wants to activate the Goddess Array will be aware of the dangers of overusing the BlackBerry at home. He will make time, from time to time, even if it does not come naturally to him, to gaze deeply into his wife's or lover's eyes.

## TALK TO HER, LISTEN TO HER

A day-to-day stressor for straight women living with men they love is male silence. I don't mean hostile silence or antagonistic silence—I mean just plain old garden-variety male-brain quiet.

Many studies have confirmed the difference between male and female brains when it comes to verbal processing: women have far greater levels of activity between the two hemispheres of their brains, thus leading women to have a far higher interest in talking, to use greater vocabulary ranges, and to be far more interested in discussing emotions.[30] For straightforward neurobiological reasons, these activities are of far less interest to men. They aren't trying to be rude or dismissive; their brains simply don't light up in those activities in the same way. Add to this the factor that many men come home from jobs at which they have had to spend all day verbally processing and reading people's emotions—those post-industrial-revolution jobs that require men's brains, in effect, to act more like women's. Many men walk in the door at the end of the day completely exhausted in terms of brain activity. All they want is to recover—to rest the male brain.

This, I believe, is why so many marital fights take place just when both members of a couple have entered the house after a day's work—her brain is agitated and desperate to talk things through, which is how it calms down and feels better, while his is desperate to have some downtime doing nothing, or in front of the TV, which is how his brain calms down and feels better. She feels bored, thwarted, if he won't or can't just keep talking to her—and he feels invaded by her need to talk.

Dr. Louann Brizendine, in her book *The Male Brain,* points out that the male brain does not engage in as much verbal processing as the female brain.[31] The female brain is always on, verbally. So, often, when women ask men, "What are you thinking?" and men answer, "Nothing," women assume the man is withholding, or denying them access to their inner lives, because the female brain existentially, hermeneutically, cannot imagine a brain state in which verbal processing is less prominent, at least while a person is still conscious. But men actually do go into a less verbal brain state—and need to, in order to recover their equilibrium.

This is a difficult reality for women, with their ever-restless brains, to accept.

In virtually every culture outside the West, many women spend some time, usually on a daily basis, only with other women (and children). Women run markets in West Africa; do the washing daily at the riverbed in the Valley of Roses in Morocco; spend lunchtimes visiting one another on the verandas in suburban Delhi. While women in these societies face immense hurdles and inequities, they often seem to be much less irritated with the men they live with than women tend to be in the West. (I am not addressing here physical abuse.) The burden is not on the husband to somehow, heroically, alone, fill that deep neural need for talk, which his brain chemistry makes difficult to impossible.

In contemporary Western society, in contrast, men and women in couples or as parents of families are expected to spend most of their leisure time with one another, when they are not at work. So men and women rarely have a break, either at work or at home, from this inevitably neurobiologically stressful, because verbally mismatched, togetherness.

To manage social arrangements, as we do in the West, in such a way that a woman has to get most of her touch, gaze, and attention needs met in the few hours after work, and by only one person—and, most implausibly of all, by a tired *male* person at that, who just as desperately needs the opposite, for a while at least—is a recipe for conflict and frustration.

Dr. Daniel Goleman, in his 1995 book, *Emotional Intelligence,* and psychologist John Gottman, in his 2001 book, *Seven Principles for Making Marriage Work,* both explore the differences in the genders' stress response and its role in marital conflict. In his chapter "Intimate Enemies," Goleman notes that men are "the vulnerable sex" because they tend on average to "flood . . . at a lower level in intensity" than their wives do, and "[o]nce flooded, men secrete more adrenaline into their bloodstream . . . [so] it takes husbands longer to recover physiologically from flooding."[32] These important books advise women to understand the male stress response—men get "flooded" by too much emotional processing, and need to withdraw—and adjust for it. This is good advice. But I believe it is also very, very important for us to understand the female stress response and adjust for it. Gottman assigns the woman the role of moderating her approach to conflict, since he points out that biologically, she handles stress in conflict better. This is true short term, and both authors equitably give male readers good guidance on how to keep their wives or girlfriends' stress levels from hijacking the discussion as well. But I think this excellent advice could be complemented with a discussion of the long-term effects on women—especially sexually—of certain kinds of chronic stress that can inevitably arise from living in Western-model close, isolated contact with even the nicest of men.

## STROKE, DON'T SNAP

Stress affects each gender differently. In a kind of tragic misalignment, during a fight men tend to get "flooded" with stress hormones in a way that leads them to long to shut down, withdraw, and detach—the "flight or fight" response to adrenaline—in order to regain neuroendocrine equilibrium; whereas women react to the same stress by needing to talk more and connect more—the "tend and befriend" response, which lowers their own stress levels. Gottman and Goleman both based their bestsellers on this data, and both advise couples to adapt their argument styles to account for this gender difference.

Data do confirm that women have a higher neurochemical tolerance for having difficult discussions than men do. John Gottman notes that this is why men tend to "stonewall" in stressful marital or relationship conversations. They can't really help it: the male body takes far longer—as long as twenty minutes—to subside from that negative arousal.

Gottman's data show that women's stress hormones spike when men stonewall. Male stonewalling certainly leaves women negatively aroused and in a state of anxiety, even if the spikes are less dramatic.

However, Dr. Gottman, in what is generally a very pro-woman book, tends to put the "housekeeping" role on women—since the data show that women do not "flood" as much or as destructively as men. He notes that natural selection favored women who could stay calm—thus benefiting from the boost to lactation of poxytocin—while evolution favored men whose adrenaline could spike quickly: "To this day," he writes, "the male cardiovascular system remains more reactive than the female and slower to recover from stress." Dr. Gottman is right about the different effects on the male and female body of fights, pointing out that because of men's slower recovery from stress, men tend to stonewall to avoid emotional discussions, and women are more likely to initiate talking about the couple's issues, since they can handle such discussion without such sharp adrenaline spikes. But he did not address the lower-level, longer-term, less immediately dramatic ways in which a man can stress a woman out in a couple's dynamic.[33]

Women may not get flooded in the same immediate way as men do in a conflict, but without looking at the more holistic and subtler ongoing interactions of everyday life, rather than at moments of conflict, something important may be being missed. In these other less-dramatic interactions, I believe that some women experience less dramatically measurable, but perhaps more chronic states of being stressed out by men. In other words, the very behaviors that Gottman flags as symptoms of male "flooding" during an argument—male withdrawal, silence, turning attention to another subject, and so on—will elevate some women's heart rates over time, send catecholamines into their bloodstreams, and stress some women out in a lower-key but still significant ongoing way, unless their men regularly do some simple things to calm women down. They can do these things at other times than during the fight itself, since soothing behaviors during conflict itself are very difficult for male neurobiology to accomplish.

In research on the female brain and how women process stress, there is some intriguing scientific data confirming that women respond to touch differently than men do. In Roger Dobson and Maurice Chittenden's 2005 *Sunday Times* article, "Women Need That Healthy Touch," they report on psychiatrist Kathleen Light's findings. Light, at the University of North Carolina's Medical Center, and her team, found that after only ten minutes of stroking, a woman's body produces oxytocin—the chemical that, you recall, strengthens affection and trust. The women's blood pressure levels also dropped significantly as they were being stroked.[34]

Light and her researchers tested fifty-nine heterosexual couples: they asked each woman to sit for ten minutes on a loveseat as she watched a romantic movie. Her husband or boyfriend was instructed to stroke her hands, neck, or back—or whatever part of her body he chose. Before and after the stroking, the woman's blood pressure levels were taken. The stroking actually boosted women's affection-producing hormones by one-fifth in that brief ten-minute period. In other words, in ten minutes, one could roughly say that they liked and trusted their husbands a fifth more than they had before the stroking began. But the men, in contrast, after being stroked by their female partners, did not show any such changes in their hormone levels and blood pressure.

Kathleen Light said, of the research, "It is a new finding for humans. When a man strokes or hugs his partner it seems to stimulate an increase in levels of oxytocin which tends to lower blood pressure." The reason this finding is so groundbreaking is that it is the first such finding in humans: other studies have managed to identify the role of oxytocin following stroking only in female mammals lower on the evolutionary ladder than human beings. So, many heterosexual women really do need to be caressed by their men in order to stay calm and healthy, much more than men may think is natural or reasonable, based on their own differing physical needs.

When I presented this data online and asked women (and men) to send in their own accounts of whether stroking—male to female—changed the emotional dynamic in a heterosexual couple, I was overwhelmed with responses confirming that the act made a substantial difference.

"I have started to use this method with my practice," wrote one couples' counselor, "after I read about it here, and it has transformed my work with couples. I have been telling the man to stroke the woman when he is bringing up a subject that causes her anxiety. It has a miraculous effect on supporting her ability to listen and not close down, and the couples are able to solve conflicts much more easily, without escalation."

"When my husband rubs my feet in a nonsexual way when I am tired at the end of the day or stressed from work," wrote Theresa, from Arizona, "it makes me much more interested and open sexually at other times and makes the feeling between us much more intimate."

Christopher in Virginia wrote, "I tried what you suggested. I am able to help my wife feel better faster about things that are bothering her much more easily now, and we have stopped bickering nearly so much about little things."

Mike in Dallas wrote, "My girlfriend can hear me when we are talking about something difficult and I am stroking her hair." Many men noted, however, that they couldn't or did not wish to do this during a fight—"It's hard to want to do this when you're being told you are the bad guy," as one man put it. Women, too, cautioned that if this stroking was attempted in the context of a fight, it would seem to them manipulative.[35]

I personally can attest to the fact that my own tendency toward high anxiety and "flooding" when some subjects come up in the context of a relationship has been softened by drawing upon this practice; since I shared this finding with my partner, he has been stroking my hair and neck when a difficult subject arises between us, and it tends immediately to lower my heart rate—as well as to make me laugh.

While men reported that it was difficult to be the stroker when they felt that they themselves were under attack (a point well taken given their higher susceptibility to stress chemicals during a fight), they noted that if they could stroke their wives or girlfriends often in a natural context throughout the day, it made the women seem much happier and calmer in general. Many women, for their part (in separate responses), noted with surprise that they felt less irritated in general with their husbands or boyfriends also after the introduction of regular stroking into the relationship, the level of bickering about trivia radically deescalated, and that they felt more warmly toward their mates overall. This makes sense: if Kathleen Light found that stroking elevates women's oxytocin levels by at least a fifth, it will indeed make them feel more affectionate toward, more trusting of, and closer to their men if they are stroked every day, or even caressed many times a day. It will also make these women feel significantly more relaxed. By lowering their blood pressure, men's stroking the women they love regularly can even help protect the women from heart disease and stroke.

We saw the direct connection between women's ability to be in a relaxed state around their husbands and lovers, and their ability to "open" fully sexually. The obverse of this is that we need to take very seriously what happens physically in a relationship when a man regularly or even from time to time feels free to snap at his wife or girlfriend.

I have yet to see a relationship guide for couples that takes seriously enough the issue of men engaging in low-level snapping at their wives and children, and how that affects women physically. Plenty of women are certainly guilty of snapping at or showing irritation to their partners and children, of course—and men deserve a book of their own about what female snapping does to the male body. But my subject here is the female body and mind. There is still an often unconscious assumption in our culture that the right of men to snap or be irritable with women and children in their families is not really serious, and that this entitlement goes along with other privileges of male domestic life. There is not a great deal of cultural energy directed at urging men who are not otherwise abusing them, to stop snapping at women and children in their homes.

But in an environment in which women expect to be snapped at regularly, the female ANS closes down the channels that women need open in order to be sexually alive. It is evolutionarily negative for women to bond with violent or scarily unpredictable men. For evolutionary reasons, probably, many women react to men's sudden anger at themselves and at their children (whom they are wired to protect) in immediate ways, with raised heart rate, adrenaline response, and so on; if the snapping is chronic, the woman's "bad stress" levels will be chronically raised and her sexual response will suffer. Men who want a more passionate sexual response from their wives or girlfriends may wish to try a no-snapping week on their part, and see what good things begin to happen to them when their partner's ANS can be activated fully, having gotten used to an emotional environment without those stressors.

## FIND HER "SACRED SPOT," THEN HANG OUT THERE FAR LONGER THAN YOU THINK REASONABLE

I asked Mike Lousada what advice he had for heterosexual men. What was the takeaway from all the experience he had had successfully sexually arousing and awakening women—even those who had had great difficulty with orgasm or great problems with low libido?

"It's very simple, in a way," he said. "It's not rocket science. I want men to have two pieces of advice. One: be patient and compassionate. The other thing men should remember is that women have *two* sexual centers, the clitoris and the G-spot." (There are actually many, as we saw, but two is a good start.)

As noted earlier, the average man climaxes in four minutes whereas the average woman requires sixteen. This average time differential is worth taking very seriously. Women are often expected to 'adapt' to men sexually but this is one way in which such expectations are pointless. Many women may have taken for granted that, sadly, it is just not easy for them to climax when they are with a man; but this is an unnecessarily bleak conclusion, one that the latest data do not support. The right kind of stimulation—which is most successful when it combines clitoral, G-spot, and other kinds of stimulation—brings the success rate for female orgasm to almost 90 percent. In one study, Milan Zaviacic at Comenius University in Bratislava, Slovakia, found a G-spot in every one of the twenty-seven women he studied; every single woman, who had her "sacred spot" massaged, had an orgasm: ten of them ejaculated. In another study, an additional 40 percent of 2,350 respondents also experienced ejaculation.[36] So the low levels of satisfaction and desire that American and Western European women report are a sign of a major schism between the levels of pleasure and orgasmic capacity that women are capable of in the right conditions, and their actual experience; it is a sign that they are not being treated in an ideal way, either physically or emotionally.

"Vaginal Eroticism: a Replication Study," a study by Heli Alzate, in the *Archives of Sexual Behavior,* investigated "vaginal eroticism" in a group of women volunteers.[37] Alzate and the research team engaged in "systematic digital stimulation of both vaginal walls." The headline is that "erogenous zones" were found in all subjects, mainly located on the upper anterior wall and the lower posterior one. An orgasmic response was elicited by stimulation of these zones in 89 percent of the subjects. That is a darned high rate of return for women and orgasm; remember that a third to a half of women in the University of Illinois study had problems with attaining regular sexual satisfaction. When I read this study's striking results, which have been replicated elsewhere, I thought of the remarkable amounts of time—by Western standards—Tantric practitioners spend caressing the sacred spot (the actual technique is often demonstrated as a "come here" kind of beckoning gesture with an index or index and middle finger, often combined with clitoral and other stimulation).

Alzate concluded that the study supports earlier findings on the importance of vaginal eroticism and the sacred spot, or G-spot, to orgasm, though he notes that he did not find a "discrete anatomical structure" in terms of the "G-spot." Alzate also argues that the findings support the concept that there are two kinds of orgasms for women, clitorally evoked and vaginally evoked, and that some women expel fluid through the urethra during orgasm.

Many women—and Tantra gurus—report that while clitoral orgasm involves bodily tension and release (a lot like male orgasm), "sacred spot" orgasm involves relaxation. Many women learn to have sacred spot orgasms, those Tantric four-star never-ending orgasms, by actually directing themselves to relax and lose consciousness during sacred spot stimulation—to their surprise, this can make the orgasm come in sequential inexhaustible waves—rather than tensing up and focusing on sexual thoughts or fantasies, which women tend to do to secure clitoral orgasms (and which Western images of sexuality model).

We've seen throughout the course of this book that sexual satisfaction and regular orgasm foster a woman's creativity, confidence, and sense of self. The more men learn about how to bring heterosexual women to orgasm via sacred spot massage, as well as all other ways, the better for women's state of mind. Stuart Brody and Petr Weiss report that scientists from Scotland and the Czech Republic found that simultaneous orgasm in intercourse, and regular vaginal orgasm, not only contributed to women's satisfaction with their sexual lives, but correlated with their levels of happiness with their partners, their own lives, and satisfaction with their overall mental health. (Women, of course, can reach simultaneous orgasm more easily if they understand and feel a sense of control over their own sexuality, and feel that they have a right to communicate about their responses.) In other words, sexual satisfaction correlated with satisfaction in many other "unrelated" areas of women's lives.[38]

Other extraordinary but underreported recent data about vaginal satisfaction confirm that when researchers are trained, they can identify women who have vaginal orgasms *from the way the women walk,* with accuracy rates above 80 percent, a finding that Lousada believes has to do with the pelvic levator muscles. Other researchers, G. L. Gravina and colleagues, found that a thicker urethral pad made it easier for the women they studied to have vaginal orgasms— perhaps because the thicker pad made penile or other pressure on the woman's pelvic neural network more efficient. In 2008 these Italian scientists discovered the Holy Grail of understanding female sexual response when they confirmed that changes in the clitoris and G-spot during orgasm seemed to prove that the G-spot is actually *part* of the clitoris—the back of the clitoris, essentially—which in turn turns out to be much bigger, and to extend far deeper into the pelvis, than was believed to be the case.[39]

Dr. Deborah Coady and Nancy Fish's 2011 book, *Healing Painful Sex,* confirms this finding, which is now being integrated into their concept of female anatomy by researchers in the vanguard of the study of female sexual response: indeed, the clitoris and G-spot are two points on the same nerve structure.[40]

Scandinavian researcher Zwi Hoch reported, in "Vaginal Erotic Sensitivity by Sexological Examination," that 64 percent of women who identified themselves as "coitally anorgasmic"—that is, they could have orgasms through masturbation or external stimulation but not during intercourse—were able to learn to have "coital" orgasms immediately upon simply being shown what to do in terms of rhythmic pressure on what had earlier been called "the G-spot."[41]

Actually these researchers, too, refuted the idea of a discrete G-spot, and also refuted the notion of a clitoral versus vaginal reflex, and found, too—another confirmation of the new science—that what is really going on for women in orgasm involves what they, not mellifluously, call "a clitoral/vaginal sensory arm of orgasmic reflex" that includes "deeper situated tissues" that we don't even have specific names for. They found that the whole anterior wall of the vagina was sexually responsive:

> The entire anterior vaginal wall, including the deeper situated urinary bladder, periurethral tissues and Halban's fascia, rather than one specific spot, were found to be erotically sensitive in most of the women examined, and 64% of them learned how to reach orgasm by direct specific digital and/or coital stimulation of this area. All other parts of the vagina had poor erotic sensitivity. This supports our conceptualization of a "clitoral/ vaginal sensory arm of orgasmic reflex" including the clitoris, the entire anterior vaginal wall as well as the deeper situated tissues. Instead of looking for a "vaginal (coital) orgasm" distinctly different from a "clitoral orgasm," this concept speaks towards a "genital orgasm" potentially achievable by separate

*or, most effectively, combined stimulation of those different trig-*
*ger components of the genital sensory arm of the orgasmic reflex.*

Given how easily orgasmic most women are with nothing more romantic going on than a clued-in researcher minimally showing them
the ropes, it is shocking that the data on female orgasm and sexual
satisfaction currently show such relatively low levels of female sexual
happiness.

Don't be alarmed: I do not think any of these data suggest we
need to bring back the days before *The Hite Report,* when women
had to adjust their response around the pacing of male penetration.
The data above about using different kinds of stimulation to address
all of women's sexual centers show that up to 90 percent of women
can have regular orgasms if they want to—if their partners are "patient and compassionate" and a bit clued in. We could also read this
data as demonstrating that those who do attend well to their lovers'
vaginas, and so adjust their pacing, are likely to bring about clitoral/
vaginal orgasms reliably in their partners. The data may also show
that having someone like that in one's bed—or knowing these skills
for oneself with oneself—correlates positively to satisfaction in all
other areas of one's life—including to good mental and physical
health.

### TELL HER SHE'S BEAUTIFUL

This is not trivial. There are evolutionary reasons, as I noted above,
that women need to be told regularly by their mates that they are
beautiful—indeed, "the most beautiful"—in order to truly sexually
release.

When I was in college, a friend was dating a man who was very
nice, but who absolutely never told her she was pretty. They had lots
of sex, but she was never completely at ease afterward. He would
leave, and then the three of us young women who hung out in the
apartment used to sit together around the kitchen table, drink pots

of dark coffee with cream, and listen to this roommate fantasize. She would regularly imagine locking him into an unused room in the flat and not releasing him until, a hungry day or two later, she finally heard his grudging voice mutter, "Fine, okay. You're *pretty.*"

Was she a bitch? Or was she dealing with a terribly uncomfortable ANS? There was not a woman who passed through our apartment who did not understand this fantasy.

We saw that it stands to evolutionary reason that women would respond sexually to what they see as "investment behavior" from their partners—signs that he is in for the long haul. If a woman thinks her partner sees other women as more attractive, she will not be able to relax fully, because she will be anticipating competition for resources and protection that she needs for her own offspring. (This one aspect of female sexuality alone is a reason that men's looking at pornography often affects women's arousal levels negatively.) But if a man assures a woman often that she is, to him, "the most beautiful," a woman's ANS can send the message: it is safe here. Then it can let go of the stress of vigilance about the threat of another woman's potential encroachment on her caretaker team.

Because of the role of the ANS in female sexual response, to release completely into the sexual trance state, a woman must, to a certain degree, feel permitted to indulge in a kind of self-absorption that can feel to contemporary women like narcissism; she must feel unselfconscious. She can't worry about her cellulite or how long she is taking to climax or about her smell "down there." All of that is easier if a woman feels admired and cherished, which is where "You are so beautiful" comes in.

In the Cambridge Women's Pornography Collective's half-joking anthology, *Porn for Women,* a sexy male model gazes deeply into the eyes of the camera and the caption reads: "You get more beautiful every time I look at you."[42] Another page shows another male model looking surprised: "You're telling me there's pornography on the Internet?" the caption reads. For the ANS to be completely activated, a women ideally should feel, in short, not just beautiful, but *actually,* ideally, like "the most beautiful"—and this is where that unfamiliar "Goddess" language comes in.

Why do Mike Lousada and other Tantric gurus say, at the very start of their sexual contact with a woman: "Welcome, Goddess," and engage in seduction rituals that address "the Goddess" in the woman? Why did scores of women who don't actually believe in this kind of New Age mumbo jumbo respond with transformationally different orgasms, or have orgasms for the first time, after being addressed in this way? What magic did this seemingly obscure or slightly ridiculous honorific confer? Did it operate, I wondered, on some kind of physiological level?

The more I learned about the ANS, the more I realized that addressing a woman as "Goddess"—or addressing the Goddess in her, if the former is just too much to attempt—is a way of allowing her a transcendental sexual response, or even an orgasm for the first time.

Why a Goddess? Goddesses are powerful; those around them hold them in reverence. Goddesses do not need to doubt themselves, their value, or their allure—they can even be a bit self-absorbed—so they can allow permission to go on the trance journey inward identified by Georgiadis's team. And Goddesses are entitled, without anxiety or guilt or self-reproach, to high levels of attention and pleasure.

I put this hypothesis, and Mike Lousada's experience with his clients around the Goddess language, with some trepidation, in my online and face-to-face interviews with women. Again I received very surprising confirmation of this aspect of the Goddess Array, which I think of as the erotics of reverence—or at least of admiration.

"I tried what you wrote about," wrote one reader. "We were in our hot tub in the backyard. . . . I love [my husband] and our sex life is usually okay, but with jobs, commuting, etc. it has been kind of mundane for quite a while much of the time.

"I told my husband about the 'Goddess' hypothesis," she continued, "and about the information in your article. He was amused, but seemed interested, I think especially at the prospect of its possibly changing my own response. He started to try to become sexual with me, and I wasn't really in the mood yet—it felt kind of porny and not really engaging. I could do it, and climax, but felt I would sort of be going through the motions. I was ready for that slight sense of disappointment you feel at those times. But I kind of pushed him back a little, playfully, and said, 'You should address the Goddess.'

"He laughed and said, really awkwardly, 'You're a cute Goddess.' It sounds crazy, but something in me opened up. I think he saw this, so he added, making the most of the moment, 'You have a cute yoni.' I laughed too—he said it in such a goofy way, and it was very funny—but there was something there that was also sincere. When we made love after that it was as if gates that had been rusted shut had opened. When we were done with our lovemaking, I felt different about myself. I felt differently toward him afterwards because of what he had said. It wasn't about some fake flattery. It is hard to put into words. I felt *seen* somehow."

I am not suggesting that everyone who reads this will or even should manage to address his lover, even in passing, as "Goddess." The ridiculousness meter each of us carries inside may not allow it to happen. But it is obvious from putting the recent science of female sexual response side by side with Tantra 101 that when heterosexual men treat women like Goddesses—overtly—in various ways, even very everyday and manageable ways, simply verbalizing their admiration, telling them how uniquely precious they are, how beautiful they are—"the most beautiful," in their eyes—or making gestures that show that they cherish them, this helps open up even tired, depressed, and hurt women.

## DON'T BE SCARY, BUT DON'T BE BORING

There is a continuing duality in the representations of men that heterosexual women desire, which resurfaces in culture from decade to decade and even century to century. Consider (bad, haughty, unkind) Darcy in Jane Austen's *Pride and Prejudice* (1813) and (good, kind) Darcy revealed later in the novel. Think about (nice) Edgar

Linton versus (dangerous) Heathcliff in Emily Brontë's *Wuthering Heights* (1847). Look at the (dangerous) Rochester before the fire in Charlotte Brontë's *Jane Eyre* (1847), vs. the (safe, nice) St. John, and the (safe, nice) Rochester who is blinded, after the fire. Look at (nice, boring) Ashley Wilkes vs. (bad, enthralling) Rhett Butler in Margaret Mitchell's *Gone with the Wind* (1936). Look at the (safe, nice) early Beatles versus the (bad, dangerous) Rolling Stones in the 1960s.

This is more than a good parlor game; these dual heroes are, I believe, archetypal for heterosexual women. Romance novels, which are the biggest-selling category of any fiction at all, tend to center on a repeated narrative arc involving an apparently bad man—a lead character who seems emotionally troubled, or arrogant, or dangerous—who turns out to be a good man, and a stable, loving, and committed husband. The enduring appeal of reading romances with this plotline—a plotline that women who read romances consume over and over with minimally changed details—may have to do with how fantasy can resolve, at least temporarily, painfully unresolvable real-life physiological tensions.

Just because women, to be sexually fully alive, need to feel safe doesn't mean they can sexually tolerate being bored. Dr. Pfaus, as you may recall, emphasized the negative role of "bad stress" and the erotic potential of "good stress." I would tease this out as excitement and "safe danger." A profound dilemma—that looks at first like a paradox—in female consciousness may be built into female neurobiology. The data we saw above on hormone fluctuations during the menstrual cycle show that when we are ovulating, we are attracted to high-testosterone, risk-taking, unpredictable males—and when we are not ovulating, we are drawn to nurturing, safer, more reliable mates.[43]

This dualism, of course, makes perfect evolutionary sense, from the perspective of Dr. Helen Fisher's theory: women are not, she argues, by nature monogamous, though it is in their interest to pair-bond with a safe, reliable male for at least the first two years of a child's life. But she also argues that adultery can be evolutionarily valuable to women because they get the sperm competition, as scientists call a situation in which more than one man's ejaculate is inside a not monogamous woman, and this aids conception. A woman can raise the baby, for at least the vulnerable first two years of its life, with the (reliable) helpmate provider. This unresolvable, even tragic tension—the sexy drive to be impregnated by the unpredictable stranger, and the equally compelling emotional drive to "marry" the predictable, nurturing man—may be built into our evolutionary wiring as women; and it is certainly built into our monthly variability. Rochester or St. John? Brett or Ashley? It may depend on the time of the month, and on our baseline SNS levels.

This tension may also explain an enduring problem within female heterosexuality, which is so tenacious but so shameful that we tend to shy away from discussing it. And this is the problem of the obvious and enduring appeal to many heterosexual women of the "bad boy" and of themes in female sexual response around domination, submission, and power. The slightly S&M novel series *Fifty Shades of Grey,* by E. L. James, sold millions of copies to women in 2012. These themes are great feminist unsayables of female sexuality. But if you look at the dozens of these scenes in, say, Nancy Friday's collection of women's erotica, *My Secret Garden,* or similar scenes of being "swept away" by a dominant male in any Harlequin romance or Mills and Boon novel, one must confront the fact that there can be something magnetic about, not force in men, but about a kind of capacity for mastery.

The really beloved bad boys of women's literature don't bully or abuse the heroine, but they continually provoke and tease her—they are teasing her to release her own latent wildness. And one thing the romantic heroes of women's fiction, even the bad boys, who can be brusque or verge on rudeness, never, ever do is actually snap at, that is, negatively startle, the heroine; think of the edgy but grudgingly respectful repartee of Darcy and Elizabeth. Virtually every woman's genre romance novel follows a script of a man who seems bad—insensitive, corrupt, womanizing—but turns out to be good. It also often features a heroine who begins demure and unripe—"Poor, obscure, plain and little" in Jane Eyre's speech—but who becomes herself, grows into herself, under the provocation of this bad boy who is secretly good.

This seeming paradox or politically incorrect fantasy is, I would argue, an essential archetype of the female heterosexual journey. A skilled, even at times slightly dangerous, male provocateur can help the female sexual journey to begin. "Badness" is not literal badness—it is otherness, wildness, the dimensions of the unknown. The motorcycle boots, the Harley—they are about *her* adventures, *her* penchant for the open road, erotically and in terms of her own creativity and subversiveness, that society has generally repressed in her and forbidden her to claim as a longing, let alone as part of her "good girl" identity. His male "badness" is simply the projected dark anima of her own unacknowledged wild self.

The difficult secret is that there is something about power—or skill, or mastery of a situation—in men that is erotic to many heterosexual women, and that probably has to do with that hormonal variation that leaves us alert to high-testosterone signals, as well as the "good stress" of SNS activation in a context a woman can ultimately control. Old-fashioned, male-centered theories of evolutionary biology have popularized notions such as the one espoused by Richard Dawkins in *The Selfish Gene,* which support the idea that men who are old, rich, and powerful can attract young, beautiful women seeking security; and that women will always be at a disadvantage in the mating dance, because they desire commitment whereas men want to spread their seed. But Dr. Helen Fisher's theory tells a very different story about male attractiveness to women: it is not the males who are sexually selecting but the females—which is the case throughout the mammal kingdom. In this scenario, a woman isn't looking for an old guy with a gold MasterCard. She is looking for a helpmate, and she is looking for high-quality sperm—a dual mission that can lead to pair-bonding with simultaneous female adultery. Could her hormonal fluctuations, and the "good stress" appeal of a man who can be dangerously exciting but not actually injurious, also intensify the duality of this mission and help explain why male fantasy figures in women's films and books manifest such opposing, even irreconcilable traits?

I have been listening to the language of women who have left their marriages or who have committed adultery. The following is another cultural secret: a substantial theme that surfaces when women say why they left solid, stable marriages, or committed adultery against good, devoted, faithful men, is that they *were bored*. Our cultural script tells us that women never leave or stray unless the men they married have done something awful to them, but I cannot count how many perfectly nice, reasonable, sane, considerate women have confided to me that the reason they left or strayed is that they "couldn't stand" the sexual boredom caused by the good, safe, nice, predictable man. They are not proud of what they have been driven to do, but they use the language of survival in explaining this: "I thought I would die if I didn't ever get this again in my life," said one adulteress, referring to the erotic chemistry of her affair. Others remarked, "I thought I would die if I stayed," and "I was dying inside." The men who were being left, or deceived, by the women who told me their stories were all incredibly nice; but they had stopped relating intellectually to the women in their lives from a condition of growth or adventure. They had stopped bringing seduction and drama into the marital bed. They had stopped seeing the women in their lives as if the women themselves needed excitement and drama within the relationship and were themselves not to be taken for granted. This seemed to have a knock-on effect: the women stopped treating the men as if their needs for excitement and novelty mattered, and started to treat them as if they were uninteresting. I believe that women's monthly need for drama in intimate settings means that when men do not provide it in positive forms, heterosexual women tend to become provocative and bitchy so they will get the stimulation they crave from men even if it arrives in a negative form such as an argument. By becoming so changeless, so predictable, many husbands lock themselves into the staid, less sexy, provider role in women's psyches, and they abandon the provocateur role—leaving nothing to fire the imagination or the SNS during the times of the months when a woman craves adventure, the "dance," and excitement. Could these women have married the men who provide for half of the need sets that our hormones prime us for—but that ignore the other half—the high-risk, unpredictable half?

Is there also something about the unpredictability of the "bad boy" that boosts the female SNS? Yes. When "bad stress" takes over the SNS, it focuses the woman's attention on anxiety rather than sexual arousal. But, as Dr. Pfaus puts it, "Good stress can sometimes be good for your sex life." Vacation sex is so arousing because of the novelty and unpredictability of the setting, which boost the SNS in a sexual way rather than an anxiety-producing way. "Some women can't quite reach orgasm without activation of the SNS produced by, say, a spanking or by hair pulling," explains Dr. Pfaus. He notes that these tastes have often been construed as evidence of these women's innate masochism, but they can simply result from the fact that these women's baseline SNS needs a bit more activation than is typical.[44]

It strikes me that this nonweird explanation for a bit of aggression being exciting to some women may explain many women's attraction to rape fantasies and other kinds of role playing, all of which heighten the SNS. (Knowing that these tastes may not derive from any psychological masochism does not mean, though, that I believe one should ignore the risk of habituation to violent sexual imagery or practices, and the risk of escalation through habituation, that I discussed in Chapter 12, "The Pornographic Vagina.")

The SNS-activating excitement and unpredictability that is good for female arousal can come from more gentle surprises, too. I know a very happily married couple; they have every stress other long-married couples have: bills, commutes, jobs, two kids who sometimes whine and who need braces and who will need college tuition eventually. But the wife is sparkling and "in the Goddess" well into her forties, and the man is very pleased with his life. For her birthday, at a time when they had very little money, the husband booked a cheap long-weekend flight to a second-class Caribbean resort.

They could have been like every other bored couple: standing in line at security together; reading magazines together; arriving at the resort tired and hungry and putting away their clothes with all the usual stresses and familiarities of every other long-married marital unit. But that is not what happened to them. Because the husband never told his wife where they were going—he only told her to pack some clothes for warm weather, and a swimsuit. He went ahead of her to the gate to explain the surprise to the bemused airline personnel. Then he went back to where she was waiting, opened a bottle of champagne, took out a dish of strawberries, poured her a glass, handed her some fruit, and then, with her permission, blindfolded her while they got onto the plane. Though her blindfold came off once they were seated, she had no idea where she was going and wouldn't find out until she landed and disembarked. Her husband said she was grinning the entire flight.

His steadiness, combined with his sense of fun, risk taking, and surprise, activate both sets of her needs at all times of the month.

Does that mean that nice, overscheduled, hardworking men reading this should despair, or take stupid lessons from seduction con men, as in Neil Strauss's *The Game,* about how to be mean to women? No. But it may mean that one way to keep a woman interested and faithful for life, if you are a man, is to never give up your role as seducer, and to never stop growing, changing, and finding little and big ways to surprise her.

Both archetypes of the male are there to provoke her, to get all her complex and continually shifting carnal and evolutionary needs met; and it may be her challenge in her real life to build enough excitement and unpredictability into her "safe" relationship, or to secure enough safety and emotional commitment in contexts in which the risky mastery that may attract her is what prevails.

## DO WHATEVER SHE LIKES TO HER NIPPLES

Whatever she likes you to do to her nipples—do it the way she likes it, and as much as she likes. As we saw earlier, nipple stimulation releases oxytocin, which will make a woman feel that the world is a good place, that love exists, that it is meaningful, and that her circumstances can be trusted (men also can have nipple stimulation during sex, but it is less sustained and frequent, in general). It may also help her see the connections between things and help her to read subtle emotional cues better—making her a more sensitive partner, a better leader, a more gifted creative artist within the circumstances of her own life, and a more tender mother. I find it very interesting that when I ask women to reflect on when they encourage nipple stimulation from their lovers, what I find anecdotally is that women want their nipples touched, pinched, or sucked by men they love or like. They can have very hot sex with men they do not like, but many women reported to me finding those men's touches of, or suckling upon, their nipples unbearable. You may have to trust your partner already to want to encourage your body to feel even more trust.

As we saw, it is scientifically well established that a baby's sucking on a mother's breasts releases oxytocin in the mother, which in turn firms the bonded feelings the mother has toward the baby. A man's sucking on a woman's breasts would also release oxytocin—generating that chemical response in women that makes them feel relaxed and affectionate, making the woman, in short, feel bonded to the person suckling her nipples. Given this possibility, women would be well advised not to let those men (or women) to whom they do not wish to feel attached and trusting, engage with their breasts. Oxytocin appears to play a big role in easing "neophobia" or "fears of the new" and anxiety; the more a lover sucks on your breasts, the more like "home" he will feel. Because of oxytocin, women are both aroused and relaxed by a lover's sucking on their nipples. In this way, too, women become "hooked" on sexual attention from their lovers, "hooked" on love.

Women may wish to be aware that if they want to have hot anonymous sex with some guy they may not trust, but don't want to fall in love with him—they would be well advised to discourage him from interacting with their nipples.

## EJACULATE

Does male ejaculate affect women's feelings? Dr. Helen Fisher takes so seriously the psychological effect of sex on women that she warns that, since antidepressants can suppress ejaculation, men who are prescribed the medications should be told that if they can't ejaculate, they may "lose the ability to send courtship signals." [45]

Receiving his ejaculate during lovemaking may make a woman feel differently about a man than does lovemaking in which she does not receive his ejaculate. Semen has sugar, sperm, and some aromatic compounds. Because it is viscous, it is sexually stimulating to more parts of a woman's vagina and cervix than penile thrusting can manage alone; a woman actually ingests the sugar in an ejaculation through the walls of her vagina. If she feels energized and "up" after sex with ejaculation, it may also be because she is on a minor sugar high, combined with the deeper stimulation she receives from hot viscous liquid. Dr. Cindy Meston and David M. Buss, in *Why Women Have Sex,* assert that semen contains trace mood elevators: "Semen contains hormones including testosterone, estrogen, follicle-stimulating hormone, luteinizing hormone, prolactin, and several types of prostaglandins. All of these hormones," they claim, "have potential mood-altering abilities and can be absorbed into a woman's bloodstream through the vaginal walls." [46] If people practice safe sex, then sex without a condom can signal that lovemaking is taking place in the context of a secure, committed relationship that is conducted with safe sex practices—boosting still more the oxytocin and opioids she may experience. Many women reported to me that they did indeed feel differently about a man after making love with ejaculation, without a condom, than they had felt before. They felt closer to him, more satisfied, and more joyful, and little things that had annoyed them before seemed less bothersome.

I conducted informal interviews with groups of women with whom I met both in person and online. I told them about the possible effects of semen, and then I asked them to remember back to a relationship in which they had at first religiously used condoms, and then after they had taken their STD tests—this was a group of very sexually responsible women—had stopped using condoms. Same guy, same sexual style, same scent: any difference?

I saw looks of shocked recognition cross my interviewees' faces. "Totally different," said Julia, a graphic designer. "Oh my God. Once we stopped using condoms—the little things [a boyfriend] did that had annoyed me were cute. He looked better! His geeky shirts didn't bother me! I felt the relationship was somehow more serious and not just because of the commitment implied by not using condoms anymore. . . . I can't believe this."

"I felt different afterward," confirmed Anastasia, a student in New York City. "I felt much more involved. I had seen him with some detachment before. After we stopped using condoms—I felt connected to him, fired up about him, motivated."

"Different. I felt different with him when we stopped using condoms," confirmed Dianne, an operations manager. "I felt more in love. I felt more satisfied. Happier. More connected."

"Our relationship completely escalated when we stopped using condoms," said Nina. "And now that I think of it our best times were right after we had made love. My mood lifted right up at those times. I hadn't felt he was that great before, when he wasn't ejaculating inside of me—I hadn't felt he was the right guy for me. But when we stopped using condoms, that coincided with my feeling that he could be the one."

Many women tried hard to remember if they had the same emotional alteration of mood upon swallowing semen after giving oral sex; several reported that they believed, in retrospect, this may have affected their mood to some extent—the sugar rush, perhaps—but that the effect was much less obvious than it had been with ejaculate in the vagina, with its opioid-boosting, and possibly other kinds of mood-elevating, action.

I am in no way seeking to undermine the important message of always practicing safe sex. But I do think it is important to understand what may happen to the female mind when we do take in semen. Think of a time when you were falling in love with a man, and using condoms. Then, after you committed to each other exclusively, you may have stopped using condoms; you were making love frequently, intoxicated by his nearness and smell, and it may also be that your sense of safety was enhanced by the exclusivity this implies, which as we now know boosts female orgasm. Think of the emotional exaltation after such lovemaking. Now think of a time when, for whatever reason, you reentered the dating scene and made love again using condoms. Did you feel a letdown, a sense of distance, and did you feel emotionally very different, after the act?

When a man comes in a woman's mouth, she may feel energized; when he comes in her vagina, it can boost her tenderness and, if Meston and Buss are right, help elevate her mood. Women's responses to men's ejaculate varies immensely from one man to another, and science has yet to explain why some men's semen feels so much more "right" than that of others. Many women have told me that some men's semen right away felt "wrong": many heterosexual women I heard from confirmed that a turning point in any number of otherwise promising early relationships was the moment when they realized they did not like—sometimes it was could not tolerate—the semen of a new lover. It is very possible that this issue is part of what women refer to when they speak of a man who is otherwise a good potential mate having "no spark" with them, or "no chemistry." When odors are aversive, people avoid coming into contact with them; it is the same with tastes. A first-time ejaculation without a condom, in a couples context, introduces a new smell and taste. At this point, many women may find they like or love the ejaculate, or at least its effect on them; other men's tastes and scents are offputting.

"So are you suggesting," many of my interviewees asked, in one way or another, completely unprompted, "that even when things are not going that well—I should get myself some of his semen to feel better?" Many of them laughed when they asked me this, but they were understandably quite serious, too. It seems that the old folk wisdom of "just have sex till you want to have sex" may have some biochemical foundation to it. The extra opiate boost provided by an ejaculation in women, and potentially other kinds of mood elevators—if their mates are doing other nice things for them, too—may indeed help get some couples through tough moments.

## YOU WILL INADVERTENTLY DRIVE HER CRAZY
## IF YOU IGNORE THE GODDESS ARRAY

In our culture, the woman is tasked with "keeping the fire alive" sexually in a relationship—showing up at the door wearing nothing but Saran Wrap, as women were counseled to do in the 1970s in Marabel Morgan's bestseller, *The Total Woman,* or exhausting herself with costumes and novelties to get his attention. But practitioners of Tantra think this model is backward. In their worldview, it is the man who must tend the fire; the man who, in Mike Lousada's terms, must "hold" the woman. Many Western men, sadly, ignore the Goddess Array unless they want sex—and often even then—and allow what Tantrists call "the fire" to subside in their wives or girlfriends to almost nothing. Then, misguidedly, they reach for their wives' or girlfriends' vaginas— as if that were part of lovemaking's beginning, instead of the end result of a long and complex sexual and emotional process. A vagina eager and ready for lovemaking is the by-product of a complex and dynamic process between two people, a process that unfolds over all twenty-four hours of the day, in which the man has, in Tantric terms, done many other apparently nonsexual things to "stoke the fire."

A straight woman who lives day to day in close relationship to a man who attends well to the Goddess Array—who, in the midst of all the other responsibilities of his life, doesn't forget to give her a strong, warm hug when he comes home from work in the evening, who doesn't skip taking the trouble to tell her she looks beautiful in a new dress, who finds the energy, even when he is tired too, to stroke her hair—this woman is, even when she is just watering her garden or opening her mail, living inside a positive, exciting sexual and emotional, yet physical, environment that her mate has created for her. Because of the idiosyncracies of the female system, creating this uniquely relaxing and stimulating environment is more the task of the man than of the woman (she has other emotional responsibilities if his biochemistry is to be taken into account). In this atmosphere, she is living with a calm SNS, which allows her circulatory system to lubricate and flush with blood easily; in turn, the hormones that elevate her mood and create confidence in her and attachment to him are steadily replenished. So when the time comes to make love, she already wants to; for she is, on all the levels that are so completely interconnected in women, eager to *and able to*—two different things for women—open up to her husband or lover.

Indeed, Dr. Pfaus's lab has found evidence—at least in lower female mammals—that there is a physiological "point of no return" for females experiencing bad sex with males—a vanishing point, if you like, related to female sexual disappointment, after which a positive connection with a mate is not physiologically recoverable. Remember the experiment in which the female rats were made "horny" through hormone injections, and one group was allowed to get pleasure from mating with males, while the other group was injected with naloxone that inhibited their experience of pleasure?

The negative results of the experiment lasted long after the actual experiment, in the reactions of the female rats who experienced disappointing sex. After the fifth experience of bad sex, the female rats begin not just ignoring the males—they start actively fighting them. They do so even if they are now injected not with naloxone, but with saline; in other words, even though now they *can physically* experience pleasure, they don't want to bother with having sex at all.

Dr. Pfaus explained: "These female rats are fighting the males, not soliciting, not showing full-intensity lordosis (meaning not arching their backs to signal a desire for sex). There is no naloxone on board, so what has happened? The female rats have formed an expectation that sex sucks—they have gone through the motions, but they won't get off. So despite the hormone priming, they still don't want to have sex! They have had five prior experiences of bad sex! They seem to have psychologically concluded: 'This is just painful. Why should I do this anymore?' (We are now looking at how long that effect lasts.)

"So female rats can conclude: 'He is a crappy lover.'

"Female rats are not blaming themselves—they are looking at an external cause for their sexual disappointment. The conclusion? There is some point at which your female partner won't want to have sex with you in the not-distant future if you give her bad sex enough in the recent past." [47]

It is pointless for a man to wonder why his female lover climbed on top of him enthusiastically last Tuesday after the very same touch from him—but pleads a headache tonight—if he is unwilling to look at how he has attended to the Goddess Array that day or that week. But if he understands how the Goddess Array really works, he will understand that, say, his having taken a moment to look deeply into her eyes before kissing her good-bye that morning before work, or picking up the laundry off the bedroom floor that evening before he turns to her with a sexual intention—even his running the wash cycle and folding a load of the laundry—can be, later on, extremely seductive to his wife or girlfriend. If this issue has been a source of stress for her, his having taken action about it in a way that lowers her stress levels associated with it (and him) will literally make her more ready to lubricate, and her vagina will be better able to flush with blood.

I would go further: his gazing at her, or praising her, or even folding a load of laundry, is not merely rightly thought of as highly effective foreplay; it is actually, from the female body's point of view, an essential part of good sex itself.

### "SHOWERS OF STARS"

The latest science, indeed, comes full circle to where we began, and shows that women themselves, given the opportunity to initiate naming, name some kinds of orgasms with language that reflects transcendental experience.

Dr. Irv Binik at McGill University in Montreal, Canada, has developed an "orgasm checklist" for women, with twenty-four descriptors; this multiplicity of available names for women's experience has led to his team's discovery that there are different kinds of orgasms in women, as women define them subjectively: some feel very "physiological" to women; for other kinds, women use more "all-encompassing," "evaluative," "subjective" terms. Binik found that women tend to use the physiological descriptors more often for masturbation—and to draw upon the emotional, subjective descriptors more often for intercourse.[48]

Beverly Whipple and Barry Komisaruk took this insight even further; they found, in 2011, that women use different kinds of language—amounting, really, to different kinds of poetry—to describe, when invited to do so, different kinds of orgasms resulting from the stimulation of clitoris, vagina (G-spot), or cervix and various combinations. This study made me recall how sex educator Liz Topp had said sadly, about the girls she had counseled who did not understand their own anatomy—"they don't know that they have worlds inside of them."

Fascinatingly, Whipple and Komisaruk found that vulval orgasms are commonly triggered by the clitoris, the major nerve involved is the pudendal nerve, and the muscle response is mostly in the PC muscle; whereas uterine orgasm is commonly triggered by the G-spot, the major nerve involved is the pelvic nerve, and the muscle response is mostly uterine. "Blended orgasms"—most women's favorite kind, statistically—involved several trigger points, and both major nerve branches, pudendal and pelvic, as well as muscle responses in both areas.[49]

Perhaps it is not surprising that it is a team made up of a female researcher, working in tandem with a male researcher, that has identified one category of female orgasm that takes us back—or forward—to the language of mysticism. A Gnostic would say that when the experience of the Divine or the transcendental harmonizes what we see outside, with what we feel inside, that is "the God" or "the Goddess."

What new name, among many, did some women, given the chance to categorize their own orgasms in their own language, give to one kind of sexual experience?

The name: "Showers of stars."

# Conclusion:
# Reclaiming the Goddess

*It feels like home.*

—Madonna, "Like a Prayer"

*I* didn't expect to have such a shift in my own vision just from having explored dimensions of the vagina that had been unknown to me. But just as I was drawn to the subject matter because I suspected that a book about the vagina would be a book about something much greater and different than a "mere" sex organ, so the change in my understanding is not just about the vagina, but seems to include a shift in how I see the world.

To finish the book, my children and I went, with another family, to a rented house, near the Greek town of Eressos, in a chain of what had been the Minoan islands. We were heading there for a week, at the start of a new summer. Two years had passed since I first began my journey.

Physically, though I had a dramatic scar running the length of the small of my back, I was well healed in every way. I was able to swim and hike again, though sadly I will never again be able to turn my spine completely—so sports, such as tennis and some kinds of dancing, are out, forever. While sometimes this causes me a bit of a pang, I am so grateful to not be in a body brace—and, just as important, so unspeakably grateful to have all my neural systems working again, to have all aspects and dimensions of my consciousness back—that these are momentary flickers, overwhelmed by the joy of knowing I have regained what I could have lost forever. My gratitude to Dr. Coady, Dr. Cole, Dr. Babu, and the other physicians who helped me, is unbounded.

Psychologically, I feel that I have discovered, through the research I did for this book, a kind of treasure for myself as well. I am surprised at how this manifests, as I keep seeing aspects of reality that had been hidden to me before.

On the last day of the writing, I took my computer in a shoulder sack and made my way to the seaside village near our rental house. The day before, I had gone out on a sail on a little white catamaran; a British teenage girl, who was working in the village for the summer, took my friend from the other family, and me, out on the water. The morning was clear and bright, lucid with white glassy heat. The water had that quality that only the Aegean possesses, somehow—a purple tinge under the blue surface, which led Homer to call it, mysteriously to me until I saw it, "the wine-dark sea." Hidden richness, hidden treasure, depths under depths.

The young woman was confident with her sailing skills: she maneuvered into the wind. Within minutes we were in the center of the harp-shaped bay, looking back at the shore and the village. When we had arrived, tired and jet-lagged, busy with children's needs and making sure everyone was settled in, we hadn't yet acclimated to the reality that we were culturally, as well as physically, in Greece. I had not seen before how the simple housing we were staying in had been built into a hollow at what was the foot of a low range of golden hills, backed by even higher hills and, in turn, by rounded, gray-gold mountains. I looked at the landscape with a start: there was majesty all around us, and a steady soft wind was blowing. The hills undulated and yielded as if the earth itself were a feminine body.

Looking back at the landscape in all its majesty and softness, I felt a kind of smudge in my vision—which had been there for my entire conscious adult life—lift for a moment, and suddenly things sparkled. The dark, obscuring smudge, I realized in a flash, was the shame and disrespect that we assign to the feminine, and it does not just converge on the vagina, though that is its archetypal center; it washes over the whole world, with a darkness or wrongness that colors our perception of it, and our relationship to it. How extraordinary everything looked when for a flash, an instant, it was lifted. How harmoniously I could see our relationship to one another, and to the earth, becoming, in this gentle, earlier light.

We were due north of Crete, I realized with a start; we were close to the beginning of the journey. This bay, this island, was near the epicenter of Goddess worship of the ancient Minoan civilizations— the civilizations that antedated the ascent of the Aryan male-dominated pantheon of the gods of classical Greece, and that also antedated the harsher patriarchal worship of the Hebrews.

The very landscape was the color of the clay out of which dozens of Minoan snake-goddesses I had seen—sex goddesses—had been crafted. Indeed, I realized, I had unconsciously registered aspects, hints, traces of that goddess throughout the island; a schematized version of the Minoan snake-goddess, holding curled snakes out before her breasts, was the official symbol of the island—on the post office, on the town hall. On every cottage and villa, I had noticed a ruddy clay statuette of a female face, framed inside a vulval shell-like enclosure, very much like the mandorla shell that enclosed the Virgin Mary in the New College manuscript, facing outward from each roof corner, an invocation for protection. Traces of the acknowledgment of the sacredness and power of the feminine energies were still here, on this island.

Earlier in the week we had visited Molyvos, a beautiful hillside town. As we explored a Byzantine castle on the crest of the hill, my friend had said, "Look!" Across the valley great plumes of scarlet and orange flame leaped hundreds of feet into the sky, and massive sheets of white and steel-gray smoke, fissured at times with coal-black smoke, poured skyward. It was a forest fire, threatening the neighboring town of Petra. We ran down to the harbor, where we watched planes pour water on the licking, devouring wall of flame. The townspeople told us that the fires had begun to recur every summer; they could not be easily subdued. Dozens of people had died in the fires the summer before. It was so dangerous now, they said, because it was the driest summer in years, for the weather was extreme; it was changing.

In an instant, I realized that original sin did not, as the Judeo-Christian tradition has it, originate in human sexuality. Our species' original sin was in deviating from our earliest tradition of reverence for the feminine and for female sexuality, and all that it represented for us. Our original sin lies in five thousand years of shaming it, stigmatizing it, controlling it, subduing it, splitting it off from women, from men, compartmentalizing it, insulting it and selling it. Great dislocations and alienations in civilization and in human development have followed from that original sin, and the results are everywhere around us. In a flash I saw waves of tragedy—for women, for men, and for a now unbalanced, now plundering civilization that followed from this original alienation.

All these moments and insights now seemed connected to me.

I remembered educator Liz Topp, who had described the teenage girls in the high school in Manhattan. These girls had told her that they were so fed up with the disrespect accorded to them sexually, and with being so kept in the dark and silenced about their own desires and development, that one day they went to the school assembly in a group, and asked for a chance to speak. They then stood up, and shouted, in unison:

"Vagina vagina vagina!"

I smiled when I thought of this, and of these girls' impulse: that their own strength and development depended on this reclamation—as impulsive a gesture as it was.

They were right.

The final day of my writing, I stole away by myself into the center of Eressos, farther down the bay. She-goats lay peacefully under the olive trees, and their kids butted horns in the shadows. The path I followed wove parallel to the Aegean, which was on my right; the great soft hills were to my left. My path led over a small bridge; dozens of fish and turtles swam in the green river that ran beneath it. Beside the path, many-colored flowers bloomed in abundance: bright pink oleander, orange trumpet-vine flowers, soft purple thistles. In every other flower, it seemed, a bee was busily working. Flowers, of course, are the sex organs of plants; I had eaten this honey at breakfast, every morning of our stay.

I smiled. Wherever I looked around me I saw the undimmed, unsullied feminine energy, creating and giving. Female sexuality was everywhere, doing nothing less than nurturing and sustaining the entire world; doing nothing less than nurturing and sustaining us, humanity.

*Vagina vagina vagina,* I thought with amusement.

# Notes

## Introduction

1. Christopher Ryan and Cacilda Jethá, *Sex at Dawn: The Prehistoric Origins of Modern Sexuality* (New York: HarperCollins, 2010).

2. Shere Hite, *The Hite Report: A Nationwide Study of Female Sexuality* (New York: Seven Stories Press, 2004).

3. Catherine Blackledge, *The Story of V: A Natural History of Female Sexuality* (New Brunswick, NJ: Rutgers University Press, 2004).

4. William James, *The Varieties of Religious Experience* (New York: Barnes and Noble Classics, 2004), 366.

5. Ibid., 329–71.

6. Ibid., 366.

7. William Wordsworth, "Ode on Intimations of Immortality from Recollections of Early Childhood," in *The Major Works, Including the Prelude*, Stephen Gill, ed., (New York: Oxford World Classics, 2000): "There was a time when meadow, grove, and stream / The earth, and every common sight / To me did seem / Apparelled in celestial light. . . . trailing clouds of glory do we come / From God, who is our home."

8. James, *The Varieties of Religious Experience*, 370.

9. Sigmund Freud, *Civilization and Its Discontents* (New York: Penguin Books, 2002).

10. Janniko R. Georgiadis and others, "Regional Cerebral Blood Flow Changes Associated with Clitorally Induced Orgasm in Healthy Women," *European Journal of Neuroscience*, vol. 24 (2006): 3305–16.

11. Blaise Pascal, *Pensées* (New York: Penguin Books, 1996), 148.

12. Kamil Dada, "Dalai Lama Talks Meditation with Stanford Scientists," *The Stanford Daily*, www.stanforddaily.com/2010/10/18/dalai-lama-talks-meditation-with-stanford-scientists.

# One / Does the Vagina Have a Consciousness?

## *Chapter 1: Meet Your Incredible Pelvic Nerve*

1. Netter image 5101. "Innervation of Female Reproductive Organs," www .netterimages.com/image/5101.htm, and 2992; compare "Innervation of Male Reproductive Organs," 2910, www.netterimages.com/image/2910.htm.

2. "Innervation of External Genitalia and Perineum." Ibid.

3. www.netterimages.com/image/3013.htm.

4. "Innervation of Internal Genitalia," www.netterimages.com/image/ 3093.htm.

5. Ibid.

6. Naomi Wolf, *Misconceptions: Truth, Lies and the Unexpected on the Journey to Motherhood* (New York: Doubleday, 2001), 165–67.

## *Chapter 2: Your Dreamy Autonomic Nervous System*

1. Cindy M. Meston and Boris B. Gorzalka, "Differential Effects of Sympathetic Activation on Sexual Arousal in Sexually Dysfunctional and Functional Women," *Journal of Abnormal Psychology,* vol. 105, no. 4 (1996): 582–91.

2. Herbert Benson, M.D., *The Relaxation Response* (New York: Avon, 1976).

3. Janniko R. Georgiadis and others, "Regional Cerebral Blood Flow Changes Associated with Clitorally Induced Orgasm in Healthy Women," *European Journal of Neuroscience,* vol. 24, no. 11 (2006): 3305–16.

4. Naomi Wolf, *Misconceptions: Truth, Lies and the Unexpected on the Journey to Motherhood* (New York: Doubleday, 2001), 165–67.

5. Ina May Gaskin, *Spiritual Midwifery* (Nashville, TN: Book Publishing Company, 2002), 86, 440–41.

6. Carter, 1998, cited in Mark R. Leary and Cody B. Cox, "Belongingness Motivation: A Mainspring of Social Action," in *Handbook of Motivation Science,* ed. James Y. Shah and Wendi L. Gardner (New York: Guildford Press, 1998), 37.

7. Wolf, *Misconceptions,* 118, 141.

8. Netter image 3093, www.netterimages.com/image/3093.htm.

9. William H. Masters and Virginia E. Johnson, *Human Sexual Response* (New York: Ishi Press, 2010), 69.

10. Rosemary Basson, "Women's Sexual Dysfunction: Revised and Expanded Definitions," *CMAJ,* 172, no. 10 (May 2005): 1327–1333.

11. The female pelvic neural structure is so complex that at least one researcher, Hanny Lightfoot-Klein, found that Sudanese women who have been clitorally excised and even infibulated still report having some kinds of orgasms. Hanny Lightfoot-Klein, "The Sexual Experience and Marital Adjustment of Genitally Circumcised and Infibulated Females in the Sudan," *Journal of Sex Research,* vol. 26, no. 3 (1989): 375–92.

12. Barry R. Komisaruk and others, "Brain Activation During Vagino-Cervical Self-Stimulation and Orgasm with Complete Spinal Cord Injury: fMRI Evidence of Mediation by Vagus Nerves": "Women diagnosed with complete spinal cord injury . . . have been reported to perceive, and respond with orgasms to, vaginal and/or cervical mechno-stimulation." *Brain Research* 1024 (2004): 77–88. www.sciencedirect.com/science/article/piis0006899304011461.

## Chapter 3: Confidence, Creativity, and the Sense of Interconnectedness

1. George Eliot, *The Mill on the Floss* (London: Penguin Classics, 2003), 338.

2. Ibid., 573.

3. Christina Rossetti, "Goblin Market," *Poems and Prose* (Oxford: Oxford World's Classics), 105–19.

4. Hunter Drohojowska-Philp, *Full Bloom: The Art and Life of Georgia O'Keeffe* (New York: W. W. Norton, 2004), 115, 135; Sarah Greenough, ed., *My Faraway One: Selected Letters of Georgia O'Keeffe to Alfred Stieglitz,* vol. 1, *1915–1933* (New Haven, CT: Yale University Press, 2012), 127, 217.

5. David Laskin, *Partisans: Marriage, Politics and Betrayal among the New York Intellectuals* (New York: Simon and Schuster, 2000), 151.

6. Kate Chopin, *The Awakening and Other Stories* (Oxford: Oxford University Press, 2000), 219.

7. Hermione Lee, *Edith Wharton* (New York: Alfred A. Knopf, 2007), 327.

8. Chopin, *The Awakening,* 82.

9. Edith Wharton, *The House of Mirth* (New York: Barnes and Noble Classics), 177.

10. Gordon Haight, *George Eliot: A Biography* (Oxford: Oxford University Press, 1978), 226–280; Greenough, *My Faraway One,* 216; Candace Falk, *Love, Anarchy and Emma Goldman: A Biography* (New Brunswick, NJ: Rutgers University Press, 1990), 66.

11. Greenough, *My Faraway One,* 56–57, 217.

12. Isabel Allende, *Inés of My Soul* (New York: HarperPerennial, 2006), 8.

## Chapter 4: Dopamine, Opioids, and Oxytocin

1. See Stanley Siegel, *Your Brain on Sex: How Smarter Sex Can Change Your Life* (Naperville, IL: Sourcebooks, 2011).

2. Marnia Robinson: Dopamine Chart.

3. Dr. Jim Pfaus, interview, Concordia University, Montreal, Quebec, January 29, 2012.

4. Ibid.

5. David J. Linden, *The Compass of Pleasure: How Our Brains Make Fatty Foods, Orgasm, Exercise, Marijuana, Generosity, Vodka, Learning, and Gambling Feel So Good* (New York: Viking, 2011), 94–125.

6. Dr. Helen Fisher, *Anatomy of Love: A Natural History of Mating, Marriage, and Why We Stray* (New York: Ballantine Books, 1992), 162.

7. Ibid., 175.

8. Cindy M. Meston and K. M. McCall, "Dopamine and Norepinephrine Responses to Film-Induced Sexual Arousal in Sexually Functional and Dysfunctional Women," *Journal of Sex & Marital Therapy*, vol. 31 (2005): 303–17.

9. Claude de Contrecoeur, "*Le Rôle de la Dopamine et de la Sérotonine dans le Système Nerveux Central,*" www.bio.net/bionet/mm/neur-sci/1996 -July/024549.html.

10. Ibid.

11. Dr. Pfaus interview, January 29, 2012.

12. See Mary Roach, *Bonk: The Curious Coupling of Science and Sex* (New York: W. W. Norton, 2008).

13. Ibid., and Susan Rako, *The Hormone of Desire: The Truth About Testosterone, Sexuality, and Menopause* (New York: Harmony, 1996).

14. Linden, *The Compass of Pleasure*, 94–125.

15. Ibid., 94–125.

16. Marnia Robinson and Gary Wilson, "The Big 'O' Isn't Orgasm," www.reuniting.info/science/oxytocin_health_bonding.

17. Ibid.

18. Navneet Magon and Sanjay Kalra, "The Orgasmic History of Oxytocin: Love, Lust and Labor," *Indian Journal of Endocrinology and Metabolism* Supp. 3 (September 2011): 5156–61.

19. Agren, 2002, cited in Beate Ditzen, *Effects of Romantic Partner Interaction on Psychological and Endocrine Stress Protection in Women* (Gottingen, Germany: Cuvillier Verlag, Gottingen, 2005), 50–51.

20. C. A. Pedersen, 2002 and Arletti, 1997, cited in Robinson and Wilson, "The 'Big O' Isn't Orgasm," http://www.reuniting.info/science/oxytocin_health_bonding.

21. R. W. B. Lewis and Nancy Lewis, *The Letters of Edith Wharton* (New York: Scribner, 1988), 324–36.

22. James G. Pfaus, and others, "Who, What, Where, When (and Maybe Even Why)? How the Experience of Sexual Reward Connects Sexual Desire, Preference, and Performance," *Archives of Sexual Behavior* 41 (March 9, 2012): 31–62:

> Although sexual behavior is controlled by hormonal and neurochemical actions in the brain, sexual experience induces a degree of plasticity that allows animals to form instrumental and Pavlovian associations that predict sexual outcomes, thereby directing the strength of sexual responding. This review describes how experience with sexual reward strengthens the development of sexual behavior and induces sexually-conditioned place and partner preferences in rats. In both male and female rats, early sexual experience with partners scented with a neutral or even noxious odor induces a preference for scented partners in subsequent choice tests. Those preferences can also be induced by injections of morphine or oxytocin paired with a male rat's first exposure to scented females, indicating that pharmacological activation of opioid or oxytocin receptors can "stand in" for the sexual reward-related neurochemical processes normally activated by sexual stimulation. Conversely, conditioned place or partner preferences can be blocked by the opioid receptor antagonist naloxone. A somatosensory cue (a rodent jacket) paired with sexual reward comes to elicit sexual arousal in male rats, such that paired rats with the jacket off show dramatic copulatory deficits. We propose that endogenous opioid activation forms the basis of sexual reward, which also sensitizes hypo-thalamic and mesolimbic dopamine systems in the presence of cues that predict sexual reward. Those systems act to focus attention on, and activate goal-directed behavior toward, reward-related stimuli. Thus, a critical period exists during an individual's early sexual experience that creates a "love map" or Gestalt of features, movements, feelings, and interpersonal interactions associated with sexual reward.

23. www.guardian.co.uk/science/2011/nov/14/female-orgasm-recorded-brain-scans and Barry R. Komisaruk, PhD, and Beverly Whipple, PhD, "Brain Activity During Sexual Response and Orgasm in Women: fMRI Evidence," presentation, International Society for the Study of Women's Sexual Health, 2011 Annual Meeting, Scottsdale, Arizona, February 10–13, Program Book, 173–184.

24. Ian Sample, "Female Orgasm Captured in a Series of Brain Scans," *The Guardian*, November 14, 2011, www.guardian.co.uk/science/2011/nov/14/female-orgasm-recorded-brain-scans.

25. Dr. Pfaus interview, January 30, 2012.

26. Simon LeVay, *The Sexual Brain* (Cambridge, MA: MIT Press, 1993), 71–82.

27. Sappho, "Fragment," *Sappho's Lyre: Archaic Lyric and Women Poets of Ancient Greece,* trans. Diane J. Rayor (Berkeley, CA: University of California Press, 1991), 52. "Come to me now again, release me from / this pain, everything my spirit longs / to have fulfilled, fulfill. . . ."

28. "Song of Songs," 2:5–16, *The New International Version,* www.biblegate way.com.

## Chapter 5: What We "Know" About Female Sexuality Is Out of Date

1. Liz Topp, interview, New York City, April 15, 2010.

2. See Shere Hite, *The Hite Report: A Nationwide Study of Female Sexuality* (New York: Seven Stories Press, 2004); Shere Hite, *The Shere Hite Reader: New and Selected Writings on Sex, Globalism, and Private Life* (New York: Seven Stories Press, 2006).

3. Anaïs Nin, *Delta of Venus* (New York: Penguin Modern Classics, 1977), 140.

4. J. A. Simon, "Low Sexual Desire—Is It All in Her Head? Pathophysiology, Diagnosis, and Treatment of Hypoactive Sexual Desire Disorder," *Postgraduate Medicine* 122, no. 6 (November 2010): 128–36.

5. Dr. Helen Fisher and J. Anderson Thompson, Jr., "Sex, Sexuality And Serotonin: Do Sexual Side Effects of Most Antidepressants Jeopardize Romantic Love and Marriage?," www.medscape.org/viewarticle/482059.

6. In 1992, the National Health and Social Life Survey found that the prevalence of low female sexual desire in the general population in the United States was high and that low desire and arousal concerns were the category most strongly associated with dissatisfaction in women: http://popcenter .uchicago.edu/data/nhsls.shtml. The survey was updated in 2009, and it still found that 43 percent of women in the sample reported sexual dysfunction, compared to 31 percent of men: Edward O. Laumann, Anthony Paik, and Raymond C. Rosen, "Sexual Dysfunction in the United States: Prevalence and Predictors," *Journal of the American Medical Association,* vol. 281, no. 6 (February 10, 1999): 587.

7. J. J. Warnock, "Female Hypoactive Sexual Desire Disorder: Epidemiology, Diagnosis and Treatment," *CNS Drugs* 16, no. 11 (2002): 745–53. Another study found a third of premenopausal women suffered from low sexual desire: S. L. West, A. A. d'Aloisio, R. P. Agansi, W. D. Kalsbeek, N. N. Borisov, and J. M. Thorp, "Prevalence of Low Sexual Desire and Hypoactive Sexual

Desire Disorder in a Nationally Representative Sample of US Women," *Archives of Internal Medicine* 168, no. 3 (July 2008): 1441–49.

8. Corky Siemaszko, "Sex Survey Finds U.S. Men Aren't the Lovers They Think They Are—and Women 'Faking It' Is to Blame," *New York Daily News,* October 4, 2010.

## Two / History: Conquest and Control

### *Chapter 6: The Traumatized Vagina*

1. Jonny Hogg, "400,000-plus Women Raped in Congo Yearly: Study," *Reuters,* May 11, 2011, citing a study by the *American Journal of Public Health*. www.reuters.com/article/2011/05/11/US-congo-rape -idUsTRE74A79Y20110511. See also Jeffrey Gettleman, "Congo Study Sets Estimate for Rapes Much Higher," *New York Times,* May 11, 2011. www .nytimes.com/2011/05/12/world/Africa/12congo.html. The Congolese Women's Campaign Against Sexual Violence confirms lower numbers, but notes that forty women are raped daily in Eastern Congo: http://www.rdc -viol.org/site/en/node/35.

2. Jimmie Briggs, interview, New York City, May 12, 2010.

3. Douglas Bremner, Penny Randall, Eric Vermetten, Lawrence Staib, Richard A. Bronen, Carolyn Mazure, Sandi Capelli, Gregory McCarthy, Robert B. Innis, and Dennis S. Charney, "Magnetic Resonance Imaging-Based Measurement of Hippocampal Volume in Posttraumatic Stress Disorder Related to Childhood Physical and Sexual Abuse—A Preliminary Report," *Biological Psychiatry* 1, no. 41 (January 1997): 23–32.

4. Dr. Burke Richmond, interview, New York City, November 20, 2011.

5. Roni Caryn Rabin, "Nearly 1 in 5 Women in U.S. Survey Say They Have Been Sexually Assaulted," *New York Times,* December 14, 2011. www .nytimes/2011/12/15/health/nearly-1-in-5-women-in-us-survey-report-sexual -assault.html.

6. Tami Lynn Kent, *Wild Feminine: Finding Power, Spirit & Joy in the Female Body* (New York: Atria Books, 2011), 51–65.

7. Alessandra H. Rellini and Cindy M. Meston, "Psychophysiological Arousal in Women with a History of Child Sexual Abuse," *Journal of Sex and Marital Therapy* 32 (2006): 5–22. See also Cindy M. Meston and Boris B. Gorzalka, "Differential Effects of Sympathetic Activation on Sexual Arousal in Sexually Dysfunctional and Functional Women," *Journal of Abnormal Psychology,* vol. 105, no. 4 (1996): 582–91, and Cindy M. Meston, "Sympathetic Nervous System Activity and Female Sexual Arousal," in

"A Symposium: Sexual Activity and Cardiac Risk," *American Journal of Cardiology,* vol. 86, no. 2A (July 20, 2000): 30F–34F.

For more data on the link between relaxation and female sexual arousal, and the link between anxiety and female sexual inhibition, see Andrea Bradford and Cindy M. Meston, "The Impact of Anxiety on Sexual Arousal in Women," *Behavioral Research and Therapy,* vol. 44 (2006): 1067–77: "A high incidence of sexual dysfunction has been reported in women with anxiety disorders." Hannah Gola and others show that women who have been violently raped show changes in their cortisol responses in response to psychological triggers: "Victims of Rape Show Increased Cortisol Responses to Trauma Reminders: A Study in Individuals with War- and Torture-Related PTSD," *Psychoneuroendocrinology* 37 (2012): 213–20.

8. See Margaret Buttenheim and A. A. Levendosky, "Couples Treatment for Incest Survivors," *Psychotherapy,* vol. 31 (1994): 407–14. The studies that document the damage of sexual abuse, especially early sexual abuse, to female sexual response later in life are many and the correlation is strong. Most of them, however, focus on emotional and psychological trauma as the primary inhibitor of sexual response in previously victimized women. *The Abuse of Men: Trauma Begets Trauma,* edited by Barbara Jo Brothers, summarizes many studies: "Courtois (1988) has reported that 80% of the victims of childhood sexual abuse experienced some difficulty in adult relationships." Becker, Skinner, and Able, they note, cited in Sarwer and Durlak, 1996, place the range of such damaged relationships, rather, at 50 percent: "Difficulties range from hypoarousal, to aversion of genitals and painful sex. . . . Buttenheim and Levendosky confirm [this issue] when they describe the sexless marriage as another manifestation of the survivor's difficulty with sexuality." Barbara Jo Brothers, ed., *The Abuse of Men: Trauma Begets Trauma* (Binghamton, NY: Haworth Press, 2001), 20. Sandra Risa Leiblum, ed., in *Principles and Practice of Sex Therapy,* cites Levendosky and Buttenheim's 1994 study that argues that sexual dysfunction in a relationship that involves an incest or sex abuse survivor is "an elaborate mutual reenactment" of the original incest. Sandra Risa Leiblum, ed., *Principles and Practices of Sex Therapy* (New York: The Guilford Press, 2007), 361.

9. M. F. Barnes, 1995, cited in Abrielle Conway and Amy Smith, "Strategies for Addressing Childhood Sexual Abuse in the Hope Approach," *Regent University Hope Research Study,* www.regent.edu/acad/schlou/research/ initiatives.htm#hope.

10. J. Douglas Bremner, and others, "MRI and PET Study of Deficits in Hippocampal Structure and Function in Women with Childhood Sexual Abuse and Posttraumatic Stress Disorder," *American Journal of Psychiatry* 160, no. 5 (May 1, 2003): 924–32. These researchers found that women with childhood sexual abuse have measurable changes in the hippocampus

area of their brains—16 percent to 19 percent smaller hippocampal area and less hippocampal activation was found in the women who had experienced childhood sexual abuse as opposed to the controls. The hippocampus is involved in "verbal declarative memory" tasks, as well as consolidation of new memories and emotional responses—which raises an intriguing question about the possible light that this result may shed on the brain-level ability of women who have been sexually traumatized in childhood to easily experience an unmediated "I." Sexual-abuse or rape-induced PTSD could be shown in this experiment as well to break down a woman's ability to "know what she knows" and reconstitute a certain sense of self in an ongoing way:

OBJECTIVE: Animal studies have suggested that early stress is associated with alterations in the hippocampus, a brain area that plays a critical role in learning and memory. The purpose of this study was to measure both hippocampal structure and function in women with and without early childhood sexual abuse and the diagnosis of posttraumatic stress disorder (PTSD). METHOD: Thirty-three women participated in this study, including women with early childhood sexual abuse and PTSD (N=10), women with abuse without PTSD (N=12), and women without abuse or PTSD (N=11). Hippocampal volume was measured with magnetic resonance imaging in all subjects, and hippocampal function during the performance of hippocampal-based verbal declarative memory tasks was measured by using positron emission tomography in abused women with and without PTSD. RESULTS: A failure of hippocampal activation and 16% smaller volume of the hippocampus were seen in women with abuse and PTSD compared to women with abuse without PTSD. Women with abuse and PTSD had a 19% smaller hippocampal volume relative to women without abuse or PTSD. CONCLUSIONS: These results are consistent with deficits in hippocampal function and structure in abuse-related PTSD.

11. R. Yehuda, 2003, and S. M. Southwick and others, 1999, cited in Thomas Steckler, N. H. Kalin, and J. M. H. M. Reul, *Handbook of Stress and the Brain: Integrative and Clinical Aspects,* vol. 15, *Techniques in the Behavioral and Neural Sciences* (New York: Elsevier Science, 2005), 251, 272.

12. S. M. Southwick, R. Yehuda, and C. A. Morgan III, "Clinical Studies of Neurotransmitter Alterations in Post-Traumatic Stress Disorder," in *Neurobiology and Clinical Consequences of Stress: From Normal Adaptation to PTSD,* ed. M. J. Friedman, D. S. Charney, and A. Y. Deutch (Philadelphia, PA: Lippincott-Raven, 1995), 335–49.

13. Ibid.

14. K. Stav, P. L. Dwyer, and L. Roberts, "Pudendal Neuralgia: Fact or Fiction?" make Ms. Fish's point. *Obstetrical and Gynecological Survey* 64, no. 3 (March 2009): 190–99.

15. Nancy Fish, interview, Copake, New York, April 5, 2011.

16. See Stephen Porges, *The Polyvagal Theory: Neuropsychological Foundations of Emotions, Attachment, Communication, and Self-Regulation* (New York: W. W. Norton, 2011).

17. Mike Lousada, interview, London, UK, June 12, 2011.

18. Dr. James Willoughby, Faculty of History and New College, New College Archives, University of Oxford, interview, June 11, 2011.

19. Juan Eduardo Cirlot and Jack Sage, *A Dictionary of Symbols* (New York: Philosophical Library, Inc., 1971), 381.

## Chapter 7: The Vagina Began as Sacred

1. Riane Eisler, *The Chalice and the Blade: Our History, Our Future* (New York: HarperOne, 1988), 51.

2. See J. A. MacGillivray, *Minotaur: Sir Arthur Evans and the Archaeology of the Minoan Myth* (New York: Hill and Wang, 2000).

3. Rosalind Miles, *The Women's History of the World* (London: Paladin Books, 1989), 34–37.

4. Asia Shepsut, *Journey of the Priestess: The Priestess Traditions of the Ancient World* (New York: HarperCollins, 1993), 62–79.

5. Ibid., 16.

6. Ibid., 72.

7. Ibid., 69.

8. Catherine Blackledge, *The Story of V: A Natural History of Female Sexuality* (New Brunswick, NJ: Rutgers University Press, 2004), 30.

9. Erich Neumann, *The Great Mother: Analysis of an Archetype* (Princeton, NJ: Princeton University Press), 168.

10. Sigmund Freud, "Three Essays on the Theory of Sexuality," *The Freud Reader,* ed. Peter Gay (New York: W. W. Norton, 1989), 239.

11. Thomas Laqueur, *Making Sex: Body and Gender from the Greeks to Freud* (Cambridge, MA: Harvard University Press, 1990), 26.

12. Leviticus 15:19, www.come-and-hear.com/editor/america_3.html.

13. Babylonian Talmud, *Tractate Kerithoth 2B* Soncino 1961 Edition, 1, www.come-and-hear.com/editor/america_3.html.

14. Tertullian, "On the Apparel of Women," www.public.iastate
.edu/~hist.486x/medieval.html; see also Kristen E. Kvam, Lina S. Schearing, and Valarie H. Ziegler, *Eve and Adam: Jewish, Christian, and Muslim*

*Readings on Genesis and Gender* (Bloomington, IN: Indiana University Press, 1999), 131.

15. Morton M. Hunt, *The Natural History of Love* (New York: Minerva Press, 1959), 187.

16. Ibid., 207. For a full account of the rise of sexless mariolary, see Jacques Delarun, "The Clerical Gaze," *A History of Women: The Silences of the Middle Ages,* ed. Christiane Klapisch-Zuber (Cambridge, MA: Harvard University Press, 1992), 15–36.

17. Mary Roach, *Bonk: The Curious Coupling of Science and Sex* (New York: W. W. Norton, 2008), 214–15.

18. Geoffrey Chaucer, *The Canterbury Tales,* ed. Nevill Coghill (New York: Penguin Classics, 2003), 285. In "The Miller's Tale," one of the clerks tells Alison that "If I don't have my wish, for love of you, I will die." "And prively he caughte hire by the queynte, / And seyde, 'Ywis, but if ich have my wille, / For deerne love of thee, lemman, I spille.' " Foreword, 88. In "The Wife of Bath's Prologue," the Wife of Bath tells one of her husbands that "For, certeyn, olde dotard, by youre leve, / Ye shul have quente right ynogh at eve." Later she refers to her vagina as her "bele chose" (Fr. *belle chose*, beautiful thing).

19. "Case Study: The European Witch-Hunts, c. 1450–1750," www .gendercide.org/case_witchhunts.html.

20. Dr. Emma Rees, "Cordelia's Can't: Rhetorics of Reticence and (Dis)ease in King Lear," *Rhetorics of Bodily Disease and Health in Medieval and Early Modern England,* ed. Jennifer Vaught (London: Ashgate, 2010), 105–16.

21. Rees, "Cordelia's Can't," 105–16.

22. William Shakespeare, *The Compete Works,* ed. G. B. Harrison (New York: Harcourt, Brace and World, 1958), 1546.

23. Rees, "Cordelia's Can't," 110.

24. Ibid.

25. Ibid.

26. Ibid.

27. John Donne, *The Complete Poetry and Selected Prose of John Donne,* ed. Charles M. Coffin (New York: Modern Library, 2001), 85.

28. Naomi Wolf, "Lost and Found: The Story of the Clitoris," in *Promiscuities: The Secret Struggle for Womanhood* (New York: Random House, 2003), 143–53. Also Catherine Blackledge, *The Story of V: A Natural History of Female Sexuality* (New Brunswick, NJ: Rutgers University Press, 2004), 125.

29. Laqueur, *Making Sex,* 4, 239.

## Chapter 8: The Victorian Vagina: Medicalization and Subjugation

1. Michel Foucault, *The History of Sexuality,* vol 1, *An Introduction* (New York: Vintage, 1990), 12.

2. Jeffrey Moussaieff Masson, *A Dark Science: Women, Sexuality, and Psychiatry in the Nineteenth Century* (New York: Noonday Press, 1988), 63–65.

3. Erna Olafson Hellerstein, Leslie Parker Hume, and Karen M. Offen, eds., *Victorian Women: A Documentary Account of Women's Lives in Nineteenth-Century England, France, and the United States* (Palo Alto, CA: Stanford University Press, 1981), 5.

4. William Acton, *A Complete Practical Treatise on Venereal Diseases* (London: Ibotson and Palmer, 1866), cited in *Suffer and Be Still: Women in the Victorian Age,* ed. Martha Vicinus (Bloomington, IN: Indiana University Press, 1973), 82–83, 84.

5. Steven Seidman, *Romantic Longings: Love in America, 1830–1980* (New York: Routledge, 1993), 33.

6. Hellerstein, Hume, and Offen, *Victorian Women,* 3.

7. Ibid., 5.

8. Ibid.

9. Masson, *A Dark Science,* 3.

10. Ibid., 65–90.

11. Dr. Emma Rees, "Narrating the Victorian Vagina: Charlotte Brontë and the Masturbating Woman," *The Female Body in Medicine and Literature,* ed. Andrew Maugham (Liverpool: Liverpool University Press, 2011), 119–34.

12. Peter T. Cominos, "Innocent Femina Sensualis in Unconscious Conflict," and E. M. Sigsworth and T. J. Wyke, "A Study of Victorian Prostitution and Venereal Disease," in Vicinus, *Suffer and Be Still,* 77–99, 155–72. See also *A New Woman Reader,* ed. Carolyn Christensen Nelson (New York: Broadview Press, 2000).

13. See A. N. Wilson, *The Victorians* (New York: W. W. Norton, 2003). *A History of Private Life,* vol. 4, *From the Fires of Revolution to the Great War,* ed. Michelle Perrot (Cambridge, MA: Harvard University Press, 1990), 261–337. There were countercurrents to the Victorian and Edwardian hostility to the vagina: in Victorian and Edwardian France, a betrothed man would send flowers that symbolized vulval engorgement, in the days leading up to his wedding: "Following an oriental custom, some men chose flowers that gradually turned redder and redder until on the eve of the wedding, they

became purple, as a symbol of ardent love. Manuals of etiquette declared this new fashion to be in the worst possible taste." Ibid., 311.

14. George Eliot, *The Mill on the Floss* (London: Penguin, 1979), 318, 338.

15. Rees, "Narrating the Victorian Vagina," 119–34.

16. Christina Rossetti, *Poems and Prose,* ed. Simon Humphries (Oxford, UK: Oxford World Classics, 2008), 105–19.

17. See Richard von Krafft-Ebing, *Aberrations of Sexual Life: The Psychopathia Sexualis* (London: Panther, 1951); Havelock Ellis and John Addington Symonds, *Sexual Inversion* (New York: Arno Press, 1975).

18. *Freud on Women: A Reader,* ed. Elisabeth Young-Bruehl (New York: W. W. Norton, 1990), 137.

19. Wilhelm Stekel, *Frigidity in Woman,* vol. 2, *The Parapathiac Disorders* (New York: Liveright, 1926), 1–62.

## Chapter 9: Modernism: The "Liberated" Vagina

1. Steven Seidman, *Romantic Longings: Love in America, 1830–1980* (New York: Routledge, 1993), 76–77.

2. Elizabeth Sprigge, *Gertrude Stein: Her Life and Work* (New York: Harper and Brothers, 1957), 128.

3. Ibid., 94.

4. Rhonda K. Garelick, *Electric Salome: Loie Fuller's Performance of Modernism* (Princeton, NJ: Princeton University Press, 2007), 164–65.

5. Hunter Drohojowska-Philp, *Full Bloom: The Art and Life of Georgia O'Keeffe* (New York: W. W. Norton, 2004), 115, 135. Sarah Greenough, ed., *My Faraway One: Selected Letters of Georgia O'Keeffe and Alfred Stieglitz* (New Haven, CT: Yale University Press, 2012), 127.

6. Edna St. Vincent Millay, *Collected Poems of Edna St. Vincent Millay,* ed. Norma Millay (New York: HarperPerennial, 1981), 19.

7. Ellen Chesler, *Woman of Valor: Margaret Sanger and the Birth Control Movement in America* (New York: Simon and Schuster, 1992), 272, 343.

8. Remy de Gourmont, *The Natural Philosophy of Love,* trans. Ezra Pound (London: Casanova Society, 1922), 205–6.

9. Henry Miller, *Tropic of Cancer* (New York: Grove Press, 1961), 2.

10. Ibid., 24, 31.

11. Michael Whitworth, "Modernism" (lecture, Department of English Language and Literature, University of Oxford, May 10, 2011).

12. Mina Loy, *The Lost Lunar Baedeker,* ed. Roger L. Conover (New York: Farrar, Straus and Giroux, 1997), xv.

13. D. H. Lawrence, *Women in Love* (New York: Penguin, 1987), 37, 55–56.

14. Anaïs Nin, *Delta of Venus* (New York: Penguin Modern Classics, 1977), 8–19.

15. Miller, *Tropic of Cancer,* 31.

16. Paul Garon, *Blues and the Poetic Spirit* (London: Eddison Press, 1975), 69.

17. Memphis Minnie, "If You See My Rooster," Bluesistheroots, www .youtube.com/watch?v=UxSjUmGweqg.

18. Bessie Smith, "I Need a Little Sugar in My Bowl," www.lyricstime.com/ bessie_smith_i_need_a_little_sugar_in_my_bowl_lyrics.html.

19. Merline Johnson, the Yas Yas Girl, "Don't You Feel My Leg," 1938, www.jazzdocumentation.ch/audio/rsrf/high.ram.

20. Ruth Brown, "If I Can't Sell It I'll Keep Sittin' on It (Before I Give It Away)," 1940, *Essential Women of Blues,* compact disc, Hill/Razaf, Joe Davis Music.

21. See Betty Friedan, *The Feminine Mystique* (New York: W. W. Norton, 2001).

22. See Shere Hite, *The Hite Report: A Nationwide Study of Female Sexuality* (New York: Macmillan, 1976).

23. Betty Dodson, "Getting to Know Me," *Ms.* magazine, 1974, in Jeffrey Escoffier, *Sexual Revolution* (New York: Running Press, 2003), 698.

24. Germaine Greer, *The Madwoman's Underclothes: Essays and Occasional Writings* (New York: Atlantic Monthly Press, 1994), 74–89.

25. Erica Jong, *Fear of Flying* (New York: Signet, 1974), 310–11.

26. Seidman, *Romantic Longings,* 150–51.

27. Ibid.

28. Andrea Dworkin, *Intercourse* (New York: Free Press, 1997), 188.

29. Ibid.

## Three / Who Names the Vagina?

### Chapter 10: "The Worst Word There Is"

1. John Austin, *How to Do Things with Words* (Cambridge, MA: Harvard University Press, 1975), 12.

2. Sarah Forman, "Yikes! . . . Yale Edition," *Yale Daily Herald Blog*, October 24, 2010, blogdailyherald.com/tag/yale/.

3. H. Yoon and others, "Effects of Stress on Female Rat Sexual Function," *International Journal of Impotence Research: Journal of Sexual Medicine* 17 (2005): 33–38.

4. Ibid.

5. Ibid.

6. Ibid.

7. Ibid.

8. Ibid.

9. See Kate Millett, *The Prostitution Papers: A Candid Dialogue* (New York: Avon Books, 1973).

10. Matthew Hunt, "Cunt: The History of the C-Word" (PhD), abstract, www.matthewhunt.com/cunt/abstract.html; see also www.matthewhunt.com/cunt/references.html.

11. Ibid. See also encyclopedia.jrank.org/articles/pages/657/Cunt.html for an additional history of the word *cunt*.

12. Hunt, "Cunt."

13. Ibid.

14. Christina Caldwell, "The C-Word: How One Four-Letter Word Holds So Much Power," *College Times*, March 15, 2011.

15. Cited in Hunt, "Cunt." www.matthewhunt.com/cunt/abstract.html; see also www.matthewhunt.com/cunt/references.html.

16. Ibid. www.matthewhunt.com/cunt/abstract.html; see also www.matthewhunt.com/cunt/references.html.

17. Ibid. www.matthewhunt.com/cunt/abstract.html; see also www.matthewhunt.com/cunt/references.html.

18. See Gordon Rattray Taylor, *Sex in History* (New York: Vanguard Press, 1954).

19. Russell Ash, cited in Hunt, "Cunt," www.matthewhunt.com/cunt/abstract.html; see also www.matthewhunt.com/cunt/references.html.

20. "Egypt Bans Forced Virginity Tests by Military," *Al Jazeera*, December 27, 2011, www.aljazeera.com/news/africa/2011/12/20111227132624606116.html.

21. Vanessa Thorpe and Richard Rogers, "Women Bloggers Call for a Stop to 'Hateful' Trolling by Misogynist Men," *The Observer*, November 5, 2011. www.guardian.co.uk/world/2011/Nov/05/women-bloggers-hateful-trolling.

## Chapter 11: How Funny Was That?

1. Richard E. Nisbett, *The Geography of Thought: How Asians and Westerners Think Differently . . . And Why* (New York: Free Press, 2003), cited in Marcia Beauchamp, "Somasophy: The Relevance of Somatics to the Cultivation of Female Subjectivity" (PhD diss., California Institute of Integral Studies, San Francisco, 2011), 301–3.

2. Douglas Wile, *Art of the Bedchamber: The Chinese Sexual Yoga Classics, Including Women's Solo Meditation Texts* (Albany, NY: State University of New York Press, 1992), 9.

3. Sunyata Saraswati and Bodhi Avinasha, *Jewel in the Lotus: The Sexual Path to Higher Consciousness* (San Francisco: Kriya Jyoti Tantra Society, 1987), 180–81: "Only through woman can man come to enlightenment as she is the divine principle. And so in Tantra, female energy, symbolized by the Divine Mother, is worshipped."

4. See Clement Egerton, *The Golden Lotus*, trans. Lanling Xiaoxiaosheng (London: Tuttle, 2011).

5. Virginia Woolf, *A Room of One's Own* (New York: Mariner Books, 1989), 18.

6. Onlineslangdictionary.com/thesaurus/words+meaning+vulva+ ('vagina'),+female+genitalia.html.

7. Blackchampagne.com/wordpress/.

## Chapter 12: The Pornographic Vagina

1. Naomi Wolf, "The Porn Myth," *New York* magazine, October 20, 2003. nymag.com/nymetro/news/trends/n_9437.

2. Dr. Jim Pfaus, interview, January 29–30, 2012.

3. Ibid.

4. See Robert Sapolsky, *Why Zebras Don't Get Ulcers: An Updated Guide to Stress, Stress-Related Diseases, and Coping* (New York: W. H. Freeman, 1998).

5. Dr. Helen Fisher, *The Anatomy of Love: A Natural History of Mating, Marriage and Why We Stray* (New York: Ballantine Books, 1992), 182–84.

6. Dr. Pfaus interview, Montreal, Quebec, January 29–30, 2012.

7. Marnia Robinson, *Cupid's Poisoned Arrow: From Habit to Harmony in Sexual Relationships* (Berkeley, CA: North Atlantic Books, 2009), 133–66.

8. Ibid, 137–66. For more on porn addiction, see J. M. Bostwick and J. A. Bucci, "Internet Sex Addiction Treated with Naltrexone," *Mayo Clinic*

*Proceedings* 83, no. 2 (February 2008): 226–30. See also Marnia Robinson and Gary Wilson, "Santorum, Porn and Addiction Neuroscience," *Psychology Today,* March 26, 2012, www.psychologytoday.com/blog/cupids-poisoned -arrow/201203/santorum-porn-and-addiction-neuroscience.

9. Naomi Wolf, "Is Pornography Driving Men Crazy?" Project Syndicate, June 13, 2011, www.project-syndicate.org/commentary/is-pornography-driving-men-crazy.

10. Reuniting.info/science/articles/sexual_neurochemistry#reward.

11. Ibid.

12. www.psychologytoday.com/blog/cupids-posioned-arrow/201107/porn-induced-sexual-dysfunction-is-growing-problem.

13. Jason S. Carroll and others, "Generation XXX: Pornography Acceptance and Use Among Emerging Adults," *Journal of Adolescent Research* 23, no. 1 (January 2008): 6–30.

14. In Britain, the number of labiaplasties carried out on the National Health Service rose by 70 percent in 2009. http://www.guardian.co.uk/lifeandstyle /2009/nov/20/cosmetic-vulva-surgery.

15. Dr. Basil Kocur, interview, New York City, February 26, 2011.

16. John Cleland, *Memoirs of a Woman of Pleasure* (Oxford: Oxford University Press, 2008), 116–17.

17. Ibid., 139.

## Four / The Goddess Array

### Chapter 13: "The Beloved Is Me"

1. See Marcus Buckingham, *Find Your Strongest Life: What the Happiest and Most Successful Women Do Differently* (New York: Thomas Nelson, 2009).

2. Douglas Wile, *Art of the Bedchamber: The Chinese Sexual Yoga Classics, Including Women's Solo Meditation Texts* (Albany: State University of New York Press, 1992), 9.

3. Ibid., 140–41.

4. Richard Burton, trans., *The Perfumed Garden of Cheikh Nefzoui: A Manual of Arabian Erotology* (London, UK: Kama Shastra Society of London and Benares, 886), 129–59.

5. Leora Lightwoman, of Diamond Light Tantra, another Tantric teacher, offers caveats for the growing field of Tantric sexual healing for women. In an e-mail, she wrote:

Tantric massage for women, including yoni massage, is a beautiful ritual to share between lovers, and practitioners such as Michael offer this opportunity to those who are not in a couple, or whose partners are not Tantrically inclined, to receive a delicious, sacred sexual and emotional offering. This is good. Tantric massage can be profound. . . . I am, however, deeply concerned about the reputation of the whole field of Tantric massage, as it is clearly not regulated. Anyone can call himself a Tantric masseur. The difference between a Tantric massage and an erotic massage can be nebulous, even to those in the field, and I would see it more as a continuum.

She sets out what she sees as distinctions between real Tantric sexual healers and garden-variety sexual healers and cautions that the Tantric teacher should have respect for the client and should have a "sense of innocence" about the transaction.

Also, Leora Lightwoman, interview, London, UK, July 15, 2011.

## Chapter 14: Radical Pleasure, Radical Awakening: The Vagina as Liberator

1. Judith Horstman, *The Scientific American Book of Love, Sex and the Brain: The Neuroscience of How, When, Why and Who We Love* (New York: Jossey-Bass, 2012), 85.

2. Dr. Louann Brizendine, M.D., *The Female Brain* (New York: Morgan Road Books, 2006), 123: "In the male brain, most emotions trigger less gut sensation and more rational thought. The typical male brain reaction to an emotion is to avoid it at all costs. . . ."

3. Dr. Helen Fisher, *The Anatomy of Love: A Natural History of Mating, Marriage and Why We Stray* (New York: Ballantine Books, 1992), 182–84.

4. The following is a description of the instrument that measures the vaginal pulse amplitude:

Vaginal Photoplethysmography—

Embedded in the front end of the probe is a light source that illuminates the vaginal walls. Light is reflected and diffused through the tissues of the vaginal wall and reaches a photosensitive cell surface mounted within the body of the probe. Changes in the resistance of the cell correspond to changes in the amount of back-scattered light reaching the light-sensitive surface. It is assumed that a greater back-scattered signal reflects increased blood volume in the vaginal blood vessels (Levin, 1992). Hoon et al. (1976) introduced an improved model of the vaginal photometer that substituted an infrared LED (light-emitting diode) for the incandescent light source and a phototransistor for the photocell.

These innovations reduced potential artifacts associated with blood oxygenation levels, problems of hysteresis, and light history effects. The vaginal photometer is designed so that it can be easily placed by the participant. A shield can be placed on the probe's cable so that depth of insertion and orientation of the photoreceptive surface is known and held constant (Geer, 1983; Laan, Everaerd, & Evers, 1995). The photometer yields two analyzable signals. The first is the DC signal, which is thought to provide an index of the total amount of blood (Hatch, 1979), often abbreviated as VBV (vaginal blood volume). The second is the AC signal, often abbreviated as VPA (vaginal pulse amplitude), which is thought to reflect phasic changes in the vascular walls that result from pressure changes within the vessels (Jennings et al., 1980; see Figure 11.2). Although both signals have been found to reflect responses to erotic stimuli (e.g., Geer, Morokoff, & Greenwood, 1974; e.g., Hoon, Wincze, & Hoon, 1976), their exact nature and source is unknown. Heiman et al. (2004) compared, in 12 women, VPA and genital volume changes as measured using MRI, and found no significant correlations between the two. Heiman and Maravilla (2005) suggested it may be possible that at moderate levels of arousal the vaginal probe might detect changes to vaginal tissue that do not correspond with other genital blood volume changes. (Interestingly, however, the same study reported higher correlations with subjective sexual arousal for VPA than for MRI variables.) The interpretation of the relationship between the photometer's output and the underlying vascular mechanisms is hindered by the lack of a sound theoretical framework (Levin, 1992) and of a calibration method allowing transformation of its output in known physiological events. At present, most researchers describe their findings in relative measures, such as mm pen deflection or change in microVolts. Levin (1997) stated that one of the basic assumptions underlying use of the plethysmograph is that changes in VBV and VPA always reflect local vascular events. In his discussion of findings from studies on the effects of exercise and orgasm on VBV and VPA, however, he suggests that the signals are likely to reflect rather complex interactions between sympathetic and parasympathetic regulatory processes and between circulatory and vaginal blood pressure. However, Prause et al. (2004) found that, whereas VPA discriminated between sexual, sexually threatening, and threatening film stimuli, blood pressure (while increased during all three conditions) did not. The construct validity of VPA is better established than that of VBV. Researchers have reported high correlations between VPA and VBV, particularly with stronger sexual stimuli, but others have found low or no concordance between the two signals (Heiman, 1976; Meston and Gorzalka, 1995). VPA appears to be more sensitive to changes in stimulus intensity than VBV (Geer et al., 1974;

Osborn & Pollack, 1977). VPA also corresponds more closely with subjective reports of sexual arousal than VBV (Heiman, 1977). Finally, VBV changes in response to increases in general arousal, indicating that VBV is less specific to sexual arousal than VPA (Laan, Everaerd, & Evers, 1995). Two studies have directly assessed the sensitivity and specificity of VPA (Laan et al., 1995; Prause, Cerny, & Janssen, 2004). Both studies measured responses of sexually functional women to sexual, anxiety inducing, sexually threatening, and neutral film excerpts, and found maximal increases in VPA to the sexual stimulus and moderate increases to the sexually threatening film. (Participants also reported intermediate levels of sexual arousal to the sexual-threat stimulus.) On both studies, VPA did not increase in response to anxiety-inducing stimuli. These results demonstrate response specificity of vaginal vasocongestion to sexual stimuli.

From E. Janssen, N. Prause, and J. Geer, "The Sexual Response," in *Handbook of Psychophysiology,* eds. J. T. Cacioppo, L. G. Tassinary, and G. G. Berntson, 3rd ed. (New York: Cambridge University Press, 2007).

5. Dr. Louann Brizendine, *The Female Brain,* 77-86.

6. Beverly Whipple and John Delbert Perry, "Pelvic Muscle Strength of Female Ejaculators: Evidence in Support of a New Theory of Orgasm," *Journal of Sex Research* 17, no. 1 (1981): 22–39.

7. Ibid., 22–39. Whipple and Perry also looked at the neural connections in the lower spine to explain their hypothesis. Indeed, one member of the research team had suffered a sprained lower back and then found that her Kegel-type uterine contraction strength measurements were significantly lower than usual: the health and functionality of the spinal cord, in this study, was confirmed to have affected the contracting powers of the vagina.

8. Ibid., 22–39.

9. Ibid., 22–39.

10. Ibid., 22–39.

11. Janniko R. Georgiadis and others, "Regional Cerebral Blood Flow Changes Associated with Clitorally Induced Orgasm in Healthy Women," *European Journal of Neuroscience* 24, no. 11 (2006): 3305–16.

12. K. Mah and Y. M. Binik, "The Nature of Human Orgasm: A Critical Review of Major Trends," *Clinical Psychology Review* 6 (August 21, 2002): 823–56. See also R. King and others, "Are There Different Types of Female Orgasm?" *Archives of Sexual Behavior* 40, no. 5 (October 2010): 865–75:

In attempt to identify and validate different types of orgasms which females have during sex with a partner, data collected by Mah and Binik (2002) on the dimensional phenomenology of female orgasm were subjected to a typological analysis. A total of 503 women provided adjectival descriptions of orgasms experienced either with a partner (n = 276) or while alone (n = 227). Latent-class analysis revealed four orgasm types which varied systematically in terms of pleasure and sensations engendered. Two types, collectively labelled "good-sex orgasms," received higher pleasure and sensation ratings than solitary-masturbatory ones, whereas two other types, collectively labelled "not-as-good-sex orgasms," received lower ratings. These two higher-order groupings differed on a number of psychological, physical and relationship factors examined for purposes of validating the typology. Evolutionary thinking regarding the function of female orgasm informed discussion of the findings. Future research directions were outlined, especially the need to examine whether the same individual experiences different types of orgasms with partners with different characteristics, as evolutionary theorizing predicts should be the case.

13. Kevin Nelson, M.D., *The Spiritual Doorway in the Brain: A Neurologist's Search for the God Experience* (New York: Penguin, 2012), 242–43.

14. R. W. B. Lewis and Nancy Lewis, *The Letters of Edith Wharton* (New York: Scribner, 1989), 12.

15. Edith Wharton, *The House of Mirth* (New York: Barnes and Noble Classics, 2003), 177.

16. Georgiadis, "Regional Cerebral Blood Flow," 3305–16.

17. Ibid., 3305–16

18. Sally Ryder Brady, *A Box of Darkness: The Story of a Marriage* (New York: St. Martin's Press/Griffin), 114.

19. Mary Roach, *Bonk: The Curious Coupling of Science and Sex* (New York: W. W. Norton, 2008), 293.

20. Wen Zhou and Denise Chen, "Encoding Human Sexual Chemosensory Cues in the Orbitofrontal and Fusiform Cortices," *Journal of Neuroscience* 28, no. 53 (December 31, 2004): 14416–21.

21. Ibid., 14416–21.

22. Virpi Lummaa and Alexandra Alvergne, "Does the Contraceptive Pill Alter Mate Choice in Humans?" *Trends in Ecology and Evolution* 25, no. 3 (October 6, 2009): 171–79.

23. George Preti and others, cited in "Pheromones in Male Perspiration Reduce Women's Tension, Alter Hormone Response that Regulates Menstrual Cycle," *Penn News,* March 14, 2003. www.upenn.edu/pennnews/news/pheromones-male-perspiration-reduce-womens-tension-alter-hormone-response-regulates-menstrual-c.

24. Ibid.

25. Bob Beale, "What Women Need: Sweaty Male Armpits," *ABC Science Online*, June 26, 2003. www.abc.net.au/science/articles/2003/06/26/888984 .htm.

26. Dr. Daniel G. Amen, *The Brain in Love: Twelve Lessons to Enhance Your Love Life* (New York: Three Rivers Press, 2009), 50–72.

27. Dr. Daniel Goleman, *Social Intelligence: The Revolutionary New Science of Human Relationships* (New York: Bantam Books, 2006), 63–64.

28. See Naomi Wolf, *Misconceptions: Truth, Lies and the Unexpected on the Journey to Motherhood* (New York: Doubleday, 2000).

29. Ibid.

30. Brizendine, *Female Brain,* 77.

31. Louann Brizendine, M.D., *The Male Brain* (New York: Three Rivers Press, 2010).

32. Daniel Goleman, *Emotional Intelligence: Why It Can Matter More Than IQ* (New York: Bantam, 1995), 129–47.

33. John M. Gottman, *The Seven Principles for Making Marriage Work* (New York: Three Rivers Press, 1988), 38, 39.

34. Kathleen Light, cited in Roger Dobson and Maurice Chittenden, "Women Need that Healthy Touch," *Sunday Times* (London), January 16, 2005, www.thetimes.co_uk/tto/public/sitesearch.do?querystring=women+ need+that+healthy+touch8p-tto&pf-all&bl-on.

35. Naomi Wolf, Facebook Community Page, informal online survey, September–October 2011.

36. See Milan Zaviacic, *The Human Female Prostate: From Vestigial Skene's Paraurethral Glands and Ducts to Woman's Functional Prostate* (Bratislava: Slovak Academic Press, 1999).

37. Heli Alzate, "Vaginal Eroticism: A Replication Study," *Archives of Sexual Behavior* 6 (December 14, 1985): 529–37.

38. Stuart Brody and Petr Weiss, "Simultaneous Penile-Vaginal Orgasm Is Associated with Satisfaction (Sexual, Life, Partnership, and Mental Health)," *Journal of Sexual Medicine* 8, no. 3 (2011): 734–41.

> Previous multivariate research found that satisfaction was associated positively with frequency of specifically penile-vaginal intercourse (PVI; as opposed to other sexual activities) as well as with vaginal orgasm. The contribution to satisfaction of simultaneous orgasm produced by PVI merited direct examination in a large representative sample.

39. G. L. Gravina and others, "Measurement of the Thickness of the Urethrovaginal Space in Women with or without Vaginal Orgasm," *Journal of Sexual Medicine* 5, no. 3 (March 2008): 610–18.

40. See Deborah Coady and Nancy Fish, *Healing Painful Sex: A Woman's Guide to Confronting, Diagnosing, and Treating Sexual Pain* (New York: Seal Press, 2011).

41. Zwi Hoch, "Vaginal Erotic Sensitivity by Sexological Examination," *Acta Obstetricia et Gynecologica Scandinavica* 65, no. 7 (1986): 767–73.

> We studied vaginal erotic sensitivity by vaginal sexological examinations as part of the evaluation and treatment process of couples complaining of female coital anorgasmia but readily orgasmic at female self- or partner-performed external genital stimulation. The existence on the anterior vaginal wall of an anatomically clearly definable erotically triggering entity, termed "The G Spot", was refuted by our findings.

42. Cambridge Women's Pornography Collective, *Porn for Women* (San Francisco: Chronicle Books, 2007).

43. Lumaa and Alvergne, "Does Contraceptive Pill Alter Mate Choice?"

44. Dr. Jim Pfaus, interview, Montreal, Quebec, January 29–30, 2012.

45. The impact of antidepressants on sexual function is not an insignificant warning, as Anita Clayton, M.D., and Angel L. Montejo, M.D., reported in "Major Depressive Disorder, Antidepressants, and Sexual Dysfunction," *Journal of Clinical Psychiatry* 67, Suppl. 6 (2006): S33–S37:

> Sexual dysfunction is a common problem with a number of causes, including psychosocial factors, general medical illness, psychiatric disorders, and psychotropic and nonpsychiatric medications. It . . . has been strongly associated with antidepressant medications. Selective serotonin reuptake inhibitors (SSRIs) in particular have demonstrated a higher incidence of sexual dysfunction than other antidepressants that work through different mechanisms of action. Further supporting the relationship between sexual dysfunction and antidepressant mechanism of action, data from a number of studies indicate that bupropion, nefazodone, and mirtazapine alleviate symptoms of sexual dysfunction and are as effective as SSRIs at controlling depressive symptoms. Although a number of strategies besides drug substitution have been utilized to help manage antidepressant-induced sexual dysfunction, many patients remain suboptimally treated; as many as 42% of patients were found to passively wait for spontaneous remission. . . .
>
> Sexual dysfunction is a frequent problem that occurs in both healthy patients and patients with depression. According to the National Health and Social Life Survey, sexual dysfunction is more prevalent in women (43%) than men (31%); furthermore, sexual dysfunction is more prevalent in both sexes with poor emotional health than in healthy controls. Sexual dysfunction is a side effect that is particularly attributed to the

use of antidepressant medication and represents a substantial problem, especially with regard to long-term treatment compliance. Approximately 36% of patients find antidepressant-induced sexual dysfunction to be an unacceptable side effect of treatment, constituting possible grounds for treatment discontinuation. Data suggest that the mechanism of action behind antidepressants is a key contributor to sexual dysfunction. A better understanding of these data and of the physiology and etiology of sexual dysfunction will lead to more effective management strategies, which may result in better therapeutic compliance.

Dr. Helen Fisher also believes that SSRIs are part of the picture of women experiencing blunted desire. In a 2004 presentation she gave at an American Psychiatric Association Forum with J. Anderson Thomson Jr., "Sex, Sexuality And Serotonin: Do Sexual Side Effects of Most Antidepressants Jeopardize Romantic Love and Marriage?," she noted that in 2002, millions of prescriptions for antidepressants were written in the United States, most for SSRI-enhancing medication. As many as 73 percent of patients on these medications, she reported, can suffer from one or more of a range of sexual side effects:

It's well established that these drugs can cause sexual dysfunction, diminished sexual desire, delayed sexual arousal and muted or absent orgasm. . . .

The bottom line is that serotonin-enhancing antidepressants that negatively affect [the] sex drive can quite logically also negatively affect the brain circuits for romantic love. . . .

From a Darwinian perspective, orgasm also is a primary mechanism by which women unconsciously assess a mating partner. For a long time, anthropologists have thought that this is a bad design; women just don't have an orgasm every time. More recently, we came to realize that. We call it the 'fickle female orgasm' and we regard it now as a very serious adaptive mechanism that enables women to distinguish between those partners who are willing to spend time and energy on them—those we call Mr. Right— and those who are impatient or lack empathy and who might not be a good husband and father—Mr. Wrong. When women take serotonin-enhancing antidepressants that inhibit the orgasmic response, among some of these women you're jeopardizing the ability to assess the commitment level of a partner. Women also use orgasm to assess existing partnerships; women tend to orgasm more regularly with a long-term partner. With the onset of anorgasmia, this can destabilize a match.

46. Cindy M. Meston and David M. Buss, *Why Women Have Sex* (New York: Times Books, 2009), 252.

47. Dr. Jim Pfaus, interview, Montreal, Quebec, January 29–30, 2012.

48. Kurt Hahlweg and Notker Klann, "The Effectiveness of Marital Counseling in Germany: A Contribution to Health Services Research," *Journal of Family Psychology* 11, no. 4 (December 1997): 410–21.

49. Beverly Whipple, Barry Komisaruk, and Julie Askew, "Neuro-Bio-Experiential Evidence of the Orgasm," paper presented at the annual meeting of the International Society for the Study of Women's Sexual Health, Scottsdale, AZ, February 10–13, 2011, *Desert Heat: International Society for the Study of Women's Sexual Health, 2011 Annual Meeting Program Book,* 153–84.

# Selected Bibliography

Alzate, Heli. "Vaginal Eroticism: A Replication Study." *Archives of Sexual Behavior* 6 (December 14, 1985): 529–37.

Amen, Daniel G. *The Brain in Love: Twelve Lessons to Enhance Your Love Life*. New York: Three Rivers Press, 2009.

Batra, S., and J. Al-Hijji. "Characterization of Nitric Oxide Synthase Activity in Rabbit Uterus and Vagina: Downregulation by Estrogen." *Life Sciences* 62 (1998): 2093–100.

Baumgardner, Jennifer, and Amy Richards. *Manifesta: Feminism and the Future*. New York: Farrar, Strauss and Giroux, 2000.

Beauchamp, Marcia. "Somasophy: The Relevance of Somatics to the Cultivation of Female Subjectivity." PhD diss., unpublished.

Bostwicvk, J. M., and J. A. Bucci. "Internet Sex Addiction Treated with Naltrexone." *Mayo Clinic Proceedings* 83, no. 2 (February 2008): 226–30.

Brizendine, Louann, M.D. *The Female Brain*. New York: Morgan Road Books, 2006.

———. *The Male Brain*. New York: Three Rivers Press, 2010.

Brody, Stuart, and Petr Weiss. "Simultaneous Penile-Vaginal Orgasm Is Associated with Satisfaction (Sexual, Life, Partnership, and Mental Health)." *Journal of Sexual Medicine* 8, no. 3 (2011): 734–41.

Brontë, Charlotte. *Jane Eyre*. London: Penguin Classics, 2006.

Brontë, Emily. *Wuthering Heights*. New York: W. W. Norton, 1991.

Burnett, A. L., and others. "Immunohistochemical Description of Nitric Oxide Synthase Isoforms in Human Clitoris." *Journal of Urology* 158 (1997): 75–78.

Burton, Richard, trans. *The Perfumed Garden of Cheikh Nefzoui: A Manual of Arabian Erotology*. London: Kama Shastra Society of London and Benares, 1886.

Charters, Ann, ed. *The Portable Beat Reader*. New York: Penguin Books, 1992.

Chaucer, Geoffrey. *The Canterbury Tales.* Edited by Nevill Coghill. New York: Penguin Classics, 2003.

Chopin, Kate. *The Awakening and Other Stories.* Oxford: Oxford University Press, 2000.

Clayton, Anita, M.D., and Angel L. Montejo, M.D. "Major Depressive Disorder, Antidepressants, and Sexual Dysfunction." *Journal of Clinical Psychiatry* 67, Suppl. 6 (2006): S33–S37.

Cleland, John. *Memoirs of a Woman of Pleasure.* Oxford: Oxford University Press, 1985.

Coady, Deborah, and Nancy Fish. *Healing Painful Sex: A Woman's Guide to Confronting, Diagnosing, and Treating Sexual Pain.* New York: Seal Press, 2011.

Contrecoeur, Claude de. *Dopamine et Sérotonine: Le Rôle de la Dopamine et de la Sérotonine dans le Système Nerveux Central.* http://www.bio.net/bionet/mm/neur-sci/1996-July/024549.html.

Cott, Nancy F., ed. *Root of Bitterness: Documents of the Social History of American Women.* New York: Dutton, 1972.

Daley, Patricia O. *Gender and Genocide in Burundi: The Search for Spaces of Peace in the Great Lakes Region.* Bloomington: Indiana University Press, 2007.

D'Emilio, John, and Estelle B. Freedman. *Intimate Matters: A History of Sexuality in America.* New York: Harper and Row, 1988.

De Riencourt, Amaury. *Sex and Power in History: How the Difference Between the Sexes Has Shaped our Destinies.* New York: Dell, 1974.

Donne, John. *The Complete Poetry and Selected Prose of John Donne.* Edited by Charles M. Coffin. New York: Modern Library, 2001.

Drohojowska-Philp, Hunter. *Full Bloom: The Art and Life of Georgia O'Keeffe.* New York: W. W. Norton, 2004.

Dworkin, Andrea. *Intercourse.* New York: Basic Books, 1987.

Eliot, George. *The Mill on the Floss.* London: Penguin Books, 1979.

Fisher, Helen. *Anatomy of Love: A Natural History of Mating, Marriage and Why We Stray.* New York: Ballantine Books, 1992.

Freud, Sigmund. *The Freud Reader.* Edited by Peter Gay. New York: W. W. Norton, 1989.

Garon, Paul. *Blues and the Poetic Spirit.* London: Eddison Press, 1975.

Gola, Hannah, and others. "Victims of Rape Show Increased Cortisol Responses to Trauma Reminders: A Study in Individuals with War- and Torture-Related PTSD." *Psychoneuroendocrinology* 37 (2012): 213–20.

Goleman, Daniel. *Social Intelligence: The Revolutionary New Science of Human Relationships.* New York: Random House, 2006.

Gravina, G. L., and others. "Measurement of the Thickness of the Urethrovaginal Space in Women with or without Vaginal Orgasm." *Journal of Sexual Medicine* 5, no. 3 (March 2008): 610–18.

Greer, Germaine. *The Female Eunuch.* New York: HarperPerennial, 2006.

Hahlweg, Kurt, and Notker Klann. "The Effectiveness of Marital Counseling in Germany: A Contribution to Health Services Research." *Journal of Family Psychology* 11, no. 4 (December 1997): 410–21.

Hamburger, Lotte, and Joseph Hamburger, eds. *The Secret Life of a Victorian Woman.* New York: Fawcett Columbine, 1991.

Hoch, Zwi. "Vaginal Erotic Sensitivity by Sexological Examination." *Acta Obstetricia et Gynecologica Scandinavica* 65, no. 7 (1986): 767–73.

Horstman, Judith. *The Scientific American Book of Love, Sex and the Brain: The Neuroscience of How, When, Why and Who We Love.* San Francisco, CA: Jossey-Bass, 2012.

Hunt, Morton M. *The Natural History of Love.* New York: Minerva Press, 1959.

James, William. *The Varieties of Religious Experience.* New York: Barnes and Noble Classics, 2004.

Jong, Erica. *Fear of Flying.* New York: Penguin Books, 1973.

Kelsey, Morton, and Barbara Kelsey. *Sacrament of Sexuality: The Spirituality and Psychology of Sex.* Rockport, MA: Element Press, 1986.

Kent, Tami Lynn. *Wild Feminine: Finding Power, Spirit and Joy in the Female Body.* New York: Simon and Schuster, 2011.

King R., J. Belsky, and Y. Binik. "Are There Different Types of Female Orgasm?" *Archives of Sexual Behavior* 40, no. 5 (August 10, 2010): 865–75.

Klapisch-Zuber, Christiane, ed. *A History of Women: Silences of the Middle Ages.* Cambridge, MA: Harvard University Press, 1992.

Laskin, David. *Partisans: Marriage, Politics and Betrayal among the New York Intellectuals.* New York: Simon and Schuster, 2000.

Lawrence, D. H. *Lady Chatterley's Lover.* New York: Barnes and Noble Classics, 2005.

———. *Women in Love.* New York: Penguin Books, 1987.

LeVay, Simon. *The Sexual Brain.* Cambridge, MA: MIT Press, 1993.

Lewis, R. W. B., and Nancy Lewis. *The Letters of Edith Wharton.* New York: Scribner, 1989.

Mah, K., and Y. M. Binik. "The Nature of Human Orgasm: A Critical Review of Major Trends." *Clinical Psychology Review* 6 (August 21, 2001): 823–56.

Masson, Jeffrey Moussaieff. *A Dark Science: Women, Sexuality and Psychiatry in the Nineteenth Century.* New York: Farrar, Strauss and Giroux, 1986.

Masters, William H., and Virginia E. Johnson. *Human Sexual Response.* New York: Ishi Press, 2010.

Meston, Cindy M., "Sympathetic Nervous System Activity and Female Sexual Arousal." In "A Symposium: Sexual Activity and Cardiac Risk." *American Journal of Cardiology* 86 (July 20, 2000): 30F–34F.

Meston, Cindy M., and Boris B. Gorzalka. "Differential Effects of Sympathetic Activation on Sexual Arousal in Sexually Dysfunctional and Functional Women." *Journal of Abnormal Psychology* 105, no. 4 (1996): 582–91.

Miles, Rosalind. *The Women's History of the World.* London: Paladin, 1989.

Millay, Edna St. Vincent. *Collected Poems of Edna St Vincent Millay.* Edited by Norma Millay. New York: HarperPerennial, 1956.

Munarriz, R., and others. "Biology of Female Sexual Function." *Urology Clinic North America* 29 (2002): 685–93.

Nelson, Kevin, M.D. *The Spiritual Doorway in the Brain: A Neurologist's Search for the God Experience.* London: Plume, 2012.

Offit, Avodah K., M.D. *The Sexual Self: Reflections of a Sex Therapist.* New York: Congdon and Weed, 1983).

Pfaus, James G., and others. "Who, What, Where, When (and Maybe Even Why)? How the Experience of Sexual Reward Connects Sexual Desire, Preference, and Performance." *Archives of Sexual Behavior* 41 (March 9, 2012): 31–62.

Prioleau, Betsy. *Seductress: Women who Ravished the World and their Lost Art of Love.* New York: Viking, 1994.

Rellini, Allessandra H., and Cindy M. Meston. "Psychophysiological Sexual Arousal in Women with a History of Child Sexual Abuse." *Journal of Sex and Marital Therapy* 32 (2006): 5–22.

Ryan, Christopher, and Cacilda Jethá. *Sex at Dawn: The Prehistoric Origins of Modern Sexuality.* New York: HarperCollins, 2010.

Sato, Y., and others. "Effects of Long-Term Psychological Stress on Sexual Behavior and Brain Catecholamine Levels." *Journal of Andrology* 17, no. 83 (2006).

Seidman, Steven. *Romantic Longings: Love in America, 1830–1980.* New York: Routledge, 1991.

Shepsut, Asia. *Journey of the Priestess: The Priestess Traditions of the Ancient World*. New York: HarperCollins, 1993.

Stekel, William. *Frigidity in Woman*. Vol. 2, *The Parapathiac Disorders*. New York: Liveright, 1926.

Traish, A. M. and others. "Biochemical and Physiological Mechanisms of Female Genital Sexual Arousal." *Archives of Sexual Behavior* 31 (2002): 393–400.

Vicinus, Martha, ed. *Suffer and Be Still: Women in the Victorian Age*. Bloomington, IN: Indiana University Press, 1973.

Warnock, J. J. "Female Hypoactive Sexual Desire Disorder: Epidemiology, Diagnosis and Treatment." *Journal of Sexual Medicine* 3 (May 3, 2006): 408–18.

Wharton, Edith. *The House of Mirth*. New York: Barnes and Noble Classics, 2003.

Whipple, Beverly, Barry Komisaruk, and Julie Askew. "Neuro-Bio-Experiential Evidence of the Orgasm." Paper presented at the annual meeting of the International Society for the Study of Women's Sexual Health, Scottsdale, Arizona, February 10–13, 2011.

Woolf, Virginia. *A Room of One's Own*. New York: Harcourt, 1981.

Yoon, H., and others. "Effects of Stress on Female Rat Sexual Function." *International Journal of Impotence Research: Journal of Sexual Medicine* 17 (2005): 33–38.

Zaviacic, Milan. *The Human Female Prostate: From Vestigial Skene's Paraurethral Glands and Ducts to Woman's Functional Prostate*. Bratislava: Slovak Academic Press, 1999.

# Index